Praise for *Mastering Simulation*

D0731104

"Mastering Simulation *is a much-needed, timely handbook for those gettin* a reference *for those already practicing. The editors did a fantastic job of ge* contribute their knowledge. I know I will use Mastering Simulation *in my* mend it to others. I love this book!"

–KT Waxman, DNP, MBA, RN, CNL, CENP
Assistant Professor, University of San Francisco School of Nursing & Health Professions
Director, California Simulation Alliance
Project Director, Department of Defense Grant for Simulation Study

"Mastering Simulation *is a must-read for hospital leaders either currently using or in the process of implementing simulation as part of their ongoing competency development and monitoring. Ulrich and Mancini offer an excellent road map to hospital leaders. If you are pursuing or currently using simulation in your organization, stop the line. Read this book. I have no doubt it will enhance your organization's performance when using simulation.*"

–Sylvain Trepanier, DNP, RN, CENP
System Vice President & Chief Nursing Officer
Premier Health

"Mastering Simulation *by Ulrich and Mancini is a well-written tool for both academic and service-oriented educators who strive to help staff members meet their full potential. The book includes sections on how to build competence, confidence, and proficiency via consequential learning in a safe environment, using varying simulation methodologies inclusive of gamification. This book is a gift to all educators for all disciplines.*"

–Rosemary Luquire, PhD, MSN, FAAN, NEA-BC
Senior Vice President and Corporate Chief Nursing Officer
Baylor Health Care System

"This text is a must-read not only for those new to simulation but for those with a depth of experience in the domain. This book stands out from others on the topic in that it includes valuable insights into the use of simulation in the service setting, which is overlooked in many other texts. The experts in the industry are thoroughly represented. I give this book my highest recommendation!"

–Kenneth W. Dion, PhD, MSN, MBA, RN
Vice President, Healthstream

"This comprehensive primer on simulation *offers valuable information and insights for every level of simulation practitioner, from neophyte to adept. What was once a disruptive innovation has become an essential part of health care education. Whether preparing new practitioners or ensuring ongoing competence and upskilling of experienced providers,* Mastering Simulation *covers the full landscape of simulation uses and strategies. It will be a valuable addition to our resource library.*"

–Jan Jones-Schenk, DHSc, RN, NE-BC
Chief Nursing Officer and National Director
College of Health Professions, Western Governors University

Mastering Simulation

A Handbook for Success

Beth Tamplet Ulrich, EdD, RN, FACHE, FAAN
Mary E. (Beth) Mancini, PhD, RN, NE-BC, FAHA, ANEF, FAAN

Sigma Theta Tau International
Honor Society of Nursing®

The Honor Society of Nursing, Sigma Theta Tau International (STTI) is a nonprofit organization whose mission is to support the learning, knowledge, and professional development of nurses committed to making a difference in health worldwide. Founded in 1922, STTI has 130,000 members in 86 countries. Members include practicing nurses, instructors, researchers, policymakers, entrepreneurs and others. STTI's 482 chapters are located at 626 institutions of higher education throughout Australia, Botswana, Brazil, Canada, Colombia, Ghana, Hong Kong, Japan, Kenya, Malawi, Mexico, the Netherlands, Pakistan, Portugal, Singapore, South Africa, South Korea, Swaziland, Sweden, Taiwan, Tanzania, United Kingdom, United States, and Wales. More information about STTI can be found online at www.nursingsociety.org.

Sigma Theta Tau International
550 West North Street
Indianapolis, IN, USA 46202

To order additional books, buy in bulk, or order for corporate use, contact Nursing Knowledge International at 888.NKI.4YOU (888.654.4968/US and Canada) or +1.317.634.8171 (outside US and Canada).

To request a review copy for course adoption, email solutions@nursingknowledge.org or call 888.NKI.4YOU (888.654.4968/US and Canada) or +1.317.634.8171 (outside US and Canada).

To request author information, or for speaker or other media requests, contact Marketing, Honor Society of Nursing, Sigma Theta Tau International at 888.634.7575 (US and Canada) or +1.317.634.8171 (outside US and Canada).

ISBN: 9781938835032
EPUB ISBN: 9781938835049
PDF ISBN: 9781938835056
MOBI ISBN: 9781938835063

Library of Congress Cataloging-in-Publication Data

Mastering simulation : a handbook for success / [edited by] Beth Ulrich, Mary E. (Beth) Mancini.
   p. ; cm.
  Includes bibliographical references.
  ISBN 978-1-938835-03-2 (book : alk. paper) -- ISBN (invalid) 978-1-938835-04-9 (epub) -- ISBN 978-1-938835-05-6 (pdf) -- ISBN 978-1-938835-06-3 (mobi)
  I. Ulrich, Beth Tamplet, editor of compilation. II. Mancini, Mary E., editor of compilation. III. Sigma Theta Tau International, issuing body.
  [DNLM: 1. Education, Nursing--methods. 2. Patient Simulation. 3. Competency-Based Education--methods. 4. Evidence-Based Nursing--methods. WY 105]
  RT51
  610.73--dc23
          2013029466

First Printing, 2013

Publisher: Renee Wilmeth
Acquisitions Editor: Emily Hatch
Editorial Coordinator: Paula Jeffers
Cover Designer: Michael Tanamachi
Interior Design/Page Layout: Rebecca Batchelor

Principal Book Editor: Carla Hall
Development and Project Editor: Kevin Kent
Copy Editor: Charlotte Kughen
Proofreader: Barbara Bennett
Indexer: Joy Dean Lee

Dedication

To my daughter, Blythe, who inspires me in so many ways; my grandson Henry, through whose eyes I see new wonder in the world every day; my husband, Walter, who supports even my craziest ideas and projects; and to my parents, Paul and Elizabeth Tamplet, who told me I could be anything I wanted to be and encouraged me do anything I wanted to do.

To my colleagues who see no boundaries to the contributions that the nursing profession can make, who lead us into bold new worlds, who day after day serve as vocal patient advocates and, when necessary, who serve as the last line of defense to assure that patients receive high-quality care.

–Beth Tamplet Ulrich, EdD, RN, FACHE, FAAN

To David, Carla, Laura, and Jake—Love you forever; love you for always.

–Mary E. (Beth) Mancini, PhD, RN, NE-BC, FAHA, ANEF, FAAN

Acknowledgments

It takes a lot of people with many different sets of knowledge and skills to create a book such as this one.

Thanks first and foremost to our wonderful contributors. They are experts and leaders in the use of simulation in health care education and practice, and we very much appreciate their willingness to share their knowledge and expertise.

Thanks also to the fantastic Sigma Theta Tau International staff who inspire, plan, nag (when needed), organize, encourage, create, facilitate, and so much more—all to take an idea and have it become a book.

About the Authors

Beth Tamplet Ulrich, EdD, RN, FACHE, FAAN

Beth Ulrich is a nationally recognized thought leader who is known for her research studying nursing work environments and the experiences of new graduate nurses as they transition from nursing school into the workforce and for her leadership to improve the care of nephrology patients and develop the roles of nephrology nurses. Ulrich has extensive experience as a health care executive, educator, and researcher. She currently serves as the senior partner, Innovative Health Resources, and as editor of the *Nephrology Nursing Journal*, the professional journal of the American Nephrology Nurses' Association. Ulrich previously served as the vice president of hospital services for CAE Healthcare; has extensive senior executive experience in CNO, COO, and senior vice president positions in both hospitals and large health care systems; and has held graduate and undergraduate faculty positions. Ulrich has been a coinvestigator on a series of national nursing workforce and work environment studies and three studies of critical-care nurse work environments conducted with the American Association of Critical-Care Nurses.

Ulrich received her bachelor's degree from the Medical University of South Carolina, her master's degree from the University of Texas Health Science Center at Houston, and her doctorate from the University of Houston in a collaborative program with Baylor College of Medicine. She is a Fellow in the American College of Healthcare Executives, a Fellow in the American Academy of Nursing, and a past president of the American Nephrology Nurses' Association. She was recognized as the Outstanding Nursing Alumnus of the Medical University of South Carolina in 1989, as a distinguished alumnus of the University of Texas Health Science Center at Houston School of Nursing in 2002, and received the Outstanding Contribution to the American Nephrology Nurses' Association award in 2008. Ulrich is also a member of the Board of Trustees of the Foundation of the National Student Nurses Association and serves on the National Council of State Boards of Nursing Research Advisory Panel on Transition into Practice. She has numerous publications and presentations to her credit on topics including nephrology nursing, nurses' work environments, and how new graduate nurses transition into professional nurses. Her book *Mastering Precepting: A Nurse's Handbook for Success* was recognized as an AJN 2012 Book of the Year.

Mary E. (Beth) Mancini, PhD, RN, NE-BC, FAHA, ANEF, FAAN

Beth Mancini is professor, associate dean, and chair for Undergraduate Nursing Programs at the University of Texas at Arlington College of Nursing. Mancini holds the Baylor Health Care System Professorship for Healthcare Research. Prior to moving to an academic role in 2004, Mancini was senior vice president for Nursing Administration and chief nursing officer at Parkland Health & Hospital System in Dallas, Texas, a position she held for 18 years.

Mancini received a BSN from Rhode Island College, a master's in Nursing Administration from the University of Rhode Island, and a PhD in Public and Urban Affairs from the University of Texas at Arlington. In 1994, Mancini was inducted as a Fellow in the American Academy of Nursing. In 2009, she was inducted as a Fellow of the American Heart Association. In 2011, she was inducted as a Fellow in the National League for Nursing's Academy of Nursing Education.

Mancini is active in the area of simulation in health care, including having served as president of the Society for Simulation in Healthcare, past member of the Royal College of Physicians and Surgeons of Canada's Simulation Task Force, Sigma Theta Tau International's Simulation and Emerging Technologies Content Advisory Group, the World Health Organization's Initiative on Training and Simulation and Patient Safety, and cochair of the Education Task Force for the International Liaison Committee for Resuscitation.

Mancini has more than 90 publications to her credit and is a sought-after speaker at local, national, and international conferences on such topics as simulation in health care, health professions education, patient safety, teaching, retention, outcomes related to basic and advanced life-support education, emergency and critical-care nursing, nursing research, and work redesign.

Contributing Authors

Katie Anne Adamson, PhD, RN

Katie Adamson is an assistant professor in the Nursing and Healthcare Leadership Programs at the University of Washington in Tacoma, Washington. Adamson completed her dissertation research, *Assessing the Reliability of Simulation Evaluation Instruments Used in Nursing Education: A Test of Concept Study*, and earned her PhD in Nursing from Washington State University College of Nursing in 2011. Multiple researchers and educators have since employed the resources and methods she developed as part of this work for the psychometric assessment of simulation evaluation instruments. She is the coauthor of the column, "Making Sense of Methods and Measurement" for the journal *Clinical Simulation in Nursing*, as well as the author of numerous invited and peer-reviewed presentations and publications. In addition, Adamson coauthored the Advanced Evaluation course for the National League for Nursing Simulation Innovation Resource Center (SIRC). She continues to teach and do research in the area of simulation evaluation. One of her favorite roles is that of a mentor for graduate students who are pursuing careers in the area of nursing education.

Pamela Andreatta, PhD, MFA, MA

Pamela Andreatta is an associate professor in the Department of Obstetrics & Gynecology, and the founding director (emeritus) of Clinical Simulation Center at the University of Michigan Medical School. Andreatta specializes in the assessment and development of individual and team-based human performance in the provision of clinical and surgical care. Her work includes research toward optimizing team-based practices in emergent and nonemergent clinical contexts, ranging from tertiary care academic medical centers in the United States; to urban and rural ambulatory care clinics in Honduras, China, and Zambia; to remote community-based practices in Ghana and Liberia. Andreatta was awarded one of the largest medical education research grants in history by the Department of Defense for studying simulation-based training mechanisms related to performance outcomes.

Andreatta is recognized as a leading expert in the uses of simulation for health care education and serves as a member of the board of directors for the Society for Simulation in Healthcare. She is an appointed delegate to the American College of Surgeons simulation research committee and the American College of Obstetricians and Gynecologists simulation consortium. Andreatta serves as a consultant to the American College of Nurse-Midwives and to several health care and biomedical technology companies. She earned her doctorate from the University of San Francisco, San Francisco, California, after completing her master's degree at San Jose State University, San Jose, California. She has more than 60 peer-reviewed publications resulting from her research, and has presented more than 200 conference and invited addresses related to simulation-based applications in medicine, nursing, allied health, and team sciences.

Eric B. Bauman, PhD, RN

Eric B. Bauman is the founder and managing member of Clinical Playground, LLC, a consulting service focusing on game- and simulation-based learning. Bauman received his PhD from the University of Wisconsin-Madison School of Education, Department of Curriculum and Instruction, in 2007. He was one of the early Games+Learning+Society (GLS) students. Bauman is also a registered nurse, firefighter, and paramedic with more than 20 years of clinical, research, teaching, and command experience. His most recent academic appointment was as a faculty associate in the Department of Anesthesiology at the University of Wisconsin-Madison before starting Clinical Playground, LLC. Bauman is currently associate director for the Center for Simulation Excellence for DeVry, Inc., Healthcare Group and also holds the rank of division chief of Emergency Medical Services for the Blooming Grove Fire Department.

Bauman is a strong advocate for multidisciplinary education and research and continues to collaborate actively with Games+Learning+Society. His experience spans various disciplines, including adult education, human factors analysis, team dynamics, emergency medical services, firefighting, and health care. He has presented on various topics at a number of regional, national, and international conferences and has authored and coauthored book chapters and articles on game- and simulation-based education and evaluation. In addition, he is the cofounder of the Games and Simulation for Healthcare website and blog (http://healthcaregames.wisc.edu/).

Bauman is cochair of the Society for Simulation in Healthcare's (SSH) Serious Games and Virtual Environment Special Interest Group and chairs the Website Committee. He is also a member of the International Nursing Association for Clinical Simulation and Learning (INACSL), and Sigma Theta Tau International. Bauman continues to publish and present as both a vetted and invited speaker and author in the fields of simulation and game-based learning.

Deborah Becker, PhD, ACNP, BC, CCNS

Deborah Becker is the assistant dean for Innovations in Simulation at the University of Pennsylvania, School of Nursing. Becker also directs the Adult Gerontology Acute Care Nurse Practitioner, Adult Gerontology Clinical Nurse Specialist programs, and the Adult Oncology Minor. She oversees the integration of simulated activities and other innovative teaching strategies into both the undergraduate and graduate curricula in collaboration with the course faculty. She has been involved in simulation for over 20 years.

Becker is a graduate of Villanova University (BS), Thomas Jefferson University School of Allied Health (BSN), University of Pennsylvania School of Nursing (MSN and post-master's nurse practitioner certificate) and Drexel University School of Education (PhD). She is a certified acute care nurse practitioner and a certified critical-care clinical nurse specialist. She has worked in critical care for 28 years and has been teaching at the University of Pennsylvania for 18 years. She has presented locally, re-gionally, and nationally on a variety of simulation, acute care, and advanced practice issues and is a contributing author and reviewer on several nurse-related topics.

Sandra Caballero, MSN, RN

Sandra Caballero is a faculty instructor in the School of Nursing at the Texas Tech University Health Sciences Center (TTUHSC) in Lubbock. As the coordinator of The F. Marie Hall SimLife Center, she is tasked with coordination of multimodality interpro-fessional educational activities and assists with the activities at the School of Nursing's regional campuses. She is involved in the TTUHSC's Quality Enhancement Plan and coordinates educational activities involving the interprofessional teams and scenario development. Caballero was recently accepted into the National League for Nursing's Leadership Development Program for Simulation Educators. She also serves on the fi-nance committee for the International Nursing Association for Clinical Simulation and Learning (INACSL).

Caballero received her MSN and BSN from Texas Tech University Health Sciences Center. Her educational research interest relates to the utilization of simulation to en-hance student learning and promote patient safety.

Carol Cheney, MS, CCC-SLP, CHSE

Carol Cheney completed her master's degree in cognitive and communication disorders in 1995. At that time, she began her career as an acute medical speech-language pathologist for Banner Health, one of the largest nonprofit health care systems in the country, with over 36,000 employees. In 2005, she assumed the position of director of operations of the Simulation Education and Training Center (SimET) at Banner Good Samaritan Medical Center in Phoenix, Arizona, while it was still in the conceptual and development stage.

On the heels of the success of the SimET Center, Cheney led the planning, design, and development of a 55,000-square-feet simulation medical center at Banner Mesa which serves as an onboarding tool for all clinical staff to aid in the standardization of training and the highest quality of patient safety standards in all aspect of patient care by simulating a virtual patient care unit experience.

In 2011, Cheney became the senior director of Clinical Education & Simulation for Banner Health, responsible for simulation education, nursing, physician, and multidisciplinary clinical education, including electronic medical record training. She is now embarking on the development of ambulatory accountable care education models.

Cheney was among the first simulation educators to receive certification as a health-care simulation educator (CHSE), and Banner's simulation programs under her leadership are among the first internationally to be accredited as a system by the American College of Surgeons Accredited Education Institute Level 1 and Society for Simulation in Healthcare Accreditation in all five categories. She has been responsible for the development and standardization of multiple simulation curricula for physicians, residents, medical students, nurses, and allied health professionals and has presented nationally on many topics related to simulation and clinical education.

Sharon Decker, PhD, RN, ANEF, FAAN

Sharon Decker is a professor in the School of Nursing at the Texas Tech University Health Sciences Center (TTUHSC) in Lubbock. Additionally, she is the director of The F. Marie Hall SimLife Center. In this role, she has administrative oversight for the 24,500-square-feet multimodality interprofessional simulation center, as well as simulation activities at the School of Nursing's regional campuses. As the director of TTUHSC's Quality Enhancement Plan: Interprofessional Team, she facilitates the integration of activities to promote interprofessional teamwork skills among TTUHSC students from five schools on seven campuses. A member of the Standards Committee for the International Nursing Association for Clinical Simulation and Learning (INACSL), Decker is instrumental in the development of standards for simulation. As a member of the Certification Committee for the Society for Simulation in Healthcare, Decker assisted in developing the certification processes for Simulation Educators.

Decker received her BSN from Baylor University, her MSN from the University of Texas at Arlington, and her PhD from Texas Woman's University. She is a Fellow in the National League for Nursing's Academy of Nursing Education and a Fellow in the American Academy of Nursing. Decker's educational research is related to how simulation can be used to improve learning and promote professional competencies. She serves as a national and international consultant to assist nurse educators in the integration of simulation into curricula and competency assessments.

Beverly Dorney, MS, RN, NE-BC, EDAC

Beverly Dorney is a senior consultant and senior vice president for FKP Advisors. Using over 30 years of diverse leadership experience in health care operations and delivery of clinical services, she partners with providers across the country. She is a master's-prepared, board-certified nurse executive with EDAC certification. With FKP since 2000, she has worked with teams to develop evidence-based strategies for large-scale operations improvement while creating ideal care experiences for patients and providers. Her experiences include implementation of new delivery models that optimize the integration of operational and technology systems. Design teams request her guidance in operations-informed facility planning. Simulation modeling skills are included in her repertoire for process improvement. She believes in sharing knowledge as an adjunct faculty member at the University of Texas at Arlington College of Nursing and has presented at a number of national conferences. Her passion is creating innovative health care environments that will best serve patients and those who care for them. Her clients include academic medical centers, health care system hospitals, and full-service and specialty hospitals, many of which have received national recognition for successful projects and programs.

Gary L. Geis, MD

Gary Geis completed his graduate-level medical training at the University of Cincinnati College of Medicine in Cincinnati, Ohio. Geis then completed a categorical pediatric residency at Children's Hospital of The King's Daughters in Norfolk, Virginia, before completing fellowship training in pediatric emergency medicine at Cincinnati Children's Hospital Medical Center. Geis is currently an associate professor of pediatrics at Cincinnati Children's Hospital in the Division of Emergency Medicine, as well as the medical director for the Center for Simulation and Research. He has been active in simulation-based medical education and training since 2005, with special interests in teamwork's impact on resuscitative care, procedural training, and utilization of simulation to implement new teams, care environments, and care processes.

Teresa N. Gore, DNP, FNP-BC, NP-C, CHSE

Teresa Gore is an associate clinical professor and simulation learning coordinator at Auburn University School of Nursing in Auburn, Alabama. She has been a nurse for 26 years and in academia for 11 years. Gore received a BSN from Jacksonville State University in Alabama, a master's in nursing from University of Phoenix, a post-master's in family nurse practitioner and a Doctor of Nursing Practice from the University of Alabama in Birmingham. She has completed a certificate program in Simulation Education from Bryan College of Health Sciences in Nebraska and is a Certified Healthcare Simulation Educator (CHSE).

Gore is active in nursing simulation including serving on the board of directors of the International Nursing Association for Clinical Simulation and Learning (INACSL) from 2008–2013. During this time she was involved in the development of *Standards of Best Practice: Simulation*. She is a member of the Society for Simulation in Healthcare and has published and presented simulation topics both nationally and internationally. She has also served on the board of directors of the Theta Delta chapter of Sigma Theta Tau International. Gore continues her clinical practice as a nurse practitioner at the university medical clinic.

Valerie M. Howard, EdD, MSN, RN

Valerie Howard, assistant dean of External Affairs, professor of nursing, and director of the Robert Morris University (RMU) Regional Research and Innovation in Simulation Education (RISE) Center, and president of the International Nursing Association of Clinical Simulation in Nursing (INACSL), has over 17 years experience in higher education, with the past 9 years dedicated to researching, developing, and implementing simulation experiences across the curriculum. Since 2004, Howard has been responsible for integrating academically sound simulation experiences for undergraduate and graduate students and has supervised the expansion of the RMU Simulation lab into the Regional RISE Center. Howard recently created and implemented the "Leadership in Simulation Instruction and Management" online certificate program at RMU to assist with integrating this complex training methodology. Her research interests include the use of simulation and electronic health records (EHRs) in education specifically related to student learning outcomes. She is a master trainer for the TeamSTEPPS evidence-based teamwork training system developed by the Agency for Healthcare Research and Quality (AHRQ) and Department of Defense (DoD). These teamwork concepts are incorporated throughout all undergraduate and graduate simulation experiences. Howard also developed the STRIVE Model to assist faculty with the implementation and expansion of simulation services in their respective institutions.

Pamela R. Jeffries, PhD, RN, FAAN, ANEF

Pamela Jeffries, professor and associate dean for Academic Affairs at The Johns Hopkins University School of Nursing, is nationally known for her research and work in the science of learning and educational practices and outcomes. At The Johns Hopkins University School of Nursing and throughout the academic community, Jeffries is well regarded for her expertise in experiential learning, digital education, new pedagogies, and the delivery of content using emerging technologies, particularly clinical simulations in nursing education.

Jeffries has served as the principal investigator on grants with national organizations, has provided research leadership and mentorship on national projects with the National Council of State Boards of Nursing, and has served as a consultant for large health care organizations, corporations, and publishers, providing expertise in clinical and digital education and emerging technologies.

Jeffries is a Fellow of the American Academy of Nursing, an American Nurse Educator Fellow, and most recently, a Robert Wood Johnson Foundation Executive Nurse Fellow. She also serves as a member of the Institute of Medicine's Global Forum on Innovation in Health Profesional Education and, in 2013, as president-elect of the interprofessional, international Society for Simulation in Healthcare (SSH).

She has numerous publications, is sought after to deliver presentations nationally and internationally, has written over 25 book chapters, has many journal publications, and has served as editor for three books on clinical simulations in health care education. She has received federal and state grant funding to support her research focus in nursing education and the science of innovation and learning. Jeffries was inducted in the prestigious Sigma Theta Tau International Nurse Researcher Hall of Fame and is the recipient of several teaching and research awards from various national and international nursing and interdisciplinary organizations.

Karen Josey, MEd, BSN, RN, CHSE

Karen Josey is the director of simulation for Banner Health. She has been a nurse for 35 years, with a background in ICU, training center operations, and leadership. She has worked in simulation since 2007, and her scope includes leadership of three simulation centers that cover seven states. Simulations include multidisciplinary in situ scenarios, RN new-hire onboarding, physician-based simulations, curriculum for multidisciplines, and process rollouts. She learns best by doing, and simulation has been the ideal fit in her passion for learning, especially in error identification and accurate learning assessments.

Thomas E. LeMaster, MSN, MEd, RN, NREMT-P

Tom LeMaster is the program director for the Center for Simulation and Research at the Cincinnati Children's Hospital. He has been a nurse at Cincinnati Children's Hospital for over 30 years. He holds a master's degree in nursing and education through Xavier University and is a nationally registered paramedic. He has worked as a medical-surgical nurse, ED nurse, and EMS coordinator with the trauma program before joining emergency medicine. LeMaster has developed and implemented several programs at Cincinnati Children's Hospital, including the Center for Simulation and Research. Currently, he is responsible for the global operations of the Center for Simulation and Research within the hospital and the community, with 5,000 learners annually.

In 2010, LeMaster was elected as secretary of the board for the Society for Simulation in Healthcare. He is also a member of the Council for Accreditation of Healthcare Simulation Programs, chair of the Reviewer Development Committee, and a member of the Accreditation Board of Review. He has been active in the expansion of the accreditation program, participating in the development of the accreditation standards, evaluation of the overall program, selection of site reviewers, and development of the site-reviewer training program.

Lori Lioce, DNP, FNP-BC, NP-C, CHSE

Lori Lioce is a clinical assistant professor at the University of Alabama in Huntsville College of Nursing, where she serves as simulation coordinator and chair of the simulation task force. She received a BSN, master's in nursing administration, post-master's family nurse practitioner certificate from the University of Alabama in Huntsville, and her Doctor of Nursing Practice from Samford University, Ida V. Moffett School of Nursing, Birmingham, Alabama. She completed a certificate program in simulation education at Bryan College of Health Sciences in Nebraska and is a Certified Healthcare Simulation Educator (CHSE).

Lioce's clinical experience is in emergency medicine as a registered nurse and family nurse practitioner. She is active in simulation education and has presented nationally and internationally. Lioce serves as the vice-president of operations for the International Nursing Association for Clinical Simulation and Learning (INACSL), where she is a member of the Standards Committee, revising standards and developing guidelines for implementation for the INACSL *Standards of Best Practice: Simulation.*

Joseph O. Lopreiato, MD, MPH

Joseph Lopreiato received his MD from Georgetown University in 1981 and completed his pediatric internship and residency at the National Naval Medical Center in Bethesda, Maryland, in 1984. Lopreiato has held several education leadership positions, including pediatric clerkship director, director for educational affairs, and pediatric residency program director. He has completed two faculty development fellowships at Michigan State University and the University of Texas Health Science Center, San Antonio. He is the recipient of several national awards for education, including the Academic Pediatric Association's Ray E. Helfer Award for Innovation in Medical Education, the American Academy of Pediatrics National Education Award, a finalist for the Accreditation Council for Graduate Medical Education (ACGME) Parker J. Palmer Award, and the recipient of the Association of Pediatric Program Directors' Walter W. Tunnessen, Jr., MD, Award for extraordinary or innovative contributions in pediatric graduate medical education. Lopreiato is sought after as a consultant in medical education and a Grand Rounds speaker. He has conducted several consultations for pediatric training programs for the Association of Pediatric Program Directors and is a case developer for the National Board of Medical Examiners Step 2 clinical skills examination.

Lopreiato is currently the associate dean for simulation education and professor of pediatrics at the Uniformed Services University of the Health Sciences in Bethesda, Maryland. He is also the medical director of the National Capital Area Medical Simulation Center, a 30,000-square-feet facility that uses standardized patients, human patient simulators, task trainers, and virtual reality simulations to train medical students, advanced practice nurses, and several residency and fellowship programs in the Washington, DC, area. His current interests include the use of simulation technologies to teach and assess a variety of learners from medical students to faculty. He recently completed a 31-year career in the United States Navy Medical Corps.

Jody R. Lori, PhD, CNM, FACNM, FAAN

Jody Lori is a clinical associate professor and deputy director of the WHO Collaborating Center at the University of Michigan School of Nursing. Lori's professional and academic careers have focused on innovative approaches to reduce disparities in maternal and newborn health. Lori's research centers on participatory action research to develop models of care and clinical interventions to address the high rates of maternal and neonatal mortality in sub-Saharan Africa. In 2010, she was awarded one of six innovation grants by the United States Agency for International Development, Child Survival Section for a 4-year project in Liberia, West Africa, to evaluate maternity waiting homes as an intervention to increase the availability of maternal, newborn, and child health services at rural primary care health facilities. Most recently she received an NIH/Fogarty award to develop and test an innovative approach to prenatal care in Ghana. Her research has contributed to the development of sustainable community-driven, community-based models of care with influence on both policy and practice.

Lori received her bachelor's and master's degrees from the University of Michigan and her doctorate from the University of Arizona. She currently serves as chair of the Division of Global Health for the American College of Nurse-Midwives. Her extensive fieldwork experience includes Ghana, Guatemala, Ethiopia, Liberia, Mexico, and Zambia. Lori is currently working in collaboration with the American College of Nurse-Midwives on a major multiyear project addressing midwifery preservice education and faculty retention in Ghana.

Jennifer L. Manos, MSN, RN

Jennifer Manos is the associate executive director for the Society for Simulation in Healthcare (SSH). Her experience also includes serving as an education specialist at Cincinnati Children's Hospital Center for Simulation and Research. She received her bachelor's of science and master's of science in nursing from Indiana Wesleyan University.

Manos has been a pediatric critical-care and trauma resuscitation nurse for 10 years and an education specialist with the Center for Simulation and Research for 7 years. She has extensive critical-care and pediatric trauma experience, serving as an original member of the core resuscitation team at Cincinnati Children's Hospital. She is regional faculty for the American Heart Association and has served as the PALS/ACLS coordinator for Cincinnati Children's Hospital. She has developed and implemented programs at Cincinnati Children's Hospital Medical Center, including the Pediatric Emergency Management Simulation Course, Cardiac Intensive Care and Pediatric Intensive Care Serious Safety Event Reduction Courses, and the institution-wide simulation mock code program.

Manos has been involved in research surrounding patient safety, teamwork and communication, and the detection of latent safety threats through multidisciplinary simulation training. She has presented at conferences regarding simulation research, projects in simulation, and on behalf of the Society for Simulation in Healthcare. She has been an invited speaker to discuss simulation and SSH accreditation. Manos is experienced in both simulation and accreditation and provides extensive knowledge about accreditation standards and processes across multiple disciplines and organizational structures.

David Marzano, MD

David Marzano is currently an academic generalist in the Department of Obstetrics and Gynecology at the University of Michigan Medical School, where he also serves as the assistant residency director. Marzano's area of research interest involves the use of simulation in team training, including team communications, team dynamics, and patient safety. He has been actively involved in the development and implementation of simulation training for obstetrical emergencies, laparoscopic skills development, and unit-based team training. Marzano and Dr. Pamela Andreatta cofounded an interdisciplinary training program for physicians, nurses, and allied health professionals from Obstetrics, Emergency Medicine, Anesthesiology, and Neonatalogy (OBEMAN), designed to improve patient safety and quality of care for pregnant women at the University of Michigan.

Marzano received his bachelor's degree from Brandeis University. He graduated from the University of Michigan Medical School and completed his residency in obstetrics and gynecology at the University of Michigan. He has several publications and presentations on the use of simulation training in the field of obstetrics and gynecology. He currently serves as a member of the American Congress of Obstetricians and Gynecologists (ACOG) Simulations Consortium.

Chris McClanahan, MSN, RN, CEN

Chris McClanahan is a coordinator in the F. Marie Hall Sim*Life* Center and faculty instructor in the School of Nursing at the Texas Tech University Health Sciences Center (TTUHSC) in Lubbock. As a coordinator and instructor in the Sim*Life* Center, McClanahan coordinates multimodality interprofessional educational activities and assists with the activities at the School of Nursing's regional campuses. He is involved in the TTUHSC's Quality Enhancement Plan and coordinates educational activities involving the interprofessional teams and scenario development.

McClanahan is involved in developing and implementing a research project for triage nurses on selective spinal immobilization aimed at providing evidence-based procedures to change spinal immobilization protocols. He also has assisted in development of quality enhancement plan scenarios.

McClanahan received his MSN and BSN from Lubbock Christian University, Lubbock. He is a certified emergency nurse (CEN).

Janice C. Palaganas, PhD, RN, NP

Janice Palaganas is principal faculty for the Center for Medical Simulation in Boston, Massachusetts, and associate director for the Institute of Medical Simulation. Palaganas is also a Research Fellow at Massachusetts General Hospital, Department of Anesthesia. She received her PhD in nursing, exploring health care simulation as a platform for interprofessional education. She has extensive emergency department experience, including Level I trauma centers, community hospitals, and fast tracks as an emergency nurse, fast track nurse practitioner, clinical educator, clinical nurse specialist, trauma nurse practitioner, manager, and director for emergency and critical care services. Palaganas has held faculty positions in schools of medicine, nursing, management, and emergency medicine. She has worked in simulation centers in multiple roles as a professor, faculty development educator, chief operations officer, and director of research and development.

Palaganas was the implementing director of accreditation and certification for the Society for Simulation in Healthcare and continues as a member of its board of review for the Council for Accreditation of Healthcare Programs, Certification Committee. She is also chair of the Interprofessional Education Affinity Group. Palaganas has presented at multiple conferences regarding projects in simulation and has been an invited keynote speaker, nationally and internationally, to discuss simulation, interprofessional education, patient safety, and accreditation.

Shelly J. Reed, DNP, FNP, CPNP

Shelly Reed is an associate teaching professor at Brigham Young University (BYU) in Provo, Utah, where she teaches undergraduate nursing students in the maternal/child and global health courses. She received her BS in nursing from BYU, her MSN from the University of Utah in Salt Lake City, and her DNP from Case Western Reserve University. Reed has participated in simulation while maintaining NRP certification as part of her many years of employment in the labor and delivery setting. She chose to research debriefing in her DNP program as a result of an NRP debriefing experience. Reed developed a tool to evaluate the participant experience during debriefing, the Debriefing Experience Scale, and has continued her research of the debriefing experience using this tool. In addition, Reed has been able to combine her love of global health and simulation instruction by helping teach CPR and NRP courses in Tonga and Ecuador with BYU nursing students and with LDS Humanitarian Services.

John J. Schaefer III, MD

John Schaefer currently holds the position of the Lewis Blackman Endowed Chair with Health Sciences South Carolina. Schaefer's endowed chair is in patient simulation education and research. He is working to establish a statewide network of patient simulator training and research labs and directing associated research activities. There are now 10 collaborative partners and 20 affiliate partners within the state. The centers are networked and use the same systems to train medical, nursing, and allied health students each year. This approach to medical training will elevate clinical effectiveness and patient safety.

Schaefer is a professor in the Department of Anesthesia and Perioperative Medicine at the Medical University of South Carolina. He received a BA in Chemistry, BS in Chemical Engineering, and a doctorate of medicine from West Virginia University from 1981–1988, respectively.

Schaefer has been involved in human simulation with manikin-based simulators since their introduction into medical education in the United States in the early 1990s. He helped establish the first simulation training center using mannequin-based simulators at the University of Pittsburgh in the Department of Anesthesiology. He was the director of the center from 1997 to 2006 and led the multipartnered expansion of the center. Schaefer coholds patents for the development of human simulators, including the most successful mannequin-based human simulators currently on the market (Laerdal SimMan, AirMan), and has fundamentally participated in the development of hardware and software for the latest generation of human simulators of this type. He was the primary contributing author of the latest version of the operating system for this type of simulator and is participating in the beta development of the next generation of mannequin-based infant simulators. He has been at the forefront for practical simulation curriculum and applied performance assessment in this arena, including the integration of web-based curriculum to create comprehensive, practical, and quantifiable medical simulation learning systems. Schaefer is an internationally recognized educator in the field of airway management. His simulation-based airway management training learning system has been adopted by the University of Pittsburgh Medical Center and the Medical University of South Carolina as the model for patient safety programs of this type being adopted in the departments of anesthesiology, emergency medicine, and critical-care medicine. These programs include mandatory training, medical privileging licensure, competency assessment, and clinical impact through monitoring insurance claims database information.

Andrew Spain, MA, NCEE, CCP-C

Andrew Spain is the director of certification for the Society for Simulation in Healthcare. He has been a paramedic for over 20 years, first in the Denver area, then in central Missouri, doing both ground and air ambulance work. This evolved into directing an EMS education program for 5 years prior to coming to SSH. He has a master's degree in political science and is currently working on a PhD in education at the University of Missouri (emphasis in educational leadership and policy analysis). He continues to be involved in health care education and simulation, primarily with the national disaster life support programs.

Regina G. Taylor, MA CCRP

Regina Taylor obtained her bachelor's degree in psychology from the University of Dayton and a master's degree in clinical psychology from Ball State University. Taylor is currently a senior clinical research coordinator at Cincinnati Children's Hospital Medical Center. She serves as a project manager and oversees all research endeavors for the Center for Simulation and Research. Her areas of research expertise include conducting research in emergency settings, the informed consent process, research involving vulnerable populations and conducting educational research. She has been active in clinical research since 2004 and is a certified clinical research professional.

Linda Tinker, MSN, RN, CHSE

Linda Tinker is the senior manager at Banner Simulation Education and Training Center (SimET) in Phoenix, Arizona, where she is responsible for management and operations of a 6,000-square-feet simulation center that hosts almost 8,000 user visits a year. Linda has over 30 years nursing experience, including varied clinical positions, and over 20 years teaching and management experience. She is a certified healthcare simulation educator and is a member of American Nurses Association, Sigma Theta Tau International Honor Society of Nursing, and the Society for Simulation in Healthcare.

Cynthia Walston, FAIA, LEED AP

Cynthia Walston is a principal at FKP Architects, a firm specializing in health care, research, and education architecture, and also serves as its director of science and education. With translational medicine at the forefront, Walston's launch of the laboratory planning for FKP has positioned her team to work primarily in biomedical research environments and on academic health sciences campuses throughout North America, including Texas A&M Health Science Center, Rice University, Texas Children's Hospital, Baylor College of Medicine, and University of Texas Medical Branch.

Walston is a graduate of the University of Texas School of Architecture in Austin. She is an active member of BioHouston, a founding member of the American College of

Healthcare Architects, and chairman of the board of Equipment Collaborative, a laboratory and health care equipment planning company. Walston has served on several of the NIH National Institute of Allergy and Infectious Diseases (NIAD) peer review committees for the national and regional biocontainment labs and juried many *R&D Magazine* Lab of the Year awards. She speaks regularly at national conferences on the subject of education, laboratory, and equipment planning.

Table of Contents

Foreword

"I hear, I forget; I see, I remember; I do, I understand."
–Chinese Proverb

Over the course of a long career in nursing leadership, I have often contemplated what makes a *great nurse*. Not just a reasonably good, competent, and caring nurse, but a really great, *exceptional* nurse. These nurses have a highly developed ability to think critically, rapidly synthesizing a multitude of diverse inputs and data points, to quickly understand a patient's need, and to take action with full competence and confidence. Some describe this as a nurse's intuition or instinct. As I have had ample opportunities to observe many great nurses across the entire spectrum from novice to expert, it is clear to me that the development of exceptional nurses is *not* an accident, and not just a function of good instincts.

These clinical capabilities are highly developed and born out of broad and deep experience interacting in the clinical practice environment, not just the academic classroom. So it is a natural conclusion that any opportunity that provides nurses meaningful and accurate clinical experiences in advance of being confronted with an actual patient would be highly desirable. Using simulation as a laboratory for learning and experience can accelerate nurses' competence and elevate their confidence in caring for every possible clinical challenge. Patients clearly appreciate and deserve both attributes—competence and confidence.

We have high expectations of our caregivers. The academic institutions that prepare our health professions are constantly being challenged to ensure a robust educational process and training that provides diverse and comprehensive clinical experiences allowing student clinicians to become competent practitioners within the increasingly demanding patient care environment of today's health care system.

In turn, health care organizations are being equally challenged to keep their clinical workforce competent and responsive to the constant onslaught of new knowledge, complex technology, and treatment strategies. Amidst these institutional challenges is the public's increasing expectations of a flawless system of care where expertise and patient safety are guaranteed. These expectations coupled with the rapid pace of change have demanded a new and more effective knowledge transmission, acquisition, and competency development process that is both highly effective and cost efficient.

Health care organizations make significant investments in the development of nurses because it is absolutely essential to ensuring a highly capable and competent clinical team and, ultimately, highly reliable, quality patient care. As part of this organizational investment, the support of a culture of continuous learning, both in content and experience, is critical to the development of highly skilled clinical nurses. Given the cost pressures our industry faces today, it is understandable that health care organizations are in search of the most accessible and effective methods to deliver great nurses to the patients we are accountable for.

Simulation, and its use in accelerating the learning trajectory of clinicians, is what this wonderful book is about. Health care, like other high-risk/high-consequence industries, has found and eagerly embraced simulation as an effective means of providing students and practicing clinicians with realistic learning experiences and an effective vehicle for building clinical excellence and high reliability. Simulation is helping health care organizations reduce the variations in practice that contribute to process failures and less than perfect outcomes.

Simulation has become recognized as the most effective clinical teaching/learning strategy available to ensure caregiver competency in terms of clinical knowledge and critical thinking, as well as the technical application of motor skills in using technology and performing complex tasks. This book represents the many facets of simulation with a comprehensive, yet highly readable and understandable approach.

My dear colleagues, Drs. Ulrich and Mancini, have gathered together experts in simulation to provide the reader with all the current evidence on why simulation is an exceptional tool for building high performing clinicians, whether in the academic or practice setting.

What is most exciting to me is that it is clear that the true potential of simulation in transforming how we train and educate nurses and other health disciplines is yet to be seen or fully understood! It will most definitely give us a better opportunity to have many more truly *great* nurses.

–Carol Bradley, MSN, RN
Senior Vice President, Chief Nursing Officer
Legacy Health
Portland, Oregon
cbradley@lhs.org

Foreword

The first time I met Beth Mancini in her new job as associate dean at the University of Texas at Arlington (UTA), she had a papier-mâché pig with wings hanging from her office ceiling. Hmm…I knew there had to be a story about it, and there was. UTA's nursing dean had started recruiting Mancini while she was attending her doctoral program at UTA. Mancini, a CNO, was adamant that she would not leave the clinical side of nursing, throwing out that classic phrase that she'd do it when pigs fly. Well, clearly time and persuasion—and possibly those pigs—finally brought Mancini to UTA, and she never looked back. Bringing to bear her years of clinical experience at the practice, supervisory, and executive level, Mancini knew the potential for education the first time she saw a full-body high-fidelity mannequin.

Beth Ulrich came to simulation through a different route, starting when she was laboring with her first child in the teaching hospital where she also worked. Across the hall from her, she could hear two interns talking outside the door of another patient's room about who was going to do his first "laboring woman's exam." While each said he had read about it in a book, neither of them had ever done one before. From that day forward, and especially as she moved into working with new graduate nurses transitioning into professional nurses, she was committed to finding ways to make sure that, whenever possible, the first time a health care professional performed a procedure it was not on a live patient.

Though certainly some doubters may label it a fad, the use of simulation in health care education has grown exponentially over the past 10 years. Not only is it more common than not to see simulation devices in nursing schools and teaching hospitals, but also there are two thriving journals, multiple worldwide organizations, two sets of published standards, accreditation and certification opportunities, degrees, and large sums of money everywhere being dedicated to simulation. The pedagogy of simulation—note I did not say mannequins—is a paradigm shift in education, the first in 40 years (some would say 2000).

Simulation might have been a fad. But two major things happened at roughly the same time: Because of increasing political pressure, academia finally started working to adopt interprofessional education as a major teaching strategy, and hospitals adopted team training and just-in-time skills training, and began using simulation to build and test new hospital buildings and procedures as a means of improving patient safety.

Some hospitals now use simulation as a part of the hiring process and for initial and ongoing skills evaluation. Variations of the simulation theme provided a logical methodology to do all of these things, which has created an environment of longevity.

Ulrich and Mancini have assembled some of today's most recognized simulation experts—reflecting the truly interdisciplinary nature of simulation itself—to contribute their knowledge and writing to this thoughtful, up-to-the-minute reference book. It provides comprehensive and thorough coverage of the state of simulation.

–Suzie Kardong-Edgren, PhD, RN, ANEF
Assistant Professor
Washington State University
Spokane, Washington

Introduction

"Simulation is the key to patient safety and medical quality."
—*John Nance, Author,* Why Hospitals Should Fly

One of the biggest challenges we face in health care is how to educate and train health care professionals without endangering patients—especially when we are teaching the management of high stakes situations such as codes, trauma care, chest pain, and anaphylactic shock in which any delay in treatment threatens the outcome. New practitioners enter their professions often without ever having seen, much less gotten experience with, many of the high-risk/low-volume patient conditions.

The use of simulation is growing exponentially in academic and service settings. Simulation can provide students, new graduates, and experienced clinicians opportunities to develop clinical competence and confidence in caring for patients in many clinical situations—far more situations than the learner can be exposed to in live clinical environments—and can provide those opportunities in a learning environment that is safe for the learner and does not compromise patient safety or outcomes. Simulation also offers the ability to objectively assess the performance of health care professionals against a well-defined standard of practice.

In clinical settings, simulation can be used to onboard new graduate and experienced staff and assess the performance of current staff. Many organizations carefully assess the competency and performance of new staff, but—other than perhaps yearly skills fairs—often do little to assure that existing staff continue to meet standards of practice and follow evidence-based and best-practice processes and protocols. Renewing nursing or medical licenses generally only requires paying a fee and completing continuing education programs—not demonstrating continued competence. Research is changing health care practice on an almost daily basis. To assume that all professionals who renew their licenses are competent in the knowledge and skills needed to practice in the current environment is naive at best and dangerous at worst—something Florence Nightingale knew and was passionate about more than 100 years ago. It often surprises people to learn that Nightingale opposed the registration of nurses. The reason was that she thought you could not know whether a nurse was competent based on just the fact that she had finished nursing school or passed a written examination. In an 1888 letter to the probationer nurses at St. Thomas Hospital, she said,

> *"She [the nurse] may have gone to a first rate course—plenty of examinations. And we may find nothing inside. It may be the difference between a nurse nursing and a nurse reading a book on nursing. Unless it bear fruit, it is all gilding and veneering; the reality is not there, growing, growing every year. Every nurse must grow. No nurse can stand still, she must go forward, or she will go backward, every year. And how can a certificate or public register show this?"*

Simulation can be used to improve an organization's ability to ensure that all of its clinicians maintain competence.

There is also growing evidence that simulation is effective in developing, assessing, and improving the performance of health care teams. Much as the aviation industry first used flight simulators to teach the "hard" skills of piloting airplanes, such as takeoffs, landings, and handling mechanical emergencies, health care began using simulators to teach the "hard" skills of caring for patients—diagnosing and using medications and other interventions in response to a patient's physiological changes. A series of high-fatality plane crashes caused the aviation industry to look beyond the hard-skill training solutions to improve how their people worked together and communicated with each other. As a result, they developed what is now called crew resource management (CRM), redefining roles and expectations; creating a culture of transparency and learning from errors; and developing training, processes, and standards that allow team leaders to quickly create highly functional teams from a group of crew members who very often have never worked together as a team. All of these things have been integrated into the aviation industry's simulation experiences. As a result, air travel is safer than ever. Like the aviation industry, the health care industry has come to understand that how health care professionals work together can have a major impact on patient safety and improving patient outcomes. Just as aviation uses simulation to teach CRM to its professionals, health care can use simulation for developing highly functional teams.

Simulation can also contribute to risk management and quality improvement—identifying latent threats to patient and clinician safety, allowing clinicians to test "what if" scenarios (What if we used another drug? What if we did intervention B before intervention A?), and performing trial runs of new techniques, equipment, and patient care areas.

Who Should Read This Book

The primary audience for this book is health care professionals who are currently using or are anticipating using simulation, including individuals in both academic and service settings—including schools of nursing and medicine, EMT training programs, the military, and hospitals and health care systems. The availability of education for simulation professionals and others involved peripherally with simulation has not kept up with the rapid growth of simulation use in both academic and service settings. Many simulation professionals are receiving their education on simulation through the traditional on-the-job, just-in-time training.

This book is designed as a personal professional resource and also as a support text for simulation courses. It is also a book for health care leaders who want to learn more about what simulation can offer their organizations, who are looking for ways to decrease the variability on how health care is delivered, and who understand that ensuring that competency is maintained is equally or more important than determining competency when health care professionals enter their professions

This book is a handbook for individuals working in or preparing to work in simulation and for academic and service organizations that are using simulation or are planning to use simulation. The book is both evidence-based and pragmatic. It is written in a style that can be easily read by busy health care professionals and provides strategies that can be immediately integrated into practice.

Book Content

Whether you are looking for a primer on simulation or information to improve your existing knowledge and expertise in the simulation specialty, *Mastering Simulation* has content for you. The book begins with an overview of the foundations of simulation in Chapter 1, allowing the reader to become familiar with simulation terminology, philosophic foundations, and educational principles, as well as describing the range of simulator typology that is currently available. Chapter 2 discusses competence and confidence, the relationships between them, and how simulation can be used to develop both in clinical performance. Chapter 3 describes the necessity and means of creating effective simulation environments that encourage participants to suspend disbelief and fully engage in the simulation as if they were caring for a live patient. Developing and planning scenarios, the detailed scripts for simulations and simulation environments, are discussed in Chapter 4. Chapter 5 offers information on the debriefing component of the simulation experience—on how to guide simulation participants to learn through reflecting on their experiences. In Chapter 6, strategies and techniques to evaluate simulation effectiveness are described, and in Chapter 7 the use of simulation with specific learner populations is discussed. The importance of interprofessional education and practice are increasingly being recognized, and Chapter 8 is dedicated to understanding how simulation can be used to develop and enhance high functioning teamwork. Using simulation in academic environments is the topic of Chapter 9, and a discussion on how to use simulations to improve outcomes in hospitals and health care systems is found in Chapter 10. Chapter 11 addresses using simulation for risk management and quality improvement, including identifying latent threats and improving processes. Chapter 12 provides information on designing and implementing simulation-based research. Chapter 13 is a resource for individuals wanting to enter or expand their careers in the field of simulation, as well as a resource for staff requirements for simulation centers, providing descriptions of simulation roles and positions. Credentialing of individuals and simulation programs is described in Chapter 14. Chapter 15 offers the information you need to develop and build a simulation center—from the initial planning and assessment process to the details of space and design recommendations. The final chapter of the book looks to the future and describes the issues, challenges, and opportunities that are evolving around the use of simulation in health care.

Final Thoughts

We wrote this book with two goals in mind: to provide a comprehensive resource for simulation professionals and to raise the awareness of the knowledge and expertise required to utilize simulation strategies. Though there are identified best practices related to implementing simulation methodologies, no single best way to integrate simulation into health profession education or health care practice exists. Simulation has multiple "faces"—many techniques, many places to be used, many ways in which the impact can be measured.

The uses of simulation in health care are only limited by our creativity and imagination. Every week, we hear of new uses for simulation that improve patient care and patient safety. At this point in the life cycle of simulation, we need to stay nimble and innovative and be careful not to become too rigid or tied to any one method or way to do things. We also need to actively look outside the domain of health care for guidance. The lessons learned by aviation, military science, and others who use simulation successfully are applicable to health care.

Simulation has much to offer, especially in keeping patients safe. In the words of Ziv, Wolpe, Small, and Glick (2006, p. 252), "The use of simulation wherever feasible conveys a critical educational and ethical message to all: patients are to be protected whenever possible and they are not commodities to be used as conveniences of training."

–Beth Tamplet Ulrich, EdD, RN, FACHE, FAAN
BethUlrich@aol.com
Mary E. (Beth) Mancini, PhD, RN, NE-BC, FAHA, ANEF, FAAN
mancini@uta.edu

Reference

Ziv, A., Wolpe, P. R., Small, S. D., & Glick S. (2006). Simulation based medical education: An ethical imperative. *Simulation in Healthcare, 1*(4), 252-256.

"No industry in which human lives depend on the skilled performance of responsible operators has waited for unequivocal proof of the benefits of simulation before embracing it."

—David M. Gaba, MD

Foundations of Simulation

Sharon Decker, PhD, RN, ANEF, FAAN
Sandra Caballero, MSN, RN
Chris McClanahan, MSN, RN, CEN

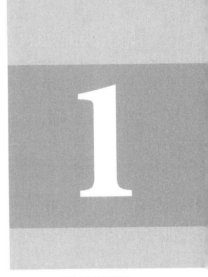

OBJECTIVES

- Describe the history of simulation including influential factors.
- Identify the philosophical framework for simulation.
- Discuss the importance of adult learning principles that pertain to simulation-based activities.
- Recognize the legal and ethical issues common to simulation-based activities.

Introduction to Simulation

Today's dynamic, complex health care environment requires nurses to demonstrate evidence-based clinical judgment while providing safe, quality patient care as a collaborative member of a health care team (Institute of Medicine [IOM], 2004a, 2011). National leaders, organizations, and accreditation agencies have challenged nurse educators to transform the current educational process to a learner-centered, active pedagogy. In 2004, the Institute of Medicine called for evidence-based revisions in the clinical education of health care professionals. Multiple IOM reports (2001, 2003, 2004a, 2011) have stressed that research is required to:

- Understand how to apply adult learning principles to clinical education
- Obtain empirical evidence to support the integration of new technologies, including simulation, into curriculum
- Explore the outcomes achieved by different types of teaching technologies
- Understand the process of translating knowledge to clinical practice

Simulation combined with other technologies provides a unique educational strategy to facilitate the development of skills, competencies, and clinical judgment that are mandatory to provide safe, quality patient care (Benner, Sutphen, Leonard, & Day, 2010; Gaba, 2004; IOM, 2004a, 2004b, 2011). For example, the 2004 IOM report *Keeping Patients Safe* stated that simulation is the most useful approach for developing skills related to unpredictable situations and crises. Similarly, Benner et al. (2010) support the development of clinical reasoning and interprofessional communication through new technologies such as simulation. Additionally, learning in a simulated environment is transferable and allows educators to monitor learner progress in a setting without risk to patients (IOM, 2011; Zigmont, Kappus, & Sudikoff, 2011). As a complex learning tool, simulation is a complement to (not a substitute for) actual patient care for promoting the learner's ability to integrate theory into a patient care situation in a safe, controlled environment (Bruce, Bridges, & Holcomb, 2003; Maran & Glavin, 2003).

History of Simulation

The history of clinical simulation has been well documented (Bradley, 2006; Cooper & Taqueti, 2004; Gaba, 2004). Although the use of mannequins to serve as simulation models is relatively new and continuing to grow with the advent of new technologies, mannequins have been utilized since the early 16th century (Bradley, 2006; Rodgers, 2007; Ziv, Wolpe, Small, & Glick, 2003). The 1911 development of "Mrs. Chase," or the Chase Hospital Doll, was the advent of the first commercially available training mannequin and was used primarily for nursing education (Decker, Gore, & Feken, 2011; Loyd, Lake, & Greenberg, 2004; National League for Nursing [NLN], 2012).

Asmund S. Laerdal further propelled clinical simulation with the advent of Resusci Anne in the 1960s, the first realistic and effective mouth-to-mouth resuscitation training aid (Cooper & Taqueti, 2004). The next leap forward came from the University of Southern California in the late 1960s with the development of SimOne, a computer-controlled, electronic mannequin capable of simulating vital signs, palpable pulses, inspiratory chest rise, eye blinking, and more (Bradley, 2006; Cooper & Taqueti, 2004). The introduction of Harvey by Dr. Michael Gordon in 1968 provided learners an anatomy-specific cardiopulmonary simulator that effectively provided 27 different cardiac pathologies (Rodgers, 2007). In the 1980s, the development of simulators for use in anesthesia training launched the movement into high-fidelity patient simulators.

Today's high-fidelity human patient simulators are capable of simulating many of the functions of the human body, its physiological variables, and its responses to pharmacological and other care interventions. In addition, the increased use of ultrasound technology in both the diagnostic and procedural arenas has led to the development of ultrasound-able human patient simulators capable of reproducing multiple pathologies or simulating human anatomy. Spurring on the continued advancement of health care simulation is the need for improved quality of care, increased urgency to advance patient safety, the transformation of how clinicians are educated, and the development of new technologies.

Influential Factors

Clinical simulation is dynamic and ever-changing, constantly morphing as new technologies are developed, clinical knowledge increases, and new evidence-based practices are implemented. New patient safety requirements and the need for innovative modalities to educate clinicians drive clinical simulation forward.

Patient Safety and Quality

The intricacy and richness characteristic of the health care profession is paralleled by the complexity of its milieus of practice (Benner et al., 2010). "New nurses need to be prepared to practice safely, accurately, and compassionately, in varied settings, where knowledge and innovation increase at an astonishing rate" (Benner et al., 2010. p. i). Evidence-based research suggests the lack of communication and collaboration within interprofessional health care teams has had a negative effect on the delivery of safe quality care (IOM, 2003; Lenard, Graham, & Bonacum, 2004). Clinical simulation centers, especially those offering interprofessional education, fill the educational gap by providing realistic, interactive, meaningful learning experiences. The result is improved skills proficiency, team dynamics, communication, and patient care (Decker, Sportsman, Puetz, & Billings, 2008; Kobayashi et al., 2008; Lewis, Strachan, & Smith, 2012; McCaughey & Traynor, 2010; Seropian, Brown, Gavilanes, & Driggers, 2004; Webster, 2009). Simulation also allows students the ability to apply Benner's concepts regarding performance characteristics and differing levels of clinical competency in a safe, yet challenging environment (Larew, Lessans, Spunt, & Covington, 2008).

For example, at the novice level learners use task trainers and role-play to develop basic technical and nontechnical skills. After competencies in these skills are attained, educators should use scaffolding to shift the learner's focus from producing replicable and predictible outcomes mastered at the novice level. With this continuous scaffolding approach, educators can facilitate the development of clinical reasoning required for competency by integrating unexpected issues within simulation-based scenarios. Development toward expertise continues as the provider transfers opportunities to exercise and implement flexible clinical judgment, ethical comportment, and formation from simulated to actual patient care situations (Benner et al., 2010).

Technology

Changes in technology, safety issues, learner attitudes, and accreditation requirements have forced changes in educational strategies and delivery. Simulation as a pedagogy includes the use of a variety of technology from low-fidelity task trainers to mid-fidelity ultrasound-compatible mannequins and high-fidelity computer-based mannequins. The development of virtual reality computer-based environments and haptic devices (defined in Table 1.1) provide realistic experiences in a risk-free environment with immediate feedback for the learner (Jenson & Forsyth, 2012). Learners are engaged in reproducible clinical environments interacting with virtual patients and interprofessional teams (Jenson & Forsyth, 2012). New integrated three-dimensional (3D) technologies immerse the learner in realistic anatomy models that can be manipulated, changing the dimension on how anatomy is learned and viewed. Ultrasound-compatible partial trainers and mannequins offer realistic representations of necessary anatomical structures facilitating proficiency in advanced skills such as central line insertion. The continued combination of low-fidelity task trainers and standardized patients (SPs) creates hybrid scenarios bringing true human interaction to the scenarios along with skills acquisition and task performance. Advances in simulator technology augment opportunities for interprofessional learning experiences, improving patient safety and patient outcomes.

Transformation in Education

The call for transformation in how health care professionals are trained is loud and clear. Critical shortages of qualified nurses and physicians have communities turning to local community colleges and universities to fill these gaps quickly with qualified, competent, safe clinicians. The Bureau of Labor Statistics (2012) has projected that registered nursing jobs will increase 26% from 2010 to 2020, faster than the average for all occupations, and forecasts indicate another nursing shortage in the near future (Juraschek, Zhang, Ranganathan, & Lin, 2012). Many factors contribute to the nursing shortage: job stress, management issues, work environment, physical demand, economy, nursing educator shortages, lack of mentoring programs, and much more. Regardless of the reasons for nursing shortages, developing innovative means of educating new nurses is paramount to combating the problem.

The IOM's (2000) report To Err Is Human identified that the lack of communication within all health care disciplines results in unnecessary increases in preventable morbidity and mortality rates. The rapid development of communication strategies was quickly followed with strategies such as TeamSTEPPS by the Agency for Healthcare Research and Quality ([AHRQ]; 2011). Because health care professionals need a way to integrate the new communication strategies in a safe environment, simulation is being utilized as a way to teach and assess competency in the newly acquired communication skills.

Additionally, the ever-increasing focus on patient safety goals and new government regulations are acknowledgments that health care professionals need to become more astute and critically analyze and think through problems while providing evidence-based care. A series of IOM reports from 1999 to 2004 identified the key components necessary to the design of a safe health care system: (1) safety, (2) quality, (3) leadership, and (4) public health (Finkelman & Kenner, 2007). The IOM reports *To Err Is Human* (2000) and *Crossing the Quality Chasm* (2001) both call for improvement in health care quality and safety by using strategies preparing clinicians to (1) work in interprofessional teams, (2) use nursing informatics, (3) maintain an improved understanding of disease processes, pathology, and outcomes, (4) provide leadership, and (5) provide safe, timely, efficient, and effective patient-centered care (Finkelman & Kenner, 2007). Simulation allows educators to deliver these expanded expectations to new and seasoned clinicians in a safe, nonthreatening environment which fosters meaningful learning.

Core Competencies for Interprofessional Collaborative Practice: The four domains of the core competencies are (1) values/ethics for interprofessional practice, (2) roles/responsibilities, (3) interprofessional communication, and (4) teams and teamwork (Interprofessional Education Collaborative Expert Panel, 2011).

Definition of Simulation

The term simulation has more than one definition:

- *Merriam-Webster Learner's Dictionary* (2013) defines simulation as "something that is made to look, feel, or behave like something else especially so that it can be studied or used to train people."

- According to Gaba (2004), "simulation is a 'technique,' not a technology, to replace or amplify real experiences with guided experiences, often immersive in nature, that evoke or replicate substantial aspects of the real world in a fully interactive fashion" (p. i2).

- Jeffries (2005) has described simulation as an educational process in which learning experiences are simulated to imitate the working environment. The learner is required to integrate skills (both technical and nontechnical) into a patient care scenario and thus demonstrate clinical judgment.

- Simulation is defined by the International Nursing Association for Clinical Simulation and Learning (INACSL) Board of Directors (BOD) (2011, p. S6) as, "A pedagogy using one or more typologies to promote improved and/or validate a participant's progression from novice to expert."

- The Society for Simulation in Healthcare (SSH) Council for Accreditation of Healthcare Simulation Programs has defined simulation as "a technique that uses a situation or environment created to allow persons to experience a representation of a real event for the purpose of practice, learning, evaluation, testing, or to gain understanding of systems or human actions. Simulation is the application of a simulator to training and/or assessment" (SSH, 2013, p. 31).

Comparing these definitions reveals similarities specific to simulation being a pedagogy that uses multiple tools (such as simulators, partial trainers, and standardized patients) to promote learning and assess learning.

For definitions approved by the Society for Simulation in Healthcare, go to http://ssih.org.

For definitions approved by the International Nursing Association for Clinical Simulation and Learning, go to http://inacsl.org.

For definitions from the National League for Nursing, go to http://sirc.nln.org/mod/glossary/view.php?id=183.

Simulation Typology

The spectrum of simulation typology varies in complexity and fidelity spanning the use of human models to high-fidelity simulators. Fidelity is defined as the "physical, contextual, cognitive, and emotional realism" (SSH, 2013, p. 32).

- **Low-fidelity mannequins** are the static tools that do not provide feedback to the learner. Low-fidelity mannequins include partial and full-body task trainers such as airway management trainers and are used predominately to develop and assess technical skills.

- **Mid-fidelity mannequins/simulators** provide learners with isolated feedback. An example of a mid-fidelity trainer is a simulator used to generate heart and lung sounds without chest movement.

- **High-fidelity simulators** provide realistic responses that can be modified to respond to the situation. These simulators provide realistic responses such as heart and lung sounds, chest movement, and palpable pulses, and they are integrated into patient scenarios requiring learners to demonstrate skill attainment while engaged in situations requiring clinical judgment (Jeffries & Rogers, 2012; Seropian, 2003).

The spectrum of simulation summarized in Table 1.1 includes a definition of the various tools or typology of simulation. The appropriate use of the spectrum of simulation typology requires strategic planning and must be appropriate for the identified learning needs and expertise of the practitioner (Decker et al., 2011; Issenberg, McGaghie, Petrusa, Gordan, & Scalese, 2005; Maran & Glavin, 2003; Seropian, 2003).

Table 1.1 Summary of and Definitions for Current Simulation Typology	
Simulation Typology	**Definition**
Task Trainers	Anatomical models or mannequins used to obtain competency in a specific skill or procedure
Peer-to-Peer	Collaboration between peers used to learn and/or master specific skills
Computer-Based Training	Computer applications (software or web-based programs) to teach, provide feedback, and assess knowledge and clinical judgment
Virtual Reality	An artificial projected environment that provides spatial dimensions and sensory stimuli through special glasses and sensors to promote authenticity
Haptic Systems	A computer-generated environment that provides tactile and visual sensations as procedures are conducted
Standardized Patients	Volunteers or paid individuals who are taught to portray a patient in a case scenario in a realistic and consistent manner
Advanced Patient Simulators	Computerized full-body mannequins that can provide realistic physiologic responses
Gaming	A simulation or program (board or computer-assisted games) that enables learners to interact, solve problems, and make decisions
Hybrid	A situation that combines more than one type of simulation typology

Sources: Decker et al., 2011; SSH, 2013

Simulation can be used to support lifelong learning at all levels from beginning novice learners to expert practitioners. In addition to assisting the practitioner in developing and maintaining competency in technical skills, simulation can assist learners with the development of nontechnical skills, such as communication and critical thinking, to acquire new knowledge and understand conceptual relationships (Cato, 2012; Gaba, 2004).

The Institute of Medicine has recognized simulation as a strategy to enhance the technical skills of health care students and professionals (IOM 2001, 2011) and the acquisition of ongoing knowledge of the practitioner (IOM, 2004). As previously discussed, multiple authorities stress that simulated experiences should:

- Be designed to replicate a realistic situation
- Have objectives that are learner dependent and state the expected outcome of the experience
- Be a complement to (not a substitute for) actual patient care to promote an individual's ability to develop competencies and clinical judgment
- Be conducted in a controlled, nonthreatening environment without risks to patients (Bruce et al., 2003; Jeffries & Rogers, 2012; Maran & Glavin, 2003)

Task Trainers

Task trainers are designed to represent a specific body part and are used for the acquisition and assessment of technical skills. Task trainers allow educators to facilitate the learner's mastery of complex skills by subdividing them into segments—for example, think about the steps involved in inserting an intravenous catheter. Partial task trainers vary in complexity from static models to trainers that provide realistic heart, lung, and bowel sounds (Decker et al., 2011; Issenberg et al., 2005; Maran & Glavin, 2003; SSH, 2013).

Standardized Patients

A standardized patient program integrates realistic case studies into role play. Individuals (paid or volunteer) are taught to portray a "patient" in a realistic and consistent manner. The learner interacting with a standardized patient is expected to demonstrate appropriate communication skills, behaviors, and attitudes while conducting interviews, performing physical examinations, and developing a plan of care (Ebbert & Connors, 2004; SSH, 2013).

Standardized patients have been a component of the competency examination of the United States Medical Licensing Examination (USMLE) since 2004. The clinical skills component of the USMLE requires the examinee to communicate effectively with a standardized patient while developing a rapport, obtaining a health history, completing a focused assessment, and documenting the results (USMLE, 2012). Standardized patients have been successfully integrated into formative and summative assessments in both graduate and undergraduate nursing programs and provide a tool to validate the learner's knowledge, skills, and clinical judgment (Ebbert & Connors, 2004).

Computer-Based Programs

Computer-based programs provide a computerized system of discovery learning in which the learner can interact with a situation and receive feedback related to performed actions. Computer-based programs are considered to be relatively inexpensive and allow learners to work independently or in groups. Navigation options allow practitioners to tailor the learning to personal needs. The competencies of practitioners can be validated through case scenarios requiring the integration of procedural and critical thinking skills. Various levels of monitoring are integrated into the software to provide educators with written documentation of the learner's performance, including multiple-choice tests and performance summaries (Issenberg et al., 2005; Maran & Glavin, 2003; Seropian et al., 2004).

Virtual Reality

Virtual reality, developed as an offshoot of video-game technology, integrates interactive computer simulation with psychomotor and cognitive learning to give the learner the feeling of being immersed in a simulated experience. Virtual reality provides cues through sensory stimulation (hearing, touch, and visual) to evoke feelings of reality. The practitioner engaged in virtual reality is required to integrate knowledge of anatomy and physiology while performing and validating clinical competency in specific procedures, such as intravenous catheter insertion, airway management, amniocentesis, endoscopy, and bronchoscopy (Agazio, Pavlides, Lasome, Flaherty, & Torrance, 2002; Loyd et al., 2004; Ziv, Small, & Wolpe, 2000).

Haptic Systems

Haptic (touch) systems have the capability of integrating the feeling of resistance when you are using instrumentation. The technology creates an illusion of having direct contact with the model. Haptic systems are used extensively with surgical training and with laparoscopic and endoscopic trainers (Kneebone, 2003; Ziv et al., 2000).

Advanced Patient Simulators

Recent advances in computer technology have produced full-body mannequins (advanced patient simulators) with various levels of complexity. The human patient simulators can be programmed to respond in real time to pharmacological and other treatment modalities. Human patient simulators have palpable pulses, audible blood pressures, and chest movements with respirations; simulate various heart, lung, and bowel sounds; and provide verbal cues to the learner. Such features add realism to clinical teaching scenarios and are supplemented with monitors programmed to provide electrocardiogram (ECG) waveforms, cardiac output, and pulse oximeter readings. Additionally, the technology allows for objective measurement of knowledge, technical skill level, and critical-thinking abilities of the learner (Maran & Glavin, 2003; Nehring, Ellis, & Lashley, 2001; Weller, 2004).

Theoretical Foundation of Simulation

"Of the many cues that influence behavior, at any point in time, none is more common than the actions of others."

–Albert Bandura, 1986

Philosophic Foundations

Learning changes behaviors and perceptions promoting insight and learning transfer (Bigge & Shermis, 2003). Research indicates that a learner develops competency in a specific area by developing a conceptual understanding of the subject. To achieve conceptual understanding, the learner must have the essential, factual knowledge needed to recognize patterns and relationships and to organize this information into a conceptual framework. After developing a conceptual framework, the competent learner can retrieve, transfer, and apply knowledge to new situations (Bigge & Shermis, 2003; Bradford, Brown, & Cocking, 2000). To promote the learning process through simulation, the experience needs to be based on adult learning principles, be evidence-based, and include three distinct phases: pre-briefing, the scenario (case study), and debriefing (INACSL BOD, 2011).

The philosophical substructure for simulation-based experiences is grounded in the works of multiple experts such as Dewey (1910, 1916, 1933), Bandura (1977, 2001), Kolb (1984), and Schön (1983, 1987). These works highlight the importance of relationships, experiential learning, and the integration of reflection into the learning process. Specifically, the relationships discussed are those among the learner, the environment, and the educator/facilitator, and reflection has been identified as critical to the development and transfer of new knowledge.

Dewey defined learning (1910) as "not learning things, but the meanings of things" (p. 176). Developing meaning or insight requires an interaction, reflective thought, and time for personal discovery (Dewey, 1933). Dewey (1933) described reflection as an active, emotional interaction that assists learners in constructing new knowledge on past experiences. According to Dewey (1933), the development of new knowledge is the outcome of a five-phase process: problem identification, data collection, interpretation, hypotheses generation, and ultimately the recognition of the new knowledge and application of this knowledge to new experiences. Dewey (1933) stressed planning the experiences and facilitating the process of discovery as the educator's responsibility. Educators can use simulation-based learning to promote the five phases of knowledge development and transfer.

Bandura (1977) also discussed the relationship between an individual's behavior and attitudes and the environment to skills acquisition. The environment, according to Bandura, includes both the physical setting and interactions with others. Social Learning (Cognitive) Theory, developed by Bandura (1997, 2001), proposes that behavior is learned through observation and imitating others and influenced by the observed consequences of initiated behavior. For example, if positive outcomes are observed, the behavior is more likely to be emulated. Bandura stressed that optimal learning requires the individual to be proactive and goal-directed and to self-regulate. The self-regulated learner has an intrinsic motivation for learning, participates actively, sets personal learning goals, and engages in reflective thought. Additionally, the self-regulated learner utilizes learning outcomes to construct new knowledge, and the process of engagement and self-regulation improves as the learner's self-confidence grows. The educator, according to Bandura (1977), functions predominantly as a role model or a facilitator and is responsible for creating an environment conducive to learning.

Simulation-based learning integrates the key concepts of the Social Learning Theory. For example, research has demonstrated that simulation enhances the self-confidence of the learner (Blum, Borglund, & Parcells, 2010; Scherer, Bruce, & Runkawatt, 2007). Educators who integrate peer observation into simulated experience should remember that observed consequences of behaviors have an effect on learning. Therefore, they need to provide feedback in a positive, constructive manner.

Kolb (1984) defined learning as a process that includes a synergetic relationship between the learner and the environment. The cycle of experiential learning according to Kolb (1984) represents the mandatory components for learning. The cycle includes the integration of concrete experience (real-life experiences), reflective observation (reflection or internalization of the experience), abstract conceptualization (looking for patterns and meanings), and active experimentation (assimilation of thoughts in an effort to develop new understandings). Finally, Kolb (1984) stressed that learning occurs best in an environment replicating a real-life situation and in situations requiring the learner to seek patterns and meaning to promote insightfulness. Educators are challenged by Kolb (1984) to use multiple active strategies to support different learning styles.

Simulation-based learning supports the cycle of experiential learning according to Kolb (1984). Simulation scenarios designed to provide realistic, concrete experiences while debriefing allow learners to reflect on the experience to make sense of their learning. In this realistic environment, simulation provides a setting for active experimentation that promotes understanding, assimilation, and changes in practice (Zigmont et al., 2011). Schön (1987) proposed the use of a "reflective practicum" (p. 18)—an active learning experience based on a realistic event and completed in a realistic environment. Schön (1983) identified two specific types of reflection: reflection-in-action and reflection-on-action.

- **Reflection-in-action** (self-monitoring) occurs while being engaged in an experience (thinking about an action while doing it). Schön (1987) described reflection-in-action as the artistry displayed when a practitioner integrates knowledge from past experiences into new situations.
- **Reflection-on-action** (cognitive postmortem) is a conscious review after the experience. The goal of reflection-on-action is to uncover new understandings with the goal of applying this knowledge to future practice.

According to Schön (1987), educators function as coaches to facilitate active learning and promote learning transfer. A simulation-based activity fulfills the requirements of a "reflective practicum" as discussed by Schön (1987). Using the principles of a reflective practicum, educators can plan the learning experience to encourage reflection-in-action through the use of Socratic questioning. The simulation-based environment allows learners to take risks and discover consequences while implementing patient care in a safe environment. Educators can facilitate reflection-on-action during debriefing.

In summary, the pedagogy of simulation is grounded in the works of Dewey, Bandura, Kolb, and Schön. These philosophers highlighted the dynamic relationships of the learner, the educator, and the environment to experiential learning. These dynamic relationships are essential to simulation-based learning.

Educational Principles

"Simulated disorder postulates perfect discipline; simulated fear postulates courage; simulated weakness postulates strength."

–Lao Tzu

Meyers and Jones (1993) identified three interrelated factors critical to experiential learning: the elements, learning strategies, and teaching resources. The elements include talking and listening, writing, reading, and reflecting. Reflection, according to Meyers and Jones (1993), assists the learner to clarify, question, and develop new knowledge. Strategies recommended by these authors to promote experiential learning include small group discussions, case studies, journal writing, and simulation. They stressed that time is needed for the individual to reflect and build upon the learning experience (Meyers & Jones, 1993).

Benner, Hooper-Kyriakidis, and Stannard (1999) further emphasized the importance of time for reflection when they incorporated the Dreyfus model of skills acquisition into the learning process. The Dreyfus model suggests that the learner progresses through five levels of learning when acquiring and developing proficiency: novice, advanced beginner, competent, proficient, and expert (Dreyfus & Dreyfus, 1980). According to Dreyfus and Dreyfus (1980), experience can facilitate progression through the stages. Benner and colleagues (1999) further stressed that the experience is not obtained through the mere passage of time, but should include the refinement of preconceived ideas through actual clinical practice.

Experiential learning, according to Benner and colleagues (1999), is defined as "clinical learning that is accomplished by being open to having one's expectations refined, challenged, or disconfirmed by the unfolding situation" (p. 568). As stressed by Benner (2000), nursing is a complex practice requiring continuous clinical knowledge development through experiential learning. Therefore, according to Benner and colleagues (1999), the nurse learning to make good clinical judgments must become engaged in a process with ongoing experiential learning and reflection.

Haag-Heitman (2008) reviewed the literature discussing the novice-to-expert continuum and identified key factors that promote expert performance. These factors include the roles of deliberate practice, risk-taking, social models, and mentoring, as well as the importance of external rewards. Simulation-based learning provides an environment that can easily integrate these factors in both the academic and practice settings. The deliberate practice model discusses the importance of time and recommends repeated intentional practice accompanied by immediate feedback to improve skill performance (Ericsson, 2004, 2006). The best results from deliberate practice are achieved when learners are self-motivated, actively participate in an experience that includes problem solving, and are given appropriate feedback (Ericsson, 2004; McGaghie, Issenberg, Petrusa, & Scalese, 2006, 2010). Additionally, educators implementing deliberate practice are expected to establish and adhere to precise measurements of performance to assess learning attainment (McGaghie et al., 2006, 2010).

The goal of deliberate practice in simulation-based learning is constant skill, knowledge, and professional improvement that progresses to the expert level of performance. Multiple studies have demonstrated that deliberate practice, grounded in behavioral theories of skills acquisition, improved the cognitive and motor components of a skill and promoted learning transfer (McGaghie et al., 2006, 2010).

To be effective, simulated experiences need to be grounded in experiential theory and adult learning principles (Jeffries & Rodgers, 2012). Learning is the process of acquiring knowledge and skills through experiences (Bigge & Shermis, 2003) or a process of change as an individual interacts with the environment to acquire habits, knowledge, and attitudes (Knowles, Holton, & Swanson, 2011). Experiences can occur in both the real or simulated environment as long as the experience is based on adult learning principles. According to Knowles (1984) and Knowles and colleagues (2011), adult learning principles that educators need to address when designing a learning experience include that adults (1) are internally motivated, (2) have past life experiences and expect these to be appreciated, (3) are goal directed, (4) expect to see relevancy of the learning, and (5) want to be respected. Simulation-based experiences provide concrete experiences (case-based clinical scenarios), reflective thought (debriefing), and experimentation. Strategies for educators to promote learning through simulation are shown in Table 1.2. Simulation educators will find many online modules available to assist in development of expertise.

Table 1.2 Incorporating Adult Learning Principles into Simulated Experiences	
Principle	**Strategy**
Internal motivation	Challenge the learner appropriately (for example, scenarios should become progressively more challenging throughout the curriculum).
	Lead the learner to inquiry through Socratic questioning.
	Actively listen to the learner.
	Provide appropriate, regular, constructive feedback
	Acknowledge goal attainment.
Life experiences	Acknowledge life experiences and help learner. connect these to the learning.
	Facilitate reflective thought.
Goal-directed	Link experiences to specific goals.
	Base learning on realistic experiences (case scenarios).
Relevancy-oriented	Allow learners to assist in designing learning experiences.
	Promote active learning and engagement by using multiple strategies.
Expect to be respected	Create a respectful, supportive environment.
	Allow learners to express ideas.
	Allow learners to participate in self and peer feedback (peer debriefing).

The ultimate goal for learning is the transfer of knowledge, skills, attitudes, and behaviors. Although limited research is available to demonstrate how and if simulation-based learning is transferred to the patient care setting, reviews of business literature (Burke & Hutchins, 2007; Merriam & Leahy, 2005) provide multiple ideas that can be integrated into health care. Some of the educational variables identified by these authors that affect transfer are presented in Table 1.3. You can see various strategies provided that you can incorporate into a simulated activity so both health care students and practitioners are promoting learning transfer.

Table 1.3   Strategies to Prompt Learning Transfer

Variables related to the learner, the experience, and the environment	Strategies for educators to initiate to promote learning transfer
Characteristics of the learner: • Intrinsic motivation • Intellectual/cognitive ability • Self-efficacy • Openness or readiness to learn (There is a direct correlation to the listed learner characteristics and the demonstrated ability to transfer learning.)	Allow learner to have input into the training. Validate usefulness of learning to current health care environment. Incorporate strategies that promote self-efficacy.
Specific stated behavioral objectives (Specific behavior objectives assisted learners in directing effort and developed strategies for learning transfer.)	Establish learning objectives for the experience that are obtainable, yet challenging.
Multiple active-learning instructional methodologies (Integration of multiple active-learning instructional methodologies improves the ability to transfer learning.)	Incorporate group work, case scenarios. Use various simulation modalities. Segment learning into manageable "chunks." Model and demonstrate the desired knowledge, skill, attitude, and behavior changes.
Perceived value and relevance of the experience	Assist learner in identifying relevance of learning. Assist learner in identifying the content to the work setting.
Degree of practice and feedback (Focused practice and integration of appropriate, regular feedback promoted learning transfer.)	Include deliberate practice into the experience. Provide positive feedback. Incorporate periodic one-on-one coaching. Incorporate peer coaching and feedback.

Table 1.3 Strategies to Prompt Learning Transfer *(cont.)*	
Variables related to the learner, the experience, and the environment	*Strategies for educators to initiate to promote learning transfer*
Opportunity to apply learning	Integrate mixture of skills and knowledge into simulations.
	Provide opportunities for learners to apply new knowledge and skills to a situation as soon as possible after the learning.
Supportive work environment and commitment of the organization (Individuals who worked in an environment that acknowledged the new knowledge and skills demonstrated greater learning transfer.)	Provide incentives and recognition of learning (financial or job-related, such as clinical ladder recognition).
	Allow individuals to provide inservice education to colleagues that highlights new learning.
	Assist learner in recognizing his or her importance to the work setting.

In summary, the goal of experiential learning is for the learner to gain new ideas and insight from an experience. Using principles of experiential learning, a simulated experience should be designed to require active participation and engagement in reflective thought in an effort to gain new ideas and insight from the experience (SSH, 2013). Simulation-based learning requires the integration of adult and experiential learning principles into a planned concrete experience (the case scenario) and into the debriefing designed to promote reflective thought (Waxman & Telles, 2009; Zigmont et al., 2011).

Legal and Ethical Issues

Health care providers face many challenges in the health care industry today. They are constantly trying to keep up with the new advances in technology. They are faced with caring for patients who have more complex disease processes and illnesses and with having to make split-second critical decisions with incomplete or inaccurate information, often because of their lack of communication and working together as a team (IOM,

2011). In 2005, the Joint Commission (TJC) linked 70% of sentinel events to the inability to communicate effectively among health care professionals (The Joint Commission on the Accreditation of Healthcare Organizations [JCAHO], 2005). Communication has been improved somewhat, but remains one of the top three root causes of sentinel events and is the leading root cause in delays in treatment (The Joint Commission [TJC], 2013). The Joint Commission's 2013 patient safety goals include the need to encourage all health care providers to work as interprofessional teams in communication and behaviors to prevent medical errors (TJC, 2012). The health care industry will never forget the publication by the IOM (2000) *To Err Is Human,* which stated that at least 44,000 people, and perhaps as many as 98,000, die in hospitals each year because of the preventable mistakes by health care providers. Our nation, at that moment, realized just how unsafe health care was. "The Quality of Health Care in America Committee of the Institute of Medicine (IOM) concluded that it is not acceptable for patients to be harmed by the health care system that is supposed to offer healing and comfort—a system that promises 'First, do no harm.'" (IOM, 2000, p. 2).

Looking at this problem prompted health care regulatory and standards organizations to investigate the causes. Where did the problem stem from? What needed to be done to decrease this outrageous statistic? The way our health care professionals are trained should have a direct effect on how health care is delivered. Was our educational training not meeting this standard? If not, what action needed to be taken? According to the Lancet Commissions, "Professional education has not kept pace with these challenges, largely because of fragmented, outdated, and static curricula that will produce ill-equipped graduates" (Frenk et al., 2010, p. 1923).

The American Nurses Association (ANA) Code of Ethics for Nurses helps nurses and guides them in pursuing ethical behavior and decisions. Nurses are to respect human dignity and are held accountable and responsible for nursing judgment and action. Above all they are responsible to provide the most compassionate and competent care to meet all the health needs and concerns of their patients (ANA, 2001). The Code of Ethics for Nurses also stresses, "Nurse educators have a responsibility to ensure that basic competencies are achieved…prior to entry of an individual into practice" (ANA, 2001, p. 18).

Is it ethical and legal to send nurses out into the clinical setting without the proper education and opportunity to practice adequately? Decker (2012) posed a question: "Are nurse educators and other health care professionals demonstrating compassion when they allow students to perform procedures for the first time on clients instead of first providing students with simulated experiences?" (p. 19). The simulated clinical setting allows learners to practice skills and different health care situations as many times as they need to achieve the level of comfort and competence needed to safely perform care in an actual patient clinical setting.

Benner et al. (2010) state that intervention requiring the credible and adequate process of assessing nurse's skills and competencies is required to prevent such incidents that can lead to patient harm. The National League for Nursing (2010) defines core competencies for nurses as "discrete and measurable skills" and says that these skills need to be the "foundation for clinical performance examination and the validation of practice competence essential for patient safety and quality care" (p. 65). The Quality and Safety Education for Nurses (QSEN) project identifies patient-centered care, teamwork and collaboration, evidence-based practice, quality improvement, safety, and informatics as quality and safety competencies (QSEN Institute, 2012).

Simulation training helps identify ethical issues that relate to the principles of beneficence, nonmaleficence, autonomy, and justice that can arise for health care providers themselves and related to patients they care for (Carlson, 2011).

- **Beneficence** "refers to a moral obligation to act for the benefit of others" (Beauchamp & Childress, 2001, p. 166). As Carlson (2011) questions, "What obligation is there to ensure that all providers, regardless of their location, have access to simulation training not only so they as providers are competent but also so the patient population they serve receives competent care?" (p. 12).

- **Nonmaleficence** is defined as doing no harm to others whether it be emotional, physical, or financial (Beauchamp & Childress, 2001). Ziv, Small, and Wolpe (2000, p. 492) stated that all educators have "an ethical obligation to make all efforts to expose a healthcare professional to clinical challenges that can be reasonably well simulated prior to allowing them to encounter and be responsible for similar real-life challenges." When students engage in simulation-based training, health care organizations see a reduction of risks (Carlson, 2011).

- **Autonomy** is respecting the right of individuals to make their own noninfluenced decisions. Pertaining to health, this autonomy includes decisions patients make only after all information is provided to them through disclosure and has been explained and understood (Beauchamp & Childress, 2001). Decker (2012) questions if autonomy is being violated when patients are not informed of the qualifications of their nurses. "Should patients be told if a student is performing venipuncture for the first time?" (p. 17).

- **Justice** is offering fair or "appropriate treatment in light of what is due or owed to persons" (Beauchamp & Childress, 2001, p. 226). Individuals have the right to equally share the risks and benefits of medical research, innovations, and practitioner training (Decker, 2012). With the increasing costs of simulation centers, not all locations are able to support the maintenance that comes along with simulation, making the opportunity for providers to equally practice impossible for those who live in an area with no center. Providers are away from their actual patients for an increased time if they are required to train with simulation and have to travel to a place that has a center (Carlson, 2011). Providers have the right to have equal opportunities to train.

Conclusion

Clinical judgment and mastery of skills (technical and nontechnical) have been identified as necessary to provide safe, competent patient care. Educators are challenged to use evidence-based teaching strategies to promote the learner's clinical judgment. As an experiential learning strategy, simulation provides a unique tool to promote clinical judgment. Simulation-based learning is consistent with experiential learning theory by requiring interactivity, building on prior knowledge, and ensuring knowledge transfer.

References

Agazio, J. B., Pavlides, C. C., Lasome, C. E., Flaherty, N. J., & Torrance, R. J. (2002). Evaluation of a virtual reality simulator in sustainment training. *Military Medicine, 167*(11), 893-897.

Agency for Healthcare Research and Quality (AHRQ). (2011). *Training guide: Using simulation in Team-STEPPS® training.* AHRQ Publication No. 11-0041-EF. Rockville, MD: Author. Retrieved from http://www.ahrq.gov/teamsteppstools/simulation/trainingd.htm

American Nurses Association (ANA). (2001). *Code of ethics for nurses with interpretive statements.* Washington, DC: American Nurses Publishing.

Bandura, A. (1977). Self-efficacy: Toward a unifying theory of behavioral change. *Psychological Review, 84*(2), 191-215.

Bandura, A. (2001). Social cognitive theory: An agentive perspective. *Annual Review of Psychology, 52*, 1-26.

Beauchamp, T. L., & Childress, J. F. (2001). *Principles of biomedical ethics* (5th ed.). New York, NY: Oxford University Press.

Benner, P. (2000). The wisdom of our practice. *American Journal of Nursing, 100*(10), 99-105.

Benner, P., Hooper-Kyriakidis, P., & Stannard, D. (1999). *Clinical wisdom and interventions in critical care: A thinking-in-action approach.* Philadelphia, PA: W.B. Saunders Company.

Benner, P., Sutphen, M., Leonard, V., & Day, L. (2010). *Educating Nurses: A call for radical transformation.* San Francisco, CA: Jossey-Bass.

Bigge, M. L., & Shermis, S. S. (2003). *Learning theories for teachers* (6th ed.). Boston, MA: Pearson Education, Inc.

Blum, C., Borglund, S., & Parcells, D. (2010). High-fidelity nursing simulation: Impact on student self-confidence and clinical competence. *International Journal of Nursing Education Scholarship, 7*(18), *1-14.* Retrieved from http://www.bepress.com/ijnes/vol7/iss1/art18(18). doi: 10.2202/1548-923X.2035

Bradford, J. D., Brown, A. L., & Cocking, R. R. (Eds.). (2000). *How people learn: Brain, mind, experience, and school.* Washington, DC: National Research Council.

Bradley, P. (2006). The history of simulation in medical education and possible future directions. *Medical Education History, 40*(3), 254-262.

Bruce, S., Bridges, E. J., & Holcomb, J. B. (2003). Preparing to respond: Joint Trauma Training Center and USAF Nursing Warskills Simulation Laboratory. *Critical Care Nursing Clinics of North America, 15*(2), 149-162.

Bureau of Labor Statistics, U.S. Department of Labor. (2012). *Occupational outlook handbook, 2012-13 edition, registered nurses.* Washington, DC: Author. Retrieved from http://www.bls.gov/ooh/healthcare/registered-nurses.htm

Burke, L. A., & Hutchins, H. M. (2007). Training transfer: An integrative literature review. *Human Resource Development Review, 6*(3), 263-296. doi:10.1177/1534484307303035

Carlson, E. (2011). Ethical consideration surrounding simulation-based competency training. *Journal of Illinois Nursing, 109*(3), 11-14.

Cato, M. L. (2012). Using simulation in nursing education. In P.R. Jeffries (Ed.), *Simulation in nursing education: From conceptualization to evaluation* (pp. 1-12). New York, NY: National League for Nursing.

Cooper, J. B., & Taqueti, V. R. (2004). A brief history of the development of mannequin simulators for clinical education and training [Electronic Version]. *Quality and Safety in Health Care, 13*(Supp 1), i11-i18.

Decker, S. I. (2012). Simulations: education and ethics. In P. Jeffries (Ed.), *Simulation in nursing education: From conceptualization to evaluation* (pp. 13-23). New York, NY: National League for Nursing.

Decker, S. I., Gore, T., & Feken, C.(2011). Simulation. In T. Bristol & J. Zerwekh (Eds.), *Essentials of e-learning for nurse educators* (pp. 277-294). Philadelphia, PA: F.A. Davis Company.

Decker, S. I., Sportsman, S., Puetz, L., & Billings, L. (2008). The evolution of simulation and its contribution to competency. *The Journal of Continuing Education in Nursing, 39*(2), 74-80.

Dewey, J. (1910). *How we think.* Lexington, MA: D.C. Heath.

Dewey, J. (1916). *Democracy in education.* Radford, VA: Wilder Publications LLC.

Dewey, J. (1933). *How we think: A restatement of the relation of reflective thinking to the educative process.* Lexington, MA: D.C. Heath.

Dreyfus, S. E., & Dreyfus, H. L. (1980). *A five-stage model of the mental activities involved in directed skill acquisition.* Berkeley, CA: University of California. Retrieved from http://www.dtic.mil/cgi-bin/GetTRDoc?AD=ADA084551&Location=U2&doc=GetTRDoc.pdf

Ebbert, D. W., & Connors, H. (2004). Standardized patient experiences: Evaluation of clinical performance and nurse practitioner student satisfaction [Electronic version]. *Nurse Education Perspectives, 25*(1), 12-15.

Ericsson, K. A. (2004). Deliberate practice and the acquisition and maintenance of expert performance in medicine and related domains. *Academic Medicine, 79*(10, Suppl.), S70-S81.

Ericsson, K. A. (2006). The influence of experience and deliberate practice on the development of superior expert performance. In K. Ericsson, N. Charness, R. Hoffman, & P. Feltovich (Eds.), *The Cambridge handbook of expertise and expert performance* (pp. 683-703). New York, NY: Cambridge University Press.

Finkelman, A., & Kenner, C. (2007). *Teaching IOM: Implications of the IOM reports for nursing education.* Silver Spring, MD: Nursebooks.org.

Frenk, J., Chen, L., Bhutta, Z. A., Cohen, J., Crisp, N., Evans, T.,…Zurayk, H. (2010). Health professionals for a new century: Transforming education to strengthen health systems in an interdependent world. *Lancet, 376*(9756), 1923-1958. doi:10.1016/S0140-6736(10)61854-5

Gaba, D. M. (2004). The future vision of simulation in health care. *Quality and Safety in Health Care, 13*(Supp 1), i2-i10. doi:10.1136/qshc.2004.009878

Haag-Heitman, B. (2008). The development of expert performance in nursing. *Journal for Nurses in Staff Development, 24*(5), 203-211.

Institute of Medicine (IOM). (2000). *To err is human: Building a safer health system.* L. T. Kohn, J. M. Corrigan, & M. S. Donaldson (Eds.). Washington, DC: National Academy Press. Retrieved from http://www.nap.edu/catalog.php?record_id=9728

Institute of Medicine (IOM). (2001). *Crossing the quality chasm: A new health system for the 21st Century.* Washington, DC: National Academies Press. Retrieved from http://iom.edu/Reports/2001/Crossing-the-Quality-Chasm-A-New-Health-System-for-the-21st-Century.aspx

Institute of Medicine (IOM). (2003). *Health professions education: A bridge to quality.* A. Grener, & E. Knebel (Eds.). Washington, DC: The National Academies Press. Retrieved from http://www.iom.edu/Reports/2003/Health-Professions-Education-A-Bridge-to-Quality.aspx

Institute of Medicine. (2004a). *Academic health centers: Leading change in the 21ˢᵗ century.* L. T. Kohn (Ed.). Washington, DC: National Academies Press.

Institute of Medicine (IOM). (2004b). *Keeping patients safe: Transforming the work environment of nurses.* A. Page (Ed.). Washington, DC: The National Academies Press. Retrieved from http://www.iom.edu/Reports/2003/Keeping-Patients-Safe-Transforming-the-Work-Environment-of-Nurses.aspx

Institute of Medicine (IOM). (2011). *The future of nursing: Leading change, advancing health.* Washington, DC: The National Academies Press. Retrieved from www.thefutureofnursing.org/IOM-Report

International Nursing Association for Clinical Simulation and Learning (INASCL) Board of Directors (2011). Standards of best practice: Simulation. Standard I: Terminology. *Clinical Simulation in Nursing, 7*(4S), s3-s7. Retrieved from http://download.journals.elsevierhealth.com/pdfs/journals/1876-1399/PIIS1876139911000612.pdf. doi:10.1016/j.ecns.2011.05.005

Interprofessional Education Collaborative Expert Panel. (2011). *Core competencies for interprofessional collaborative practice: Report of an expert panel.* Washington, DC: Interprofessional Education Collaborative. Retrieved from http://www.aacn.nche.edu/education-resources/ipecreport.pdf

Issenberg, S. B., McGaghie, W. C., Petrusa, E. R., Gordon, D. L. & Scalese, R. (2005). Features and uses of high-fidelity medical simulations that lead to effective learning: A BEME systematic review. *Medical Teacher, 27*(1), 10-28.

Jeffries. P. R. (2005). A framework for designing, implementing, and evaluating simulation used as teaching strategies in nursing. *Nursing Education Perspectives, 26*(2), 96-103.

Jeffries, P. R., & Rogers, K. J. (2012). Theoretical framework for simulation design. In P. Jeffries (Ed.), *Simulation in nursing education: From conceptualization to evaluation* (pp. 25-41). New York, NY: National League for Nursing.

Jenson, C. E., & Forsyth, D. M. (2012). Virtual reality simulation: Using three-dimensional technology to teach nursing students. *Computers, Informatics, Nursing, 30*(6), 312-318. doi: 10-1097/NSN.0b013e31824af6ae

The Joint Commission (TJC). (2012). *National patient safety goals effective January 1, 2013.* Chicago, IL: Author. Retrieved from http://www.jointcommission.org/standards_information/npsgs.aspx

The Joint Commission (TJC). (2013). *Sentinel event data: Root causes by event type 2004-2012.* Chicago, IL: Author. Retrieved from www.jointcommission.org/sentinel_event.aspx

The Joint Commission on Accreditation of Healthcare Organization (JCAHO). (2005). *Improving America's hospitals: The Joint Commission's annual report on quality and safety—2005.* Chicago, IL: Author.

Juraschek, S. P., Zhang, X., Ranganathan, V., & Lin, V. W. (2012). United States registered nurse workforce report card and shortage forecast. *American Journal of Medical Quality, 27*(3), 241-249.

Kneebone, R. (2003). Simulation in surgical training: Educational issues and practical training. *Medical Education, 37*(3), 267-277.

Knowles, M. (1984). *Andragogy in action: Applying modern principles of adult education.* San Francisco, CA: Jossey-Bass.

Knowles, M. S., Holton, E. F., & Swanson, R. A. (2011). *The adult learner: The definitive classic in adult education and human resource development.* Oxford, UK: Elsevier, Inc.

Kobayashi, L., Patterson, M., Overly, F. L., Shapiro, M. J., Williams, K. A., & Jay, G. D. (2008). Educational and research implications for portable human patient simulation in acute care medicine. *Society of Academic Emergency Medicine, 15*(11), 1166-1174.

Kolb, D. A. (1984). *Experiential learning: Experience as the source of learning and development.* Englewood Cliffs, NJ: Prentice-Hall.

Larew, C., Lessans, S., Spunt, D., & Covington, B. G. (2008). Innovations in clinical simulation: Application of Benner's theory in an interactive patient care simulation. *Nursing Education Perspectives, 27*(1), 16-21.

Leonard, M., Graham, S., & Bonacum, D. (2004). The human factor: The critical importance of effective teamwork and communication in providing safe care. *Quality, Safety, Health Care. 13*(Supp 1), i85-i90.

Lewis, R., Strachan, A., & Smith, M. M. (2012). Is high fidelity simulation the most effective method for the development of non-technical skills in nursing? A review of the current evidence. *The Open Nursing Journal, 6*, 82-89.

Loyd, G. E., Lake, C. L., & Greenberg, R. (2004). *Practical health care simulations.* Philadelphia, PA: Elsevier Mosby.

Maran, N. J., & Glavin, R. J. (2003). Low- to high-fidelity simulation—A continuum of medical education? *Medical Education, 37*(Supp 1), 22-28.

McCaughey, C. S., & Traynor, M. K. (2010). The role of simulation in nurse education. *Nurse Education Today, 30*, 827-832.

McGaghie, W., Issenberg, S., Petrusa, E., & Scalese, R. (2006). Effect of practice on standardised learning outcomes in simulation-based medical education. *Medical Education, 40*(8), 792-797.

McGaghie, W., Issenberg, S., Petrusa, E., & Scalese, R. (2010). A critical review of simulation-based medical education research: 2003-2009. *Medical Education, 44*(1), 50-63.

Merriam, S. B., & Leahy, B. (2005). Learning transfer: A review of the research in adult education and training. *Journal of Lifelong Learning, 14*, 1-24.

Meyers, C., & Jones, T. B. (1993). *Promoting active learning: Strategies for the college classroom*. San Francisco, CA: Jossey-Bass.

National League for Nursing (NLN). (2010). *Outcomes and competencies for graduates of practical/vocational, diploma, associate degree, baccalaureate, master's, practice doctorate, and research doctorate programs in nursing*. New York, NY: Author.

National League for Nursing (NLN). (2012). *Simulation in nursing education: From conceptualization to evaluation* (2nd ed.). P. R. Jefferies (Ed.). New York, NY: Author.

Nehring, W. M., Ellis, W. E., & Lashley, F. R. (2001). Human patient simulators in nursing education: An overview. *Simulation and Gaming, 32*(2), 194-204.

Quality and Safety Education for Nurses (QSEN) Institute. (2012). *Pre-licensure KSAs*. Cleveland, OH: Author. Retrieved from http://www.qsen.org/competencies/pre-licensure-ksas/

Rodgers, D. L. (2007). *High-fidelity patient simulation: A descriptive white paper report*. Charleston, WV: David Rodgers.

Scherer, Y. K., Bruce, S. A., & Runkawatt, V. (2007). A comparison of clinical simulation and case study presentation on nurse practitioner students' knowledge and confidence in managing a cardiac event. *International Journal of Nursing Education Scholarship, 4*, 1–14.

Schön, D. A. (1983). *The reflective practitioner: How professionals think in action*. Hoboken, NJ: Jossey-Bass.

Schön, D. A. (1987). *Educating the reflective practitioner*. Hoboken, NJ: Jossey-Bass.

Seropian, M. (2003). General concepts in full scale simulation: Getting started. *Anesthesia Analgesia, 97*(6), 1695-1705.

Seropian, M., Brown, K., Gavilanes, J., & Driggers, B. (2004). Simulation: Not just a mannequin. *Journal of Nursing Education, 43*(4), 164-169.

Simulation. (n.d.). In *Merriam-Webster's online dictionary*. Retrieved from http://www.merriam-webster.com/dictionary/simulation

Society for Simulation in Healthcare (SSH). (2013). *SSH accreditation process: Informational guide for the accreditation process from the SSH Council for Accreditation of Healthcare Simulation Programs*. Wheaton, IL: Author. Retrieved from http://ssih.org/accreditation/how-to-apply

United States Medical Licensing Examination (USMLE). (2012). *2013 USMLE Bulletin of information*. Philadelphia, PA: Federation of State Medical Boards (FSMB) and National Board of Medical Examiners (NBME). Retrieved from http://www.usmle.org/pdfs/bulletin/2013bulletin.pdf

Waxman, K. T., & Telles, C. L. (2009). The use of Benner's framework in high-fidelity simulation faculty development: The Bay Area Simulation Collaborative Model. *Clinical Simulation in Nursing, 5*(6), e231-e235. doi:10.1016/j.ecns.2009.06.001

Webster, M. (2009). An innovative faculty toolkit: Simulation success. *Nurse Educator, 34*(4),148-149.

Weller, J. M. (2004). Simulation in undergraduate medical education: Bridging the gap between practice. *Medical Education, 38*(1), 32-38.

Zigmont, J. J., Kappus, L. J., & Sudikoff, S. N. (2011). Theoretical foundations of learning through simulation. *Seminars in Perinatology, 35*(2), 47-51. doi: 10.1053/j.semperi.2011.01.002

Ziv, A., Small, S. D., & Wolpe, P. R. (2000). Patient safety and simulation-based medical education. *Medical Teacher, 22*(5), 489-495.

Ziv, A., Wolpe, P., Small, S. D., & Glick, S. (2003). Simulation-based medical education: An ethical imperative. *Academic Medicine, 78*(8), 783-788.

"Experience tells you what to do; confidence allows you to do it."
–Stan Smith, multiple grand slam tennis champion

Developing Clinical Competence and Confidence

Pamela Andreatta, PhD, MFA, MA
Jody R. Lori, PhD, CNM, FACNM, FAAN

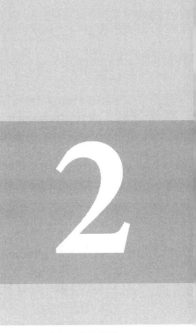

The purpose of any instruction is to affect change in a learner's knowledge, skills, or attitudes that subsequently alters his or her behaviors. The underpinnings for all human learning lay in several psychological, biological, physical, and environmental constructs. For example, the learner's self-concept of his or her ability to learn (psychological), health status (biological), and any disability (physical) all influence learning. Educators may choose to make accommodations to support these individualistic influences, but the primary role of an educator is to create an environment that facilitates learning. The environment in which instruction takes place significantly affects learning and the numerous benefits of simulation-based instruction—experiential, situated, multimodal, on-demand, safe, and so on—and is covered in Chapter 3.

The desired learning outcomes of simulation-based instruction in health care are to change (improve) a learner's behavior in applied clinical practice. The two primary factors that influence behavior in applied practice are *confidence* in the ability to perform what is required and *competence* to accurately perform what is required. Simulation-based instruction supports each of these factors and has the potential to significantly improve the

OBJECTIVES

- Discuss the relationships between confidence and competence, and how simulation can close the gaps between the two.

- Understand how simulation can be used to motivate and build confidence in clinical performance.

- Discuss the value of simulation-based methods for acquiring and maintaining competence.

- Describe the ways simulation can be used to build self-assessment skills.

- Discuss instructional considerations for simulation-based methods that support the acquisition and maintenance of clinical competency and confidence.

acquisition and maintenance of competence beyond current training systems. This chapter discusses each of these factors independently and then examines the influence of their interaction on learning and instruction.

Confidence

For the purpose of this discussion, *confidence* is defined as learners' conscious and subconscious *beliefs* about their ability to successfully perform what is required to achieve a favorable outcome in a clinical context. Conceptually, confidence is related to the theoretical constructs of self-efficacy (Bandura, 1977), self-awareness (Duval & Silvia, 2002), perceptual integration (Stemme, Deco, & Lang, 2011), critical-thinking skills (Dumitru, 2011), motivation to learn (Dweck & Leggett, 1988; Keller, 2008; Pintrich, 1999, 2003, 2004), and self-regulation (Bandura, 1991; Carver, 2006) among others. These theories explore various individual state and trait characteristics that influence a learner's self-perception of ability to perform in a specific context. These theories examine various individual factors that contribute to the learning process; however, they are difficult to address through instruction alone. Two advantages of simulation-based methods are that they may help learners gain confidence by improving their ability to accurately self-assess and they motivate learners to continue through the learning process by increasing the expectancy factor associated with motivation (Judge & Bono, 2001; Nadler, Lawler, Steers, & Porter, 1977; Vroom, 1964).

Self-Assessment

The ability of learners to self-assess is at the core of developing both confidence and competence. However, the inability to self-assess can lead to overconfidence that impedes further learning and has the potential to adversely affect patient and clinician safety. Self-assessment is defined as a process by which learners observe and evaluate their own progress toward performance objectives (Andrade & Valtcheva, 2009). Learners compare the results of their performances against explicit standards, criteria, or objectives and seek to improve, maintain, or advance their abilities depending on the quality of the performance. The ability to identify one's own performance strengths and weaknesses is essential to promote learning and achievement, as well as to inform an accurate perception of confidence.

Unfortunately, the ability for humans to self-assess is not inherent, and techniques for self-assessment are rarely taught in the health sciences. For example, the preponderance of evidence suggests that physicians have a limited ability to accurately self-assess (Davis et al., 2006). Without the mechanisms that help learners to accurately self-assess, learners are far less likely to succeed at self-regulated learning (learner-centered instruction that supports independent engagement with the learning processes). With self-regulated learning, instructional methods facilitate access to content, instructional events, and social engagements that support the learning process, but the pacing and sequencing of the instruction is left for the learner to decide. Self-regulated learning environments have several advantages, not the least of which is the ability of learners to access course material at any time and as often as they want. However, there are also disadvantages, such as learners being ill-prepared for this level of independent control of their learning processes.

Educators can help learners develop the ability to self-assess by providing explicit standards with straightforward performance metrics. In addition, timely, specific feedback about how they performed compared to the standards and recommended activities will help learners improve their performances. Nestel, Bello, and Kneebone (2012) propose seven feedback principles that support self-regulation in simulation-based instruction:

- Defining good performance
- Facilitating self-assessment
- Delivering high-quality feedback information
- Encouraging teacher and peer dialogue
- Encouraging positive motivation and self-esteem
- Providing opportunities to close the gap (between actual and desired performance)
- Using feedback to improve teaching

Feedback about performance can be provided by educators, independent assessors, peers, or through metrics provided by the performance context directly. The latter is a significant incentive for simulation-based instruction because it helps learners develop the ability to self-assess by comparing their subjective interpretation to objective metrics provided by the simulator itself. As learners further develop their ability to self-assess, their confidence level tends to correlate more closely with their performance. This in turn will encourage continued engagement (motivation) with the content domain.

Motivation

Motivation is an internal state that directs an individual's goal-oriented behavior. Learners choose to pursue what motivates them, and through that choice, they direct their attention (Wickens, 1991; Young & Stanton, 2002). Motivational factors include the intensity of the internal state (weak–strong) and the direction of the state (negative–positive). For example, one learner may be highly motivated to achieve Objective A, whereas another may desire achievement of the same objective, but desires Objective B even more. Likewise, one learner may strongly want to avoid the recriminations of failure, whereas other learners may not care whether they fail or not.

Numerous factors affect an individual's predisposition to engage in the learning process. These include:

- Biological (thirst, hunger, pain, fatigue)
- Affective (anxious, depressed, calm, happy)
- Cognitive (interest, desire to solve problems)
- Conative (dreams, desires to control life)
- Behavioral (rewards, fame, fortune, kudos)
- Spiritual (humanistic need to grow, self-actual, God-fearing)

The degree to which motivation can be influenced by instruction depends on whether the motivating patterns are a trait or state for an individual.

Motivational patterns include traits (stable) and states (unstable), each of which may be either innate or learned. Examples of innate traits include curiosity, anxiety, and sexual attraction, whereas examples of learned traits include aspiration of power, need to achieve, and desire for affiliation. Innate states include hunger, thirst, fear, etc., whereas learned states include factors such as test anxiety, overconfidence, stage fright, etc.

Further complicating the motivational soup is an individual's attribution of successes or failures; that is, what is the learner's personal agency (Bandura, 2001). Learners may have an intrinsic, extrinsic, or mixed motivation orientation (locus of control; Rotter, 1954).

- Learners with an intrinsic orientation (internal locus of control) are motivated by internal factors and rewards. They compare their current performance against their previous performance. These learners are frequently satisfied with unobservable rewards.
- Learners with an extrinsic orientation (external locus of control) are motivated by external factors and rewards and compare their performance to that of others. These learners are motivated by observable rewards.
- Learners with a mixed orientation may be intrinsically motivated in some contexts and extrinsically motivated in others.

Attribution theory describes how learners explain their successes and failures to themselves (Weiner, 2010). Similar to the concept of motivational orientation, attribution refers to the learner's beliefs about the amount of control she or he has over performance outcomes and whether those outcomes are due to internal factors or external factors. Learners who believe they have no control may attribute performance outcomes to their innate ability (internal) or luck (external). Learners who believe they have control over performance outcomes may attribute results to their efforts (internal) or the difficulty of the performance task (external).

So how do you begin to assemble these concepts in a way that helps inform instruction? The Expectancy-Value Theory of Achievement Motivation (Fishbein & Ajzen, 1975; Wigfield & Eccles, 2000) supports the organization of these multiple factors into a simple model.

$$\text{Motivation} = \text{Expectancy x Value}$$

The theory postulates that learners will be motivated by their perceptions of the likelihood that their efforts will lead to the necessary performance in a desired area, and that their performances will be rewarded. In the model, *value* is described as the present or future worth of an outcome to an individual. *Expectancy* is described as an individual's sense of confidence or efficacy that an outcome will be successful. *Motivation* can thus be viewed as a product of the learner's expectancy of achievement if the learner engages in the learning process and the value placed on the learning outcomes.

Motivating other people to engage in a learning process (instruction) is difficult because motivation is an individual thing. What motivates one person might not necessarily motivate another; worse, it might demotivate another. Ideally, instruction that provides learners with a moderate challenge has the greatest likelihood of supporting learner motivation. This is because a moderate challenge increases the expectancy factor without decreasing the value factor, and the challenge level of activities is within the educator's control.

Confidence Continuum

Motivation and the ability to self-assess influences learner confidence, but confidence is dynamic and varies depending on workload, learning curves, and acquired expertise. The relationships between confidence and expertise are illustrated in Figure 2.1. In general, novices do not possess much confidence in their abilities in an instructional domain. At an intermediate performance level, learners may be quite confident in their abilities; however, this confidence is likely the result of not knowing what they don't know. In an intraoperative study of stress levels for residents and attending surgeons, attending surgeons experienced significantly greater stress than their more junior trainees because they were able to perceive what was actually occurring during the case as well as the potential for error (Goldman, McDonough, & Rosemond, 1972). Advanced learners tend to be confident, with a minimal number preferring to remain reticent until they achieve the level of domain expert. Most expert performers are confident in their abilities to perform in their domain of expertise, and have demonstrated the ability to accurately self-assess their abilities.

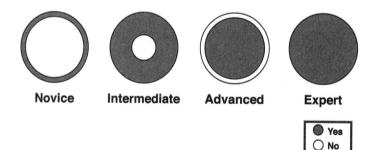

Confidence and Training Level

| Novice | Intermediate | Advanced | Expert |

● Yes
○ No

Figure 2.1   Perceived learner performance confidence at sequential levels of expertise.

The overconfidence of intermediate performers is an area of study in clinical education, primarily because of the potential risks to both patient and clinician safety. Although numerous educational studies measure confidence changes as indicative of a successful outcome, further studies evaluating the uses of retrospective self-assessment suggest the existence of a gap between intermediate and advanced learners in their ability to self-assess, and therefore their perceived confidence (Bhanji, Gottesman, deGrave, Steinert, & Winer, 2012; Hewson, Copeland, & Fishleder, 2001; Levinson, Skeff, & Gordon, 1990). Although confidence is necessary for learners to perform in a given context, it is not sufficient for assessing their abilities to perform in a domain of interest. Assessment of whether or not learners can perform competently is necessary. Fortunately, this is where simulation adds value to health care.

Competency

Confidence is one's *own belief* about one's abilities. Competence is one's *actual ability* to successfully perform what is required to achieve a favorable outcome in a clinical context. Examples of performance competencies required in clinical practice are illustrated in Figure 2.2. Determining competence, therefore, requires performance-based assessment in the clinical contexts of interest, which is easier said than done. Clinical contexts are rarely amenable to measuring the performance of multiple clinicians in the process of attending to the needs of multiple patients. Additionally, performance metrics for clinical care task completion, reasoning, and decision-making are for the most part poorly defined and rely on subjective and culturally determined parameters. In a chicken-egg type analogy, the variability of the clinical context confounds the specification of performance metrics, which in turn challenge performance in the clinical context. Simulation provides an opportunity to control some of the contextual variability by establishing parameters for clinicians even as patient characteristics remain variable.

Performance Mastery

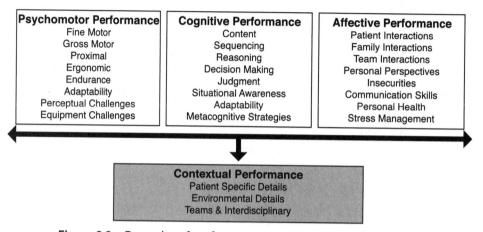

Figure 2.2   Examples of performance requirements in clinical practice.

Repetitive performance measurements by experts in a domain of interest are used to define performance metrics in the given domain (Cizek & Bunch, 2007; Hambleton, Jaeger, Mills, & Plake, 2000; McKinley, Boulet, & Hambleton, 2005). The apprenticeship model of clinical training necessitates that instructors prioritize ethical and optimal patient care over performance repetition for learners. Simulation provides a foundation from which performance can be measured because the contextual aspects of patient care can be replicated without the essential prioritization of a real patient's needs. Simulation facilitates the repetitive acquisition of performance data and at the same time it controls for extraneous variables (such as comorbidities) that might affect performance during actual patient care. Educators need to acquire these data to derive and validate the rigorous performance standards that establish the foundation of competency assessment. Simulation facilitates the ability of educators to establish standards of performance, and enables them to establish performance curves for the acquisition and degradation of abilities in a content domain. After those standards are defined, they can be used to support multilevel learning contexts that include data-driven and repeated feedback, evidence of progress toward achieving delineated standards, identification of areas of performance strength, and identification of areas where targeted remediation is needed to achieve the specific competency objectives.

Assessment

Competence is assessed through various mechanisms that allow comparison of performance against a known, expected standard. Simulation helps set those standards by providing a common platform for deriving valid and reliable performance metrics and associated assessment mechanisms. Assessment is an essential activity for gaining competence.

Formative assessment is an iterative process that provides information to learners and instructors about how well the learner is favorably progressing through the instruction. That is, it provides evidence that the learner is acquiring the requisite cognitive, psychomotor, and affective aspects of the content domain. The dependency factor for learning is therefore whether or not performance objectives are achieved at each sequential step of the learning process. Learners who are given specific feedback about their progress at regular intervals will be better able to identify what they have learned well and what requires improvement before moving to the next level (self-assessment). This affords them the opportunity to spend additional time in those areas in which performance is less than optimal so that they are fully prepared to move to the next level. Formative assessment may be formal or informal, but it always includes elements that provide the learners with specific information that enables learners to modify their performances in a way to further enhance their abilities or integrate the skills that are acquired in a more substantive or advanced way.

The intention of instruction is to aid learners in achieving proficient performance in the content domain. In addition to formative assessment, *summative assessment* provides concrete evidence that a learner has achieved specified performance requirements. Summative assessment is almost always more formal because it is considered a form of terminal evaluation that confirms the acquisition of performance objectives within the specified content domain. Summative assessment is frequently considered a high-stakes evaluation that serves a gatekeeping function. Therefore, the statistical reliability and validity of summative assessment mechanisms are more rigorous than those for formative assessment. Although considerable data must be assembled before simulation-based assessment can serve this summative function, the contextual consistency of simulation is instrumental to collecting these data and establishing accurate contextual performance standards. Thus, simulation-based methods serve to provide immediate feedback about performance against the known standard (formative), as well as inform the development of credentialing and certification requirements.

Acquiring and Maintaining Competence

Learners acquire competence by achieving explicit cognitive, psychomotor, or affective objectives under the guidance and supervision of an instructor. New learning builds upon that which has already been learned, in the same way a house is built upon a foundation. If the foundation is weak (poor prerequisite abilities), the walls of the house will also be weak (poorly learned abilities). Optimal instruction includes explicit learning objectives, specific performance criteria, and assessment opportunities that allow learners to achieve their objectives and to not lose learning time because of knowledge gaps. Numerous theoretical constructs describe the acquisition of abilities through instruction. Three have significant relevance for simulation-based learning environments:

- Experiential learning
- Deliberate practice
- Reflective practice

The foundation of experiential learning theory is that experience plays a central role in the cycle of learning—a learner has an experience, the experience promotes observation and reflection, the observation and reflection transform the experience into abstractions. The learner actively tests these abstractions, which leads to further experiences. Learning experiences may be formal or informal, directed or flexible, derived from standards, or organic in nature. The common component of all experiential learning environments is the active engagement of the learner toward assembling, analyzing, and synthesizing perceptual cues stemming from the instructional context. The theoretical supposition is that instructional designs that encourage learners to have a variety of relevant experiences will lead to improved outcomes. Simulation-based instruction presents multiple experiences of different modalities and forms, but within the desired content domain. This enables learners to consider the content through different perspectives that subsequently lead to deeper understanding while at the same time assuring patient safety.

Deliberate practice theory proposes that deep expertise is developed through highly motivated learners engaging in concentrated repetitive practice tied to well-defined objectives (Ericsson, 2004, 2011; Ericsson & Charness, 1994; Ericsson, Nandagopal, & Roring, 2009). Learners actively and incrementally refine their performances using feedback and guidance provided by an expert coach until they achieve proficiency. The key features of deliberate practice include repetition, feedback, motivation, and establishing clear challenges at the right level of difficulty. A simulated environment facilitates the iterative performance-feedback loop that is necessary for developing abilities through deliberate practice. This is especially beneficial for the acquisition of psychomotor skills, high-order cognitive processing and critical thinking, and team-based practice behaviors. Empirical evidence strongly suggests that simulation-based deliberate practice is more effective than learning procedural skills through traditional, clinical-based instruction (Andreatta, Chen, Marsh, & Cho, 2011; Andreatta, Saxton, Thompson, & Annich, 2011; Barsuk, Cohen, McGaghie, & Wayne, 2010; Issenberg, McGaghie, Petrusa, Gordon, & Scalese, 2005; McGaghie, Issenberg, Cohen, Barsuk, & Wayne, 2011; McGaghie, Issenberg, Petrusa, & Scalese, 2006; Wayne et al., 2012).

Reflective practice refers to the process by which learners deliberately think about their own individual experiences in order to learn from them. Reflection is an important part of professional development during training, and is associated with self-assessment. Reflection helps learners to adjust their performance during practical experiences (reflection-in-action), as well as to analyze their performance after its occurrence (reflection-on-action) (Schön, 1983, 1987). Reflective practice helps learners examine what they did well, what could be improved, and identify strategies for strengthening any areas of weakness. Ideally, the reflective process includes feedback from multiple sources (instructor, peers, performance outcomes, etc.).

Simulation clearly serves these theoretical models in support of acquiring domain-specific performances associated with competency. But how are these performance criteria maintained over time so that competency is sustained? Empirical evidence suggests that clinical performance abilities decline after instruction in as few as 3 weeks without use (Einspruch, Lynch, Aufderheide, Nichol, & Becker, 2007; Hunt, Fiedor-Hamilton, & Eppich, 2008; Seki, 1987, 1988; Woollard et al., 2006). Fortunately, evidence also suggests that simulation-based activities in support of professional development and maintenance of competency have a positive effect on both clinical performance and clinical outcomes (Andreatta, Perosky, & Johnson, 2012; Oermann et al., 2011).

Simulation-based instruction is necessarily learner-centered, which places the locus of control with the learner. A learner-centered approach promotes individuals to take responsibility for their learning, which is essential for developing the lifelong learning and self-assessment skills required for health care providers in every specialty. Not only do these types of post-training activities facilitate the maintenance of individual performance, they encourage the development of interdisciplinary and team-based performance that results in the types of synergistic competencies desired in health care. Much like the acquisition phases of developing competence, feedback—and its team-based correlate, debriefing—facilitate reflective practice during professional practice.

Competence Continuum

Competence is a dynamic construct that depends on acquired and maintained expertise. The relationships between competence and expertise are illustrated in Figure 2.3. Novices generally lack competence in an instructional domain. Intermediate learners might perform competently in some areas, but they likely lack sufficient competence to perform most domain-specific skills without supervision. For example, an intermediate-level nurse practitioner might demonstrate sufficient competence in placing an intravenous catheter but struggle placing a central venous catheter. Advanced learners generally demonstrate the ability to achieve most performance standards within a domain. Experts are able to demonstrate consistently competent performance in a domain.

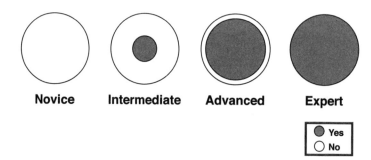

Figure 2.3   Expected performance competence at sequential levels of expertise.

The Confidence-Competence Connection

Confidence and competence are both dynamic constructs associated with different psychological processes, and therefore, each individual variably develops and maintains them. They are related, however, and this relationship can be used to design programs that individuals and groups can use to support optimal levels of both confidence and competence. The relationship between the confidence and competence at sequential levels of learner expertise is shown in Figure 2.4.

Gap Between Confidence and Competence

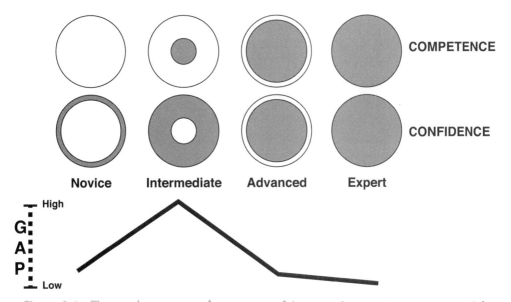

Figure 2.4   The gap between performance confidence and competence at sequential levels of expertise.

The gap between the confidence to perform in a clinical context and the actual competence of clinicians is an area of concern for learners, instructors, patients, clinicians who work with the learner during the provision of care, the responsible health care institution, and society in general. The gap is most pronounced at intermediate levels of domain expertise, where learners have acquired some domain-specific capability, but they haven't acquired sufficient expertise to accurately self-assess their abilities. As described earlier in this chapter, this is largely an interaction effect between learners having poor self-assessment skills and not knowing the influences of content they haven't yet learned. Clinical instructors can reduce this gap through simulation-based methods that provide learners with specific assessment feedback about the quality of their performance and help them to accurately self-assess. This benefits learners as they develop professional identities based on factual evidence, which subsequently supports their ability to maintain and expand their competencies.

Simulation and Clinical Competency

All instruction optimally includes detailed instructional objectives for each relevant performance area in a content domain (cognitive, psychomotor, affective, system) that collectively lead to the achievement of domain competence. These learning objectives should be explicit and measurable, stating what the learners should be able to do, the context they should be able to do it in, and the expected standard of successful performance. Segmenting and sequencing content in a logical progression so that introductory concepts precede more advanced concepts supports the construction and integration of domain-specific information, especially when formative assessment helps learners (and instructors) progress in an organized and efficient manner without exceeding the moderate challenge level that serves learner motivation. This approach helps learners engage with the content domain and progressively acquire competency.

Consulting relevant theoretical underpinnings assures that optimal instructional activities support learner achievement for each objective. For example, instructional events designed to help learners achieve an objective with significant psychomotor factors benefits from Chapman's eight steps for learning procedural skills and deliberate practice strategies (see accompanying sidebar; Chapman, 1994). Similarly, a cognitive objective requiring complex relational integration, or affective objectives tied to interpersonal relating, benefits from the application of experiential learning theory and reflective practice. Strategically facilitated formative feedback allows learners to benefit from the naïve exploration favored by experiential learning theory while still providing them the opportunity to reflect on their performances through the constructive feedback that subsequently informs their performances in succeeding activities.

Instructional events that are sequenced in accordance with a natural progression of competency from lesser to more complex abilities within the content domain ensure that learners are working at an appropriate level of challenge. Other techniques that can support learner motivation are included in the accompanying sidebar.

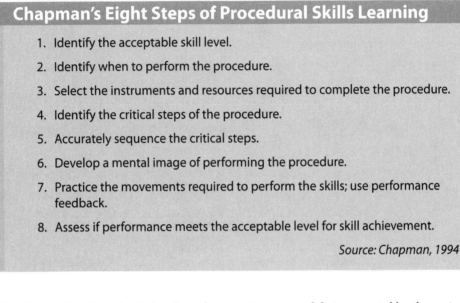

Chapman's Eight Steps of Procedural Skills Learning

1. Identify the acceptable skill level.

2. Identify when to perform the procedure.

3. Select the instruments and resources required to complete the procedure.

4. Identify the critical steps of the procedure.

5. Accurately sequence the critical steps.

6. Develop a mental image of performing the procedure.

7. Practice the movements required to perform the skills; use performance feedback.

8. Assess if performance meets the acceptable level for skill achievement.

Source: Chapman, 1994

Simulation-based methods for clinical instruction are widely interpreted by the various constituencies of users. Simulation methods are associated with the acquisition of abilities that lead to professional competency, but also with maintenance of competency and even expansion of competencies in other areas of practice. Within these various applications, simulation-based activities support procedural skills; physical and clinical assessment skills; diagnostic reasoning; psycho-social skills and history-taking; clinical management; team-based practices; communication skills (patients, families, colleagues); regulatory and administrative management; and development and refinement of clinical techniques. In other words, simulation-based methods can be—and are—used for every aspect of clinical practice. However, some uses of simulation in health care are more mature than others in terms of equipment, resource specifications, assessment mechanisms, and development of instructional scenarios and events.

Designing simulation-based instruction can be time consuming, and it is both easier and prudent to use resources developed by others if possible. After all, why reinvent the wheel? But caution is merited when criticality of the instructional goal of simulation-based instruction is considered: to facilitate the acquisition and maintenance of clinical competence performed in applied practice. If the existing instruction is not designed to achieve the specific competencies required by a learner in a given domain, it will not serve that goal. Therefore, it is essential that any instructional activities designed for other programs be thoroughly evaluated to be certain that they also support the development of competencies in the program for which they are being considered. This minimizes the likelihood that a learner successfully completes all required instructional activities without being able to perform competently in applied clinical practice.

Techniques to Support Learner Motivation

Help learners understand the value of what they are being asked to do in both the short and long term.

Inform learners about what exactly needs to be accomplished and the standard of performance.

Set short-term objectives with sequentially increased complexity.

Provide written and verbal acknowledgement of effort and outcomes.

Use formative assessment to help learners advance; summative assessment judiciously.

Capitalize on arousal value of surprise, suspense, discovery, curiosity, and exploration by occasionally doing the unexpected.

Use familiar examples with unique and unexpected contexts when applying concepts and principles.

Reinforce previous learning by including concepts in subsequent activities.

Minimize any unpleasant consequences of learner involvement or the learning environment.

Encourage a bit of fun!

As is the case with all instructional contexts, the details of the simulation environment itself influence learning. Apart from the effects of learner characteristics discussed in this and other chapters, the selection of models or simulators and setting characteristics affects not only learning within the simulated context, but also the transfer of that learning to applied practice. This concept is tied to the concept of *fidelity* in simulation. Any discussion of competencies derived from simulation-based practices must include the issue of fidelity because the more accurately a simulated context replicates the clinical context, the more sure you can be that performance will transfer between the two contexts. A simulated clinical environment that adequately reflects the contextually relevant factors influencing performance of the learning objective maximizes transfer of the acquired abilities to the applied clinical environment (Konkola, Tuomi-Gröhn, Lambert, & Ludvigsen, 2007; Sohn, Doane, & Garrison, 2006; Thomas, 2007). The quality and type of fidelity that is required for the transfer of these abilities is an active area of research, principally because the costs associated with the space, equipment, materials, and resources required to replicate a clinical context can be quite high.

The term *high fidelity* is used for simulators that are designed to replicate clinical contexts with as much visual and functional precision as possible. These also tend to be high-technology products driven by expensive computer and graphics systems. The term *low fidelity* is used to describe simulators that are less technology driven, but in many instances low-fidelity simulators have equal or greater sensorial precision when compared to high-fidelity simulators. Empirical evidence suggests that both types of simulation equipment can lead to favorable or unfavorable performance outcomes. This is because the elements of a simulated context are only as effective as the instructional design that makes use of them. If you consider the optimal instructional path for learners described earlier in this chapter, an exact replica of a clinical context is not necessary at every step of an instructional sequence. Rather, the concept of contextual fidelity is more appropriate when selecting the resources that will be included in a training program. *Contextual fidelity* is defined as a simulation activity that has sufficient detail to support the acquisition or maintenance of the skills described by the learning objective to the extent that those skills will support the acquisition of more advanced skills and will transfer to applied uses in clinical contexts.

Simulation-based instruction has many advantages over traditional, apprentice-based health care training; however, one disadvantage is that clinically embedded affective elements might be absent in a simulated context. Living patients are integral components to the apprenticeship-learning context and this, along with the demands of clinical care at a busy health care institution, places extraordinary affective demands on the learner inclusive and apart from cognitive and psychomotor demands. Because the apprenticeship-learning context includes those real factors, they must be accommodated during the instructional process if the learner is to be successful. The absence of those affective factors in simulated environments enables learners to focus exclusively on the cognitive and psychomotor competencies associated with the learning objectives for a domain. Learners might face challenges when they are required to transfer those cognitive and psychomotor competencies to an applied clinical environment, inclusive of affective factors that were not accommodated in the learning environment. Arguably, affective overload is one of the most challenging aspects of providing clinical care, yet is largely overlooked as an integral part of health care education. Although affective factors are embedded in the apprenticeship model, these factors must be conscientiously considered and built into simulation-based instruction so that transfer from the less stressful learning context (simulation) to the more stressful context (applied patient care) is supported (Andreatta, Hillard, & Krain, 2010; Langan-Fox & Vranic, 2011).

Conclusion

Simulation-based instruction that successfully alters behaviors as a result of improvements in learners' knowledge, skills, or attitudes will take into account the psychological, biological, physical, and environmental constructs that affect human learning. Educators who implement simulation-based instruction in a health care setting may optimally facilitate changes to learners' behaviors in applied clinical practice as well. Simulation-based instruction supports the development of learner confidence to perform what is required and learner competence to accurately perform what is required. The potential for simulation-based methods to significantly improve the acquisition and maintenance of competence will help clinicians achieve consistent and accurate performance assessment that will ultimately improve the quality and safety for patients and clinicians alike.

References

Andrade, H., & Valtcheva, A. (2009). Promoting learning and achievement through self-assessment. *Theory Into Practice, 48*(1), 12-19. doi: 10.1080/00405840802577544

Andreatta, P. B., Chen, Y., Marsh, M., & Cho, K. (2011). Simulation-based training improves applied clinical placement of ultra-sound guided PICCs. *Supportive Care in Cancer, 19*(4), 539-543.

Andreatta, P. B., Hillard, M. L., & Krain, L. P. (2010). The impact of stress factors in simulation-based laparoscopic training. *Surgery, 147*(5), 631-639.

Andreatta, P. B., Perosky, J., & Johnson, T. R. (2012). Two-provider technique is superior for Bimanual Uterine Compression to control postpartum hemorrhage. *Journal of Midwifery & Women's Health, 57*(4), 371-375.

Andreatta, P. B., Saxton, E., Thompson, M., & Annich, G. (2011). Simulation-based mock codes improve pediatric patient survival rates. *Pediatric Critical Care Medicine, 12*(1), 33-38.

Bandura, A. (1977). Self-efficacy: Toward a unifying theory of behavioral change. *Psychological Review, 84*(2), 191-215.

Bandura, A. (1991). Social cognitive theory of self-regulation. *Organizational Behavior and Human Decision Processes, 50*(2), 248-287.

Bandura, A. (2001). Social cognitive theory: An agentic perspective. *Annual Review of Psychology, 52*(1), 1-26.

Barsuk, J. H., Cohen, E. R., McGaghie, W. C., & Wayne, D. B. (2010). Long-term retention of central venous catheter insertion skills after simulation-based mastery learning. *Academic Medicine, 85*(10), S9-S12.

Bhanji, F., Gottesman, R., de Grave, W., Steinert, Y., & Winer, L. R. (2012). The retrospective pre–post: A practical method to evaluate learning from an educational program. *Academic Emergency Medicine, 19*(2), 189-194. doi: 10.1111/j.1553-2712.2011.01270.x

Carver, C. S. (2006). Approach, avoidance, and the self-regulation of affect and action. *Motivation and Emotion, 30*(2), 105-110.

Chapman, D. M. (1994). Use of computer-based technologies in teaching emergency procedural skills. *Academic Emergency Medicine, 1*(4), 404–407.

Cizek, G. J., & Bunch, M. B. (2007). *Standard setting: A guide to establishing and evaluating performance standards on tests.* Thousand Oaks, CA: Sage.

Davis, D. A., Mazmanian, P. E., Fordis, M., Harrison, R. V., Thorpe, K. E., & Perrier, L. (2006). Accuracy of physician self-assessment compared with observed measures of competence. *Journal of the American Medical Association, 296*(9), 1094-1102. doi:10.1001/jama.296.9.1094

Dumitru, D. (2011). Critical thinking and integrated programs: The problem of transferability. *Procedia-Social and Behavioral Sciences, 33*, 143-147.

Duval, T. S., & Silvia, P. J. (2002). Self-awareness, probability of improvement, and the self-serving bias. *Journal of Personality and Social Psychology, 82*(1), 49-61. doi:10.1037/0022-3514.82.1.49

Dweck, C. S., & Leggett, E. L. (1988). A social-cognitive approach to motivation and personality. *Psychological Review, 95*(2), 256-273.

Einspruch, E. L., Lynch, B., Aufderheide, T. P., Nichol, G., & Becker, L. (2007). Retention of CPR skills learned in a traditional AHA Heartsaver course versus 30-min video self-training: A controlled randomized study. *Resuscitation, 74*(3), 476-486. doi: 10.1016/j.resuscitation.2007.01.030

Ericsson, K. A. (2004). Deliberate practice and the acquisition and maintenance of expert performance in medicine and related domains. *Academic Medicine, 79*(19 Suppl), S70-S81.

Ericsson, K. A. (2011). The surgeon's expertise. In H. Fry and R. Kneebone (Eds.) *Surgical education: Theorising an emerging domain, Advances in Medical Education, Vol. 2* (pp. 107-122). New York: Springer Science.

Ericsson, K. A., & Charness, N. (1994). Expert performance. *American Psychologist, 49*(8), 725-747.

Ericsson, K. A., Nandagopal, K., & Roring, R. W. (2009). Towards a science of exceptional achievement: Attaining superior performance through deliberate practice. *Longevity, Regeneration, and Optimal Health: Annals of the New York Academy of Sciences, 1172*, 199-217.

Fishbein, M., & Ajzen, I. (1975). *Belief, attitude, intention, and behavior: An introduction to theory and research.* Reading, MA: Addison-Wesley.

Goldman, L. I., McDonough, M. T., & Rosemond, G. P. (1972). Stresses affecting surgical performance and learning: 1. Correlation of heart rate, electrocardiogram, and operation simultaneously recorded on videotapes. *Journal of Surgical Research, 12*(2), 83-86.

Hambleton, R. K., Jaeger, R. M., Mills, C., & Plake, B. S. (2000). Setting performance standards on complex educational assessments. *Applied Psychological Measurement, 24*(4), 355-366.

Hewson, M. G., Copeland, H. L., & Fishleder, A. J. (2001). What's the use of faculty development? Program evaluation using retrospective self-assessments and independent performance ratings. *Teaching and Learning in Medicine, 13*(3), 153-160.

Hunt, E. A., Fiedor-Hamilton, M., & Eppich, W. J. (2008). Resuscitation education: Narrowing the gap between evidence-based resuscitation guidelines and performance using best educational practices. *The Pediatric Clinics of North America, 55*(4), 1025-1050.

Issenberg, S. B., McGaghie, W. C., Petrusa, E. R., Gordon, D. L., & Scalese, R. J. (2005). Features and uses of high-fidelity medical simulations that lead to effective learning: A BEME systematic review. *Medical Teacher, 27*(1), 10-28.

Judge, T. A., & Bono, J. E. (2001). Relationship of core self-evaluations traits—self-esteem, generalized self-efficacy, locus of control, and emotional stability—with job satisfaction and job performance. *Journal of Applied Psychology, 86*(1), 80-92.

Keller, J. (August 2008). First principles of motivation to learn and e-learning. *Distance Education, 29*(2), 175-185. doi: 10.1080/01587910802154970

Konkola, R., Tuomi-Gröhn, T., Lambert, P., & Ludvigsen, S. (2007). Promoting learning and transfer between school and workplace. *Journal of Education and Work, 20*(3), 211-228.

Langan-Fox, J., & Vranic, V. (2011). Surgeon stress in the operating room: Error-free performance and adverse events. In J. Langan-Fox, & C.L. Cooper (Eds.), *Handbook of stress in the occupation* (pp. 33-48). Northampton, MA: Edward Elgar.

Levinson, W., Skeff, K., & Gordon, G. (1990). Retrospective versus actual pre-course self-assessments. *Evaluation & the Health Professions, 13*(4), 445-452.

McGaghie, W. C., Issenberg, S. B., Cohen, E. R., Barsuk, J. H., & Wayne, D. B. (2011). Medical education featuring mastery learning with deliberate practice can lead to better health for individuals and populations. *Academic Medicine, 86*(11), e8-e9.

McGaghie, W. C., Issenberg, S. B., Petrusa, E. R., & Scalese, R. J. (2006). Effect of practice on standardised learning outcomes in simulation-based medical education. *Medical Education, 40*(8), 792-797.

McKinley, D. W., Boulet, J. R., & Hambleton, R. K. (2005). A work-centered approach for setting passing scores on performance-based assessments. *Evaluation & the Health Professions, 28*(3), 349-369.

Nadler, D. A., Lawler, E. E., III, Steers, R. M., & Porter, L. W. (1977). Motivation: A diagnostic approach. *Motivation and Work Behavior* (pp. 26-38). McGraw Hill, New York, NY.

Nestel, D., Bello, F., & Kneebone, R. (2012). Feedback in clinical procedural skills simulations. In E. Molloy & D. Boud (Eds.), *Feedback in higher and professional education: Understanding it and doing it well* (pp. 140-157). New York, NY: Routledge.

Oermann, M. H., Kardong-Edgren, S., Odom-Maryon, T., Hallmark, B. F., Hurd, D., Rogers, N., …Smart, D. A. (2011). Deliberate practice of motor skills in nursing education: CPR as exemplar. *Nursing Education Perspectives, 32*(5), 311-315.

Pintrich, P. R. (1999). The role of motivation in promoting and sustaining self-regulated learning. *International Journal of Educational Research, 31*(6), 459-470.

Pintrich, P. R. (2003). A motivational science perspective on the role of student motivation in learning and teaching contexts. *Journal of Educational Psychology, 95*(4), 667-686.

Pintrich, P. R. (2004). A conceptual framework for assessing motivation and self-regulated learning in college students. *Educational Psychology Review, 16*(4), 385-407.

Rotter, J. B. (1954). *Social learning and clinical psychology.* New York, NY: Prentice-Hall.

Schön, D. (1983). *The reflective practitioner: How professionals think in action.* New York, NY: Basic Books.

Schön, D. (1987). *Educating the reflective practitioner.* San Francisco, CA: Jossey-Bass.

Seki, S. (1987). Accuracy of suture techniques of surgeons with different surgical experience. *The Japanese Journal of Surgery, 17*(6), 465-469.

Seki, S. (1988). Techniques for better suturing. *The British Journal of Surgery, 75*(12), 1181-1184.

Sohn, Y. W., Doane, S. M., & Garrison, T. (2006). The impact of individual differences and learning context on strategic skill acquisition and transfer. *Learning and Individual Differences, 16*(1), 13-30.

Stemme, A., Deco, G., & Lang, E. W. (March 2011). Perceptual learning with perceptions. *Cognitive Neurodynamics, 5*(1), 31-43.

Thomas, E. (2007). Thoughtful planning fosters learning transfer. *Adult Learning, 18*(3-4), 4-8.

Vroom, V. H. (1964). *Work and Motivation.* New York, NY: John Wiley & Sons.

Wayne, D. B., Moazed, F., Cohen, E. R., Sharma, R. K., McGaghie, W. C., & Szmuilowicz, E. (2012). Code status discussion skill retention in internal medicine residents: One-year follow-up. *Journal of Palliative Medicine, 15*(12), 1325-1328. doi:10.1089/jpm.2012.0232

Weiner, B. (2010). The development of an attribution-based theory of motivation: A history of ideas. *Educational Psychologist, 45*(1), 28-36.

Wickens, C. D. (1991). Processing resources and attention. In D. L. Damos (Ed.), *Multiple task performance* (pp. 3-34). Bristol, PA: Taylor & Francis.

Wigfield, A., & Eccles, J. (2000). Expectancy-value theory of achievement motivation. *Contemporary Educational Psychology, 25*(1), 68-81.

Woollard, M., Whitfield, R., Newcombe, R. G., Colquhoun, M., Vetter, N., & Chamberlain, D. (2006). Optimal refresher training intervals for AED and CPR skills: A randomized controlled trial. *Resuscitation, 71*(2), 237-247. doi: 10.1016/j.resuscitation.2006.04.005

Young, M. S., & Stanton, N. A. (Fall 2002). Malleable attentional resources theory: A new explanation for the effects of mental underload on performance. *Human Factors, 44*(3), 365-375.

Creating Effective Simulation Environments

3

Teresa N. Gore, DNP, FNP-BC, NP-C, CHSE
Lori Lioce, DNP, FNP-BC, NP-C, CHSE

OBJECTIVES

- Describe the levels and types of fidelity for an effective simulation environment.
- Identify the key elements required for an effective simulation environment.
- Articulate ways to identify which types and levels of fidelity are required based on the objectives of the simulation.
- Synthesize at least two strategies that can be incorporated into a simulation practice.

Simulation has been used for years in health care education. Simulation is a teaching strategy, not just technology. Fidelity is the degree to which a simulated experience approaches reality. This can range from a simple task trainer, an intravenous (IV) arm for psychomotor skill practice, to a high-fidelity mannequin that physiologically responds to participant intervention (The International Nursing Association for Clinical Simulation & Learning [INACSL] Board of Directors [BOD], 2011a). Fidelity should replicate real situations in ways that are appropriate to the learning objectives. Typically this means creating an environment that is as close as possible to reality in order for the participants to respond to the simulated situation as they would in a professional interaction with a patient, family, or community (Wickens, 2000). The fidelity of a scenario can be increased or decreased by the type of mannequins used and/or the environmental factors included. *Environmental fidelity* refers to creating an environment that is comparable to the actual setting for providing care, such as using hospital furniture and supplies that are the same as those found in the hospital, and having scripted health care provider responses relevant to the clinical situation (INACSL BOD, 2011a).

Creating effective simulation environments may allow learners to see patients holistically. The concept of holism has proven challenging for learners in a traditional clinical setting and even more difficult for educators in a teacher-centered lecture. Creating an effective simulation environment offers a solution to both and allows discovery learning through deliberate practice and guidance. Environmental fidelity is often not addressed until late in the development of the simulation program. In reality, assuring effective simulation environments can be the key to developing keen clinical assessment skills. Observational skills may be cultivated through inclusion of cues for the learner to develop effective clinical anticipation skills and focus the personal patient history. In health care simulation, effective simulation environments are referred to and measured as environmental fidelity.

Studies have shown students prefer higher levels of fidelity when reporting their level of satisfaction with simulated learning opportunities (Jeffries & Rizzolo, 2006; Lapkin, Levett-Jones, Bellchambers, & Fernandez, 2010). Many studies suggest that simulation significantly increases knowledge (Dieckman, Gaba, & Rall, 2007; Gates, Parr, & Hughen, 2012; Howard, Ross, Mitchell, & Nelson, 2010; Lapkin et al., 2010; Tiffen, Corbridge, Shen, & Robinson, 2010); competence (Butler, Veltre, & Brady, 2009; McGaghie, Issenberg, Petrusa, & Scalese, 2009); self-efficacy (Farnan et al., 2010; Kameg, Howard, Clochesy, Mitchell, & Suresky, 2010); and confidence (Cooper et al., 2012; Tiffen et al., 2010). However, other studies have shown that high-fidelity simulation does not necessarily result in increased learning of clinical reasoning skills or clinical performance (De Giovanni, Roberts, & Norman, 2009; Friedman et al., 2009; Lapkin et al., 2010; Lee, Grantham, & Boyd, 2008). With these research findings in mind, how can health care providers involved in simulation-based education create learning environments that are efficient, effective, and foster the acquisition of educational objectives?

The use of simulation should begin with activities associated with basic psychomotor skills and build in complexity to include elements of critical thinking and clinical judgment. This evidence-based approach should be used with inexperienced learners to avoid overwhelming them and to promote learning (Dieckman et al., 2007; Keene, 2009). Other studies have examined the elements of environmental and psychological fidelity in simulations, specifically, the incorporation of stressors into high-fidelity simulation training scenarios (Beaubien & Baker, 2004; Keinan, Friedland, & Sarig-Naor, 1990). This approach increased the learner-perceived realism and prepared the learners for the patient care in the real world by incorporating interference or external stressors.

There is a growing body of literature within nursing and health care to evaluate the differences in learner outcomes using low- and high-fidelity simulation experiences. Initial simulation research measured learner perceptions. More recently there has been an increase in quantitative studies. Multiple studies have reported no statistically significant differences in learner outcomes or performances when comparing varying levels of fidelity as a teaching strategy (De Giovanni et al., 2009; Friedman et al., 2009; Kardong-Edgren, Anderson, & Michaels, 2007; Kardong-Edgren, Lungstrom, & Bendel, 2009; Kinney & Henderson, 2008; Lee et al., 2008). However, other studies have revealed that the level of fidelity used in simulation increased students' self-perceived improvements and satisfaction (Grady et al., 2008; Jeffries & Rizzolo, 2006; Lapkin et al., 2010); increased knowledge (Gates et al., 2012; Howard et al., 2010; Lapkin et al., 2010; Tiffen et al., 2010); competence (Butler et al., 2009; McGaghie et al., 2009); self-efficacy (Kameg et al., 2010); and confidence (Cooper et al., 2012; Tiffen et al., 2010). Some studies revealed simulation improved patient care and clinical performance (Meyer, Connors, Hou, & Gajewski, 2011; Radhakrishnan, Roche, & Cunningham, 2007) whereas another study reported no change in self-confidence or competence (Blum, Borglund, & Parcells, 2010).

Effective simulations require the educator to use varying levels of realism and tools to meet the needs of the learners and the learning experience. Educators need to remember one important aspect: Simulation is limited only by your imagination, so think outside the box. By increasing the realism, learners can forget they are participating in a lab experience and can treat the simulation as a real-life experience. This is referred to as "suspension of disbelief" (Deckers, Doyle, & Wilkinson, 2011). All learners in the simulation will appreciate your effort and preparedness in allowing them to become immersed in the simulation experience. Through their simulation participation, learners will be exposed to various experiences and learn ways to respond to patient, family, or community needs in a safe manner, incorporating best practices. As the educator, it is up to you to decide the appropriate level of fidelity to use to achieve the objectives and goals. In order to understand and apply the concept of fidelity in ways that are effective, further definitions and examples will be provided.

Fidelity

Aspects of fidelity can include the physical, the psychological, the culture of the group, and the degree of trust (Dieckmann et al., 2007; National League for Nursing [NLN] Simulation Innovation Resource Center [SIRC], 2010). The ability of the facilitator to improve the psychological fidelity increases with the facilitator's experience and comfort in simulation (Deckers et al., 2011). The *facilitator* is "an individual who guides and supports learners toward understanding and achieving objectives" (INACSL BOD, 2011a, p. s5).

Mannequin Fidelity

Mannequin fidelity refers to the degree to which the mannequin used for simulation represents the way a patient would appear and respond. You can select various levels of mannequin fidelity based on the learner objectives (see Table 3.1).

Table 3.1   Mannequin and Environmental Selection Examples

Objective—The learner will:	Type of mannequin/trainer
Correctly insert an intravenous catheter	Task trainer
Correctly insert an IV during an urgent situation (hypertensive crisis)	Mid-fidelity mannequin with a high-fidelity environment or high-fidelity mannequin
Use effective communication skills to obtain an accurate history from a patient	Standardized patient
Use varying techniques to communicate with a family member under situational stress	Standardized patient
Recognize and correctly respond to a patient's deteriorating condition—for example, the first 5 minutes of a code	High-fidelity mannequin with high-fidelity environment

Task trainers represent anatomical human body parts that are used to practice psychomotor skills (Maran & Glavin, 2003) (see Figure 3.1). Task trainers lack realism in that they represent a section of a human body or have limited responsive capabilities. A task trainer would provide the appropriate level of fidelity when the educational objective is psychomotor skill acquisition.

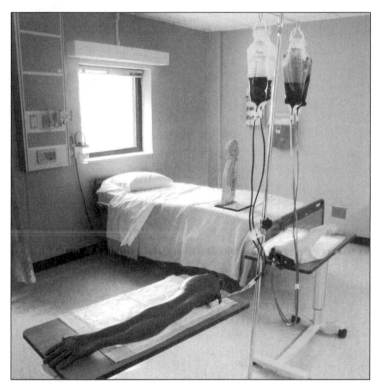

Figure 3.1   Two task trainer arms to practice venipuncture or intravenous (IV) line insertion. In the background (on the bed), a task trainer model for nasogastric (NG) tube insertion practice. Courtesy Dr. Lori Lioce, University of Alabama in Huntsville College of Nursing (UAHCON).

Static (or *low-fidelity*) *mannequins* are basic mannequins that lack pulses, heart sounds, and lung sounds and do not realistically mimic human beings (see Figure 3.2). Students can use these mannequins for training of tasks such as dressing changes for wound care, urinary catheter insertion, and bathing/linen changes (Kardong-Edgren et al., 2009).

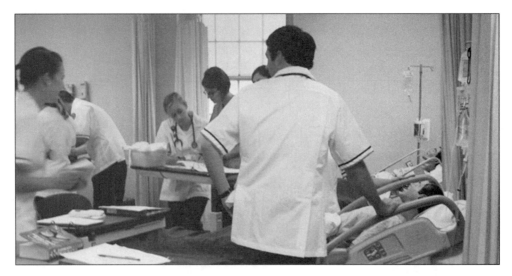

Figure 3.2 Static mannequins bed lab. Courtesy of Dr. Teresa N. Gore, Auburn University School of Nursing (AUSON).

A *mid-level mannequin* can more realistically mimic reality with pulses, heart sounds, and lung sounds, but it lacks the physiological display of chest rise and fall with breathing, blinking, or automated physiological responses to interventions (Kardong-Edgren et al., 2009). In addition to all of the features associated with a mid-fidelity mannequin, a *high-fidelity mannequin* mimics reality by blinking, by having the chest rise and fall with respirations, and by offering physiological responses to interventions (Kardong-Edgren et al., 2009).

A *standardized patient (SP)* is a "person trained to consistently portray a patient or other individual in a scripted scenario for the purposes of instruction, practice, or evaluation" (INACSL BOD, 2011a, p. s6; Robinson-Smith, Bradley, & Meakim, 2009; see Figure 3.3). Standardized patients may be actors, general community citizens who are trained, or individuals who possess previous health care work experience. Standardized patients are the best choice when communication is the main educational objective. To increase environmental fidelity, computer-based programs can generate vital signs or auscultatory sounds for abnormal findings, or moulage can be added to portray specific conditions, symptoms, or illness.

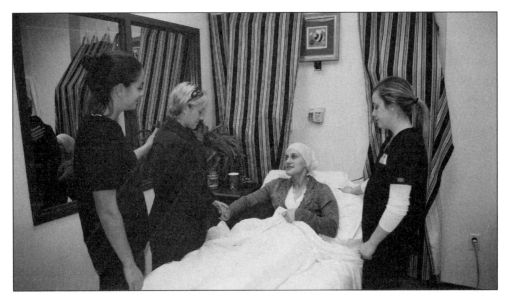

Figure 3.3 Standardized patient. Courtesy of Dr. Valerie M. Howard, Robert Morris University (RMU), Regional RISE Center.

Moulage is the art of creating the illusion of conditions, injuries, and/or physical signs for the purpose of increasing the realism of the simulation. Moulage comes from the French word *mouler* that means to mold (Merriam-Webster, 2013). The first medical moulage was the use of anatomical wax models to study the human body. Types of moulage frequently used in health care simulation are cosmetics, wigs, body art, odors, wounds, bruising, rashes, and other visual assessment cues to draw the attention of learners (see Figures 3.4, 3.5, 3.6, 3.7, and 3.8). Moulage promotes increased realism by engaging all the senses to suspend disbelief (Alinier, 2007; Beaubien & Baker, 2004; Rudolph, Simon, & Raemer, 2007) and supports critical thinking (refer to Table 3.1). This can assist learners in preparing to provide quality, safe patient care. However, moulage does have its constraining factors including cost, knowledge/imagination, manpower (personnel and time), supplies, and storage. Still, moulage can increase the fidelity of simulation and is key to engaging learners in simulation. Providing the clinically appropriate moulage ensures the details are provided for learners to view a clinical simulation, to observe objective-based cues provided through moulage, and to then take an action. Moulage allows learners and educators the opportunity to discuss the clinical reasoning that led to learner actions and the benefits or consequences of those actions.

A great resource and low-cost option for moulage supplies is a Halloween store, especially when supplies can be purchased during after-Halloween sales.

Table 3.2 shows examples of moulage techniques to engage the senses, and the nearby sidebar provides a list of resources that can be used as a foundation for various moulage techniques.

Table 3.2   Moulage to Engage the Senses

Sense	*Moulage Techniques*
Visual	
Infected urine	Chalk dust to produce sediment
	Vanilla pudding for sediment
	Liquid hand or dish soap to produce cloudy urine
Hematuria	Add a couple of drops of meat blood for positive urine dipstick.
	Ground up cherries for clots
Olfactory	
Infected amniotic fluid	Can of mackerel; pour some of the juices onto a pad under the patient. Take some small pieces of the mackerel and spread onto pad.
Feces or Flatus	Fecal spray
Infection	Parmesan cheese
	Limburger cheese
	Bleu cheese
	Gel adhesive remover (yellow/orange)

Sense	Moulage Techniques
Olfactory	
Acetone breath	Liquid fruit scents
	Juicy Fruit gum
	Fruity-smelling car air freshener
	Fruit-flavored lip balm
	Acetone spray
	Fruit-scented body spray
Tactile	
Subcutaneous Emphysema—Place under the skin of the mannequin	Crisped-rice cereal in a zip-top bag
	Chocolate syrup and kitty litter
	Bubble wrap
Auditory/Psychological	Call bell and alarms in background noise
	Crying
	Upset and demanding family member or health care team member

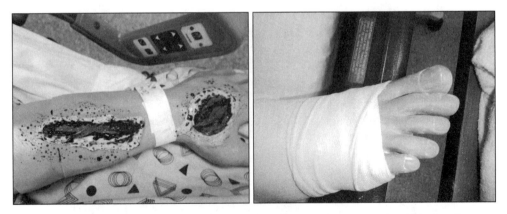

Figure 3.4   Picture left: Wounds with "glass." Picture right: Baby powder added to the toes for "fungal" diabetic foot. Courtesy of Dr. Lori Lioce, UAHCON.

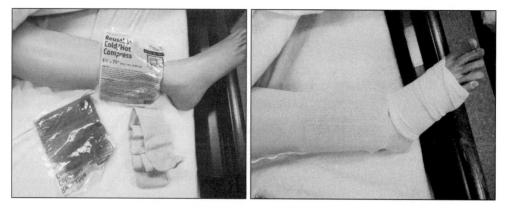

Figure 3.5 Picture left: Materials to create pitting edema. Modeling clay or gel pack under a bandage/stocking. Picture right: Pitting edema. Courtesy of Dr. Lori Lioce, UAHCON.

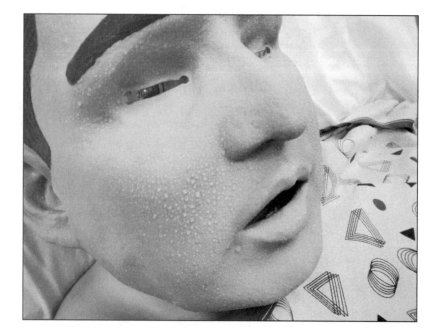

Figure 3.6 Shock-diaphoresis created with spray bottle (filled with water) and cyanosis from blue eye shadow over petroleum jelly on the lips. Courtesy of Dr. Lori Lioce, UAHCON.

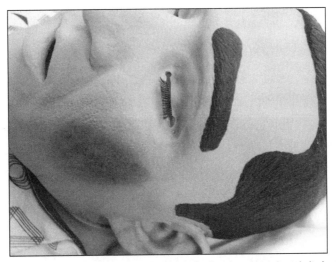

Figure 3.7   Pale complexion with contusion on left check created with light foundation makeup and layered red/brown/black makeup applied to the cheek and patted with a stipple sponge. Eyelashes added to METIman for increased fidelity and to humanize the simulator. Courtesy of Dr. Lori Lioce, UAHCON.

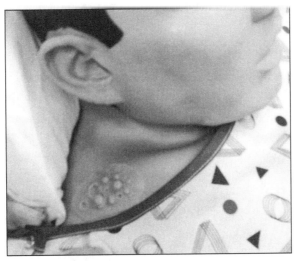

Figure 3.8   Lesion on the shoulder area from a purchased moulage kit. Courtesy of Dr. Lori Lioce, UAHCON.

Moulage Internet Resources

http://www.sickkitchen.com/

http://www.moulage.net/

http://www.militarymoulage.com/

http://www.healthysimulation.com/28/moulage-bridging-the-gap-in-simulation/

http://www.soimmature.com

http://www.nursing.louisiana.edu/learning-resource-center/Moulage%20Recipes.pdf

http://www.cert-la.com/education/moulage-recipes.pdf

http://www.unco.edu/nhs/nines/pdf/Hands_on_care.pdf

http://www.moulageconcepts.com/index.html

http://www.youtube.com/watch?v=HHBAxhNOPA0

http://www.freetechebooks.com/file-2011/moulage.html

https://caehealthcare.com/home/eng/product_services/product_details/meti_fx#

http://www.behindthesimcurtain.com/

Environmental Fidelity

A hospital-based scenario can also include hospital sounds (call light, alarms, background noises); patient care devices; and equipment. The educator must determine the level of fidelity required to accomplish the overall educational goal depending on the objectives and level of learners. A list of sound-effects resources is provided in the "Sound-Effects Resources" sidebar.

Sound-Effects Resources

http://www.youtube.com/watch?v=OEWbNeOfL9U&feature=fvsr

http://www.hark.com/collections/yjldqtzkcm-hospital

http://www.techsmith.com/download/camtasia/default.asp

http://www.healthysimulation.com/1263/voice-changers-in-your-sim-lab/

Low-level environmental fidelity uses pictures of equipment used in patient care, not actual equipment. If you need to have a patient-controlled analgesia pump and one is not available, then you can print off a life-size colored picture of the pump and paste it to a box, run tubing into the pump, and write the dose in ink (Kamp, Gore, Brown, Hoadley, & Smith, 2012). The growth of technology and the Web has greatly increased access to sources of material to create environmental fidelity. Figures 3.9 and 3.10 show examples of low- and high-level fidelity equipment and settings.

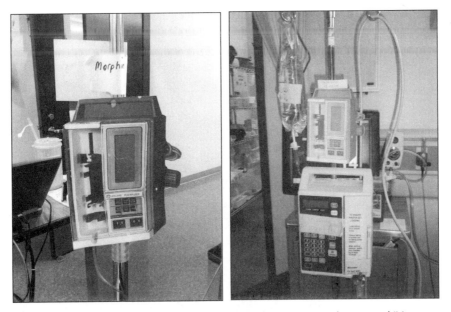

Figure 3.9 Printed paper copy of a morphine PCA pump and an actual IV pump. Courtesy of Fran Kamp, Georgia Baptist College of Nursing of Mercer University.

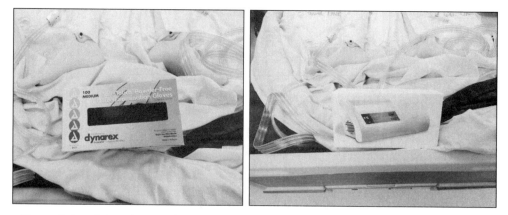

Figure 3.10   Printed copy of sequential compression device (SCD) pasted on an empty glove box. Courtesy of Dr. Teresa N. Gore, AUSON.

Mid-level environmental fidelity incorporates a furnished hospital room with actual equipment (see Figure 3.11).

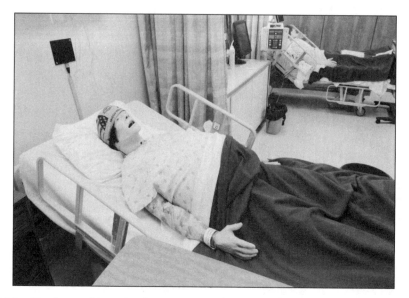

Figure 3.11   Moulage with a wig, do-rag, tattoo sleeves, and Santa Belly for a liver failure patient with ascites. This moulaged patient is used in assessment and skills lab. Learners are asked where to administer a TB skin test. Courtesy of Dr. Teresa N. Gore, AUSON.

Mid-level fidelity mannequins and props can also be used to teach concepts, such as infection control and isolation precautions. In a scenario, Glitter Bug lotion was applied to the work surface and common areas of contamination prior to beginning the simulation. The Glitter Bug was used to show how contamination occurs in an isolation situation. Under a black light, the Glitter Bug showed contaminated areas on the mannequin, bed, clothing, light switches, handles, faucet, paper towel dispenser, and the actual learners (see Figure 3.12). Learners were amazed to see the contaminated surfaces and verbalized that even if they performed everything correctly, it only takes one person not following evidence-based practices to contaminate everything. Several learners readjusted their masks and hair after touching the patient and transferred the Glitter Bug to their mask, hair, gowns, and gloves. This was a "lightbulb" moment for the learners to see the contamination.

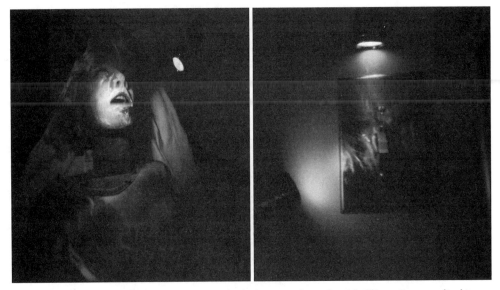

Figure 3.12   Pediatric mannequin in isolation moulaged, with Glitter Bug applied to mannequin, bed, gown, light switch, door handle, and so on. This technique was used to make this an effective simulation environment for learners to visualize isolation precautions. Courtesy of Dr. Teresa N. Gore, AUSON.

High-level environmental fidelity portrays an actual patient setting with appropriate working equipment as in a real-world setting. Figures 3.13 and 3.14 demonstrate examples of high environmental fidelity and moulage to increase the realism of the simulation. This can be applied to community settings as well as hospital or clinic settings. Figure 3.15 shows a simulated "supply room."

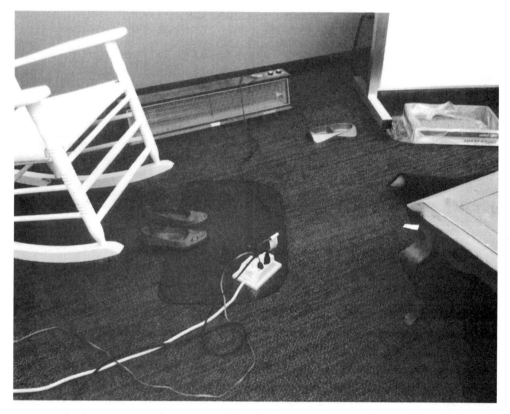

Figure 3.13   Community setting with a focus on safety and conducting a functional geriatric assessment. Courtesy of Fran Kamp, Georgia Baptist School of Nursing at Mercer University.

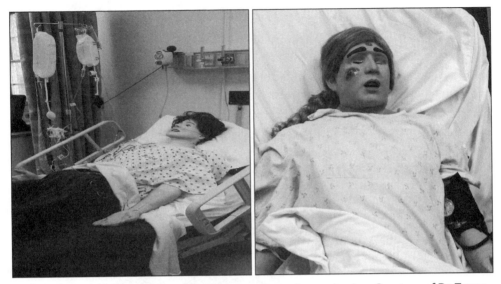

Figure 3.14   Left picture: Prepared for hemodynamic monitoring. Courtesy of Dr. Teresa N. Gore, AUSON. Right picture: Elderly female with makeup and moulage for trauma. A blood pressure cuff is located on the left arm. Courtesy of Dr. Lori Lioce, UAHCON.

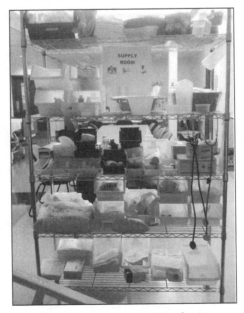

Figure 3.15   Illustration of a supply cart or a cart to depict a supply room. Courtesy of Fran Kamp, Georgia Baptist College of Nursing at Mercer University.

Psychological Fidelity

Successful simulation requires facilitators to provide a trusting, psychologically safe environment. Psychological fidelity refers to "psychological factors such as emotions, beliefs, and self-awareness of learners; social factors such as learner and instructor motivation and goals; culture of the group; degree of openness and trust, as well as learners' modes of thinking" (INACSL BOD, 2011a, p. s5). The educator should incorporate psychological factors to increase the simulation fidelity. Figure 3.16 shows an illustration of creating psychological fidelity, and Table 3.3 shows some examples of ways to increase psychological fidelity.

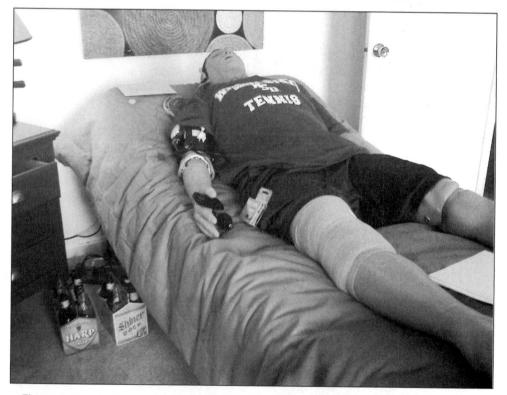

Figure 3.16   A 19 year-old patient with beer and condoms discovered during a home health visit of his grandmother. The objective is to deal with the social issues of substance abuse, underage drinking, and what referrals need to be made and what patient education needs to be conducted. Courtesy of Dr. Sherrill Smith, Wright State University College of Nursing and Health.

Table 3.3 Psychological Fidelity	
Dimensions	*Improving Fidelity*
Developmental	Place shopping bag of children's toys and a diaper bag near the bedside of a 27-year-old roofer who was admitted for a fractured femur after he fell off a roof. Does the learner explore family needs, addressing patient's anxiety related to care of the family?
Spiritual	Place a tattoo of a faith icon on patient's arm or rosary beads in the hand of a 42-year-old female patient with recent diagnosis of breast cancer post-mastectomy. Does the learner recognize the need for spiritual support and follow through with a call for consultation?
Sociocultural	Place dirty clothes and a sleeping bag with fecal and ammonia odor in a backpack at bedside of a 53-year-old homeless patient. Does the learner explore financial resources related to interventions, such as contacting a homeless shelter or social worker?
Psychological	Place a football jersey at the bedside of the 22-year-old simulated patient post-op knee surgery. Does the learner explore how the patient feels about loss of ability to participate in the sport?

Source: Howard, Leighton, & Gore, 2013

Starting Point

Regardless of the level of fidelity in a simulation environment, the facilitator needs to intentionally create a *safe learning environment*. The definition of a safe learning environment is:

> "*The emotional climate that facilitators create by the interaction between facilitators and participants. In this positive emotional climate, participants feel at ease taking risks, making mistakes, or extending themselves beyond their comfort zone. Facilitators are thoroughly aware of the psychological aspects of learning, aware of the effects of unintentional bias, aware of cultural differences, and attentive to their own state of mind in order to effectively create a safe environment for learning*" (INACSL BOD, 2011a, p. s6).

Learning and testing environments differ in several important ways. For example, in the learning environment, opportunities for variation and personalization of the experience are encouraged. Multiple approaches can be taken to all for formative feedback to be given. In the testing environment the goal is to standardize all aspects of the experience to create an equivalent activity for all participants to evaluate their knowledge, skills, and abilities.

The *simulation learning environment* is:

> "An atmosphere that is created by the facilitator to allow for sharing
> and discussion of participant experiences without fear of humilia-
> tion or punitive action. The goals of the simulation learning envi-
> ronment are to promote trust and foster learning" (INACSL BOD,
> 2011a, p. s6).

The *simulation testing environment* is:

> "An atmosphere that is created by the facilitator to allow for forma-
> tive and summative evaluation to occur. The goals of the simula-
> tion testing environment are to create an equivalent activity for all
> participants in order to test their knowledge, skills, and abilities in a
> simulated setting" (INACSL BOD, 2011a, p. s6).

Safe Learning Environment

Orientation and educator buy-in are required to develop a safe learning environment. Educators are seen as the experts in their specialties. However, when educators are placed in the simulation lab for a scenario the first time, their inexperience at that point makes them feel more novice and out of their comfort zone (Waxman & Telles, 2009). This environment is unfamiliar to the educators as compared to the patient setting. In human patient care, the educators cannot allow the learners to make errors and learn the consequences of the actions or inactions. Therefore, using simulation is a new skill even for experienced educators to develop. To facilitate educator development, educators should undertake simulation education to learn evidence-based or best practices for the best learner outcomes.

In order to create a safe learning environment, all learners should be oriented to the equipment, surroundings, environment, and fidelity of all equipment to be used in the simulation. Orientation for learners should occur prior to any requirement to perform and address any equipment that is not high-fidelity or working the same as it would in the real environment. An example of this would be an intravenous (IV) pump that is actual patient equipment but is turned off and instead has a piece of tape on the display screen as a visual cue of the rate of infusion. Orientation may be required for assessment findings also. An example is applying anti-embolism stockings stuffed with cushioning or towels to a mannequin's lower legs to depict edema. This could be confusing to the learners in the simulation because without explanation they might assume it is just the stockings and not edema.

After the simulation has been developed, educators should rehearse with simulation personnel or other simulation educators to determine the flow and accuracy, and note any deficiencies prior to learners participating. If the institution has developed scenarios, then peer review these for incorporating evidence-based practices, accuracy, and appropriateness for the level of the learner, and for ensuring the objectives can be accomplished within the timeframe stated.

As they will with any new activity, learners will face a learning curve. The learners should be oriented to the lab and equipment along with the expectations. Learners need to understand this is not a "play time," but a chance to practice the role of a health care professional providing evidence-based care to a human. The more suspension of disbelief that occurs, the more immersed the learner can become in the simulation. Educators must explain clear expectations of the performance as well as the behaviors that are allowed and others that will not be tolerated. The learner's first simulation experience should be formative as a learning experience before he or she is subjected to any testing, such as skills validation or summative performance.

Learners must also understand the need for academic integrity. The simulation information must remain confidential, and learners should understand that the sharing of any information is viewed as academic dishonesty (INACSL BOD, 2011b). Educators need to explain the relationship between the Health Insurance Portability and Accountability Act (HIPAA) and academic integrity in the simulation setting. Learners must understand that by discussing the simulation experience with others not directly involved in the same simulation session they are sharing privileged information.

Academic Integrity Example: Professional Integrity and Confidentiality for Simulated Clinical Experiences in Academic Settings

Professional integrity, including confidentiality of the performances, scenario content, and experience, is expected to be upheld. Professional integrity is expected for all components and learners in the simulation environment. Failure of the learners to maintain professional integrity related to simulation could undermine the benefits of the simulated clinical experience.

Privileged information of any kind can bias an individual's performance and interfere with the group's dynamics, thereby interfering with learning outcomes. Sharing of events and individual performances occurring during the simulation sessions with those not involved in the event may decrease the safe environment of the simulation setting. Sharing of events and correct action in the simulation with those not involved in the event may negatively alter future learners' learning outcomes. Failure to comply with this is an act of academic dishonesty. Please refer to the academic dishonesty section of the course syllabus.

I, _____, promise to adhere to the
(Print Name)

_____ Professional Integrity and Confidentiality for
(Insert Name of School)

Simulated Clinical Experiences statement. I will not provide or share any information after completion of a simulated clinical experience, ask for information about the simulated clinical experience prior to participating in a simulated clinical experience, and/or provide any cues or hints to other learners until all learners have participated in the simulation experience. Failure to comply with this is an act of academic dishonesty. The _____ Academic Dishonesty Policy will be followed.   (Name of School)

_____   _____
Date   Student's Signature

_____   _____
Course   Witness Signature

Courtesy of Dr. Teresa N. Gore, AUSON

One intervention that can assist with maintaining the academic integrity of the simulation is to have the learners sign a confidentiality agreement after offering them a detailed explanation of the need for self-discovery of a problem. An example of such an agreement is shown in the accompanying sidebar.

Educational Objectives

Scenarios need to be evidence-based. An effective simulation environment is one intentionally linked to the educational objectives. As shown earlier in the chapter in Table 3.1, educators should select the type of mannequin and degree of fidelity based on the goal and objective of the simulation, not just the type of equipment and fidelity available (INACSL BOD, 2011c).

Objectives determine the focus of the simulation and specify what the learner will be able to perform when the simulation is complete. The objectives guide all simulation planning, including cues for fidelity, the scenario end point, debriefing, and evaluation. Objectives must be clear and measurable to guide the educator to consistent and reliable evaluation of outcomes.

Planning

Educators should begin simulation planning and development by reviewing the learning objectives. If you do not know where you are going, how can you plan to get there? After the goal and objectives are determined, educators need to determine the level of fidelity required (mannequin, environment, psychological). Ideally, this process should begin at least 2 weeks prior to each simulation. Simulation centers should develop checklists for simulation that staff and facilitators use for scenario preparation to ensure an appropriate level of fidelity is created and consistency is maintained between learning sessions. Checklists are also helpful in ensuring the many details are brought together. A sample checklist is shown in Table 3.4.

Table 3.4   Sample Checklist for Simulation

SIMULATION CHECKLIST

Course #:_____ Educator_____ Date of Simulation _____
Learners/Groups _____/_____

(Date/Initial)	2 Weeks Prior to Scheduled Simulation (Confirm with Director/Coordinator)
_____	Contact faculty member Left Message _____ Email _____
_____	Verify date/time _____ , confirm # of learners _____ and # of groups _____
_____	Ask if created a schedule YES NO Collaborated with SIM Coordinator YES NO
_____	Confirm scenario numbers _____ and _____
_____	Create rotation schedule/scenario packet and email to educator Date:_____
_____	Request/Copy pretest and posttest (w/ 1 answer key)
_____	Prepare scripts for patient, lab, etc.
_____	Create a schedule w/room #s for simulation and debriefing and confirm with course manager
_____	If > 1 group per simulator, plan rotations, stations, and consult director for room assignments
(Date/Initial)	**1 Week Prior to Scheduled Simulation**
_____	Prepare patient tray(s) with all needed supplies
_____	Label IV bags/medications with correct dosage and expiration
_____	Prepare medical record with SBAR, Provider orders (scan)
_____	Create patient armband

_____	Make a list of any props that may be needed (e.g., glasses, street clothes, cigarettes) (scan)
_____	Simulated wounds, stitches, feces, urine, sputum, blood
_____	Check if simulator needs to be filled with distilled water, blood, urine

Initial	**Day Before Scheduled Simulation**
_____	Make copies of pre-/posttest, observation and evaluation forms
_____	Set up room, trays, and mannequin (needed supplies on tray, 1 tray per group of 4)
_____	Place patient charts, copies, and scripts in the control room by the computer (scan)
_____	If more than one patient, make sure you indicate which room the patients are in
_____	Make signs for rooms with patient names and educator last name on SIM and debriefing room

Initial	**Day of Simulation (Remind learners to leave all belongings in the locker area except for pencil and paper)**
_____	Ask faculty to inspect moulage and fidelity upon arrival to ensure objectives will be met
_____	Make sure all needed materials are in the room and sign-in sheet at desk for attendance
_____	Check simulator (fill with distilled water if scenario calls for it)
_____	Turn on the mannequin; turn on the computer
_____	Post room/rotation assignments for educator and learners
_____	Set up video camera (student workers can help with this)
_____	Provide technical support for educator
_____	Ensure debriefing area, screen, and computer are ready for video replay and paperwork is present
_____	Between scenarios, clean up and remove anything applied to mannequin in preparation for the next group

Table 3.4	Sample Checklist for Simulation *(cont.)*
Initial	**Following the Simulation**
_____	Collect evaluation forms, pre-/posttests (scan and place in online course folder)
_____	Label file with the scenario number, course number, educator name, and date
_____	Place all created documents *including this completed checklist,* into a patient chart with a blank pretest/posttest answer sheet
_____	Tabulate evaluation results and email to SIM coordinator, educator, and course manager (placing comments into an Excel spreadsheet)
_____	Please save file name as Course #, Scenario #, date, time, and educator last name
_____	Please email course manager, Director, and SIM Coordinator when e-file of all documents is uploaded to Charger Hospital Faculty Simulation Course

Staff Name: _____

Courtesy of Dr. Lori Lioce, UAHCON

Developing a clinically specific simulator set-up list of moulage, learners, props, and equipment available in the simulation lab enables educators to clearly and consistently communicate their needs while providing examples that will stimulate their imagination. This tool helps simulation staff to ensure clinically significant cues are in place for the learner. These tools and other simulation documents may be archived in an online faculty simulation course to increase faculty access and use. A sample simulation set-up request form is shown in Table 3.5.

Online educator simulation courses can be developed in any electronic classroom management system such as ANGEL, Blackboard, or WEBCT for academic institutions and an intranet system for health care institutions. They serve as a wonderful repository for moulage recipes, faculty-accessible scenarios, documents used in simulations such as patient files, simulation framework, simulation education updates, forms, and simulation policies and procedures.

Table 3.5   Simulator Set-Up Request Form

Simulator Set-Up
Please circle your preference below:

Gender	Male / Female
Foley	Yes / No
Urine	Clear / Bloody / *Other:* _____
Skin	Rash / Lesion scaly / papule / macule
	color _____size_____ shape _____ distribution _____
	Contusion / Lac / Burn / Abrasion / Bruise / *Other:*_____
Location	head / neck / chest / back / arm / abdomen / groin / buttocks / leg / foot / *Other:* _____
	Right / Left / Center / Side / Proximal / Distal Bilateral / Unilateral *Other:* _____
IV	Y / N Gauge: 14 16 18 20 22 24
Location	A/C Radial Central Line IJ Art Line
Fluids	Y / N Infusion Pump PCA KVO
	Normal Saline LR D5W *Other:* _____
	Rate: _____ @ _____ /LPM *Other:* _____
Monitor	Pre-set Simulator Scenario Name: _____
EKG	_____ lead(s)
ABP	_____
Pulse	_____
Beginning Vitals	Within Normal Limits Abnormal (select below)
HR	_____BPM NSR
SpO_2 CO_2	_____% RR _____ *Other:*_____
BP	_____
Equipment	12 lead EKG

Table 3.5	Simulator Set-Up Request Form *(cont.)*	
	CPAP BIPAP	
	X-ray of _____	
	Crash Cart	
Special Medications	Please specify: _____	
Special Props	Please specify: _____	
Learners	Nurse EMS Provider Respiratory *Other:* _____	
Family Member	Mom Dad Brother Sister Wife Husband Girlfriend Boyfriend Significant Other *Other:* _____	
Room Set-Up	Hospital Clinic Community Home *Other:*_____	
Lab results:	CBC CMP BMP ABG POC Glucose _____	
Other special request:	Other:_____	

Courtesy of Dr. Lori Lioce, UAHCON

Educators should plan to arrive early for their scheduled simulation and check the simulation environment for simulation cues and clinical accuracy. Photographing the set-up and moulage of each scenario is also recommended. Photographs provide visual cues to stage the simulation consistently every time, thereby increasing the reliability and validity, and potentially improving outcomes. This is especially true for courses with a large number of learner groups in which the same simulation is conducted over a period of time, requiring the scenario to be set up multiple times. These photographs can be digitally stored, printed, or kept with the scenario.

Planning, managing, and organizing moulage and props can be challenging. Stacking plastic boxes with lids and inventory lists for each scenario may provide a manageable solution. Creating a basic moulage kit is a great starting point. This kit should include basic makeup such as blue, brown, and black non-shimmering eye shadows or powders, which may be used as eye shadow or to simulate cyanosis or bruising. Be sure to check with the simulator manufacturer regarding what products may damage or permanently stain the simulator. (Application tips can usually be found on the manufacturer's web page.)

Kits range from basic to extensive for wounds or replication of trauma victims. Suggested resources to include in a simulation kit are listed in the accompanying sidebar.

Simulation Kit Resources

Educator's Corner: Recipes For Emergencies: Moulage: http://www.emsvillage.com/articles/article.cfm?id=969

Simulaids: Training Aids for Emergency, Medical and Rescue Personnel: http://www.simulaids.com

Image Perspectives (Training & Supplies): http://www.moulage.net/

Common Cents EMS Supply: http://www.savelives.com/department/moulage-makeup-kits-14231.cfm

Bound Tree Medical: https://www.boundtree.com/moulage-kits-subcategorynode-239-0.aspx

Evaluation

The evaluation used for simulation should also include feedback on the simulation environment, props, and moulage. Learners can readily recommend items that would have enhanced the reality of the simulation immediately after participating. Evaluation should include the educator in addition to the learner for continuous quality improvement. The purpose of these evaluations is to identify whether the objectives and overall goal of the simulation were met, providing opportunities for environmental improvements to the fidelity of the simulation. Evaluating simulation effectiveness is discussed further in Chapter 6.

A simulation scenario usually needs minor adjustments several times until everyone involved deems it "perfect." The scenario template tool shown in Table 3.6 depicts how these elements can be incorporated into a single tool.

Conclusion

After reviewing the information provided in this chapter, it is time to explore how simulation educators should use this teaching strategy and which learners can benefit from this approach. Simulation educators can create effective simulation environments to educate undergraduate students, graduate students, practitioners from all disciplines and experience levels, new faculty, clinical adjunct faculty, and any health care providers who wish to continue professional development or want to be lifelong learners. Increasing the depth to which learners can become immersed in the simulation environment through strategies that facilitate the suspension of disbelief increases the potential for learning. Through incorporation of psychological factors throughout the simulation, and through mannequin moulage and equipment, suspension of disbelief can be achieved, allowing learners to find the relevance in the situation.

Simulation can be used in all areas in which patient care is performed or in which educating health care providers occurs. In the clinical practice world, effective simulation can be used during the hiring process to evaluate critical thinking and practice and during annual competency evaluation for experienced health care providers, as long as organizations use valid and reliable simulations and evaluation tools conducted by proficient simulation educators. In academia, simulation can be used to educate clinical adjunct faculty, or for faculty development, by teaching techniques and strategies to handle supervision of students in the clinical area.

The use of simulation is only limited by the simulation educator's imagination. So, dream big, reach for the stars, and improve health care one provider at a time.

Table 3.6   Scenario Template

MAPPING OUT SCENARIO PEDIATRIC CYSTIC FIBROSIS AND ISOLATION

Template Courtesy of Kim Leighton, Bryan College of Health Sciences 2008, and Dr. Teresa N. Gore, Auburn University School of Nursing 2012.

Objectives:

- Identify and implement infection control (isolation) and safe patient care environment
- Develop and implement developmentally appropriate care for a school-aged child with chronic illness (pediatric cystic fibrosis) after age-appropriate assessment
- Utilize therapeutic communications with all members involved

Pre-Simulation Exercises:

- Describe the pathophysiology of cystic fibrosis (CF).
- What are the effects of CF on the respiratory and GI systems?
- What are the primary interventions in the management of respiratory distress in CF?
- What is the effect of chronic conditions, such as CF, on the growth and development of the school-aged child?

Post-Simulation Exercises:

Reflective journal

- **Evaluation of Learner:** Formative Assessment SLS Observer Evaluation Rubric
- **Evaluation Tool of Simulation:** METI and Leighton CLECS tool
- **Facilitation:** Partial Instructor Lead
- **Level of Learner:** Medical-Surgical/Pediatric
- **Minimal Number of Learners:** 1
- **Maximum Number of Learners:** Goal 2 with max 3
- **Scenario Time:** 40 minutes   **Pre-brief:** 10 minutes   **Simulation:** 15 minutes
- **Debriefing Time:** 15 minutes   **Video Recording:** No
  Will recording be retained: End of Semester
- **Designers:** LRC Coordinator and Sim Coordinator
- **Validation and Peer Review:** Pediatric and Med-Surg Faculty

Table 3.6   Scenario Template   *(cont.)*

You arrive to precept with your nurse at Baptist East today. You are assigned to Jason Bright, a 9-year-old male patient diagnosed with cystic fibrosis who was admitted to the progressive care unit with pneumonia yesterday. He presented with fever (max 102.6), dehydration, and increased secretions (thick greenish). His WBC is 13.3, O_2 saturation 90% on 4 L/min, and has blood and sputum cultures pending. CXR reveals RLL pneumonia. Other lab work is within normal limits. He is receiving Vancomycin every 12 hours with pharmacy calculating dosage based on Ht. 4'5" and Wt. 62#. He is on unit dosed nebulizer treatments, IPPB, CPT every 6 hours per respiratory therapy. He is currently on isolation pending culture results.

State #1	Interventions	State #2
Admitted 1 day with pneumonia and cystic fibrosis	Conduct an appropriate assessment and evaluate findings	Patient must be talked into cooperating with interventions
Patient sitting with HOB elevated, O_2 not applied (worn appropriately)	Recognize abnormal findings	Vital signs unchanged
HR 110, BP 104/68, RR 30 and labored (short of breath when talking), SaO_2 90%, & Temp 99.8° (T max 102.6°)	(If learners asks) cap refill 4 seconds	If appropriate interventions, improving shortness of breath
If monitor available, ST without ectopy	Respiratory toilet (HOB elevated, O_2 reapplied, consult respiratory therapy for CPT and breathing treatment using ISBARR via phone or intercom with Unit Secretary)	If not, continue uncooperative and SOB
RLL crackles and wheezing throughout	Utilization of PPE and appropriate hand hygiene	Phone call for sputum culture results— pseudomonas and WBC 15.4
"NURSE, HELP ME!! I am short of breath some. What are you going to do for me?"	Uses isolation stethoscope, BP cuff, thermometer	Use ad lib communication depending on learners' comments and interventions
"I don't like to wear the oxygen."	Using developmentally appropriate therapeutic communication w/pt	
"Just make it better. Do you know what you are doing?"		

Interventions	**State #3**
Continues to monitor and interact with patient to increase oxygen saturation level	HR 108, BP 102/68, RR 24, SaO$_2$ 93%, Temp 99.8° "I am feeling a little better." "Thanks." Black light room and learners' hands/ clothing to see contamination using Glitter Bug

Table 3.6   Scenario Template   *(cont.)*

State #1	*Interventions*	*State #2*
Props	*Props*	*Props*
Pediatric mannequin of 9-year-old male, Jason Bright		
Boys PJs, wig, baseball cap, shorts, socks, stuffed animal and football in the bed.		
Saline lock		
O$_2$ nasal cannula and venti-mask		
Isolation cart with PPE, stethoscope, BP cuff, and thermometer		
Pulse oximeter		
Hand washing/hygiene equipment		
Urinal w/ dark concentrated urine		
Suction equipment		
Call light		
High-caloric protein snacks		
Glitter Bug on side rails, door handle, patient, football, stuffed animal, and miscellaneous areas		
Black light—handheld		

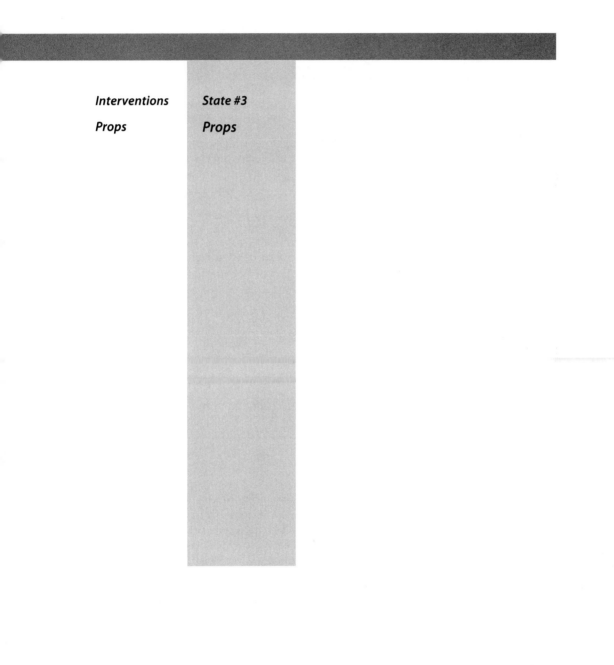

Interventions

Props

State #3

Props

Table 3.6   Scenario Template   *(cont.)*

Debriefing: (Ask at least one from each section)

Aesthetic Questions:

"I would like each of you to talk to me about the problem(s) Jason was experiencing today."

"What was your main objective during this simulation?"

"How did patient safety and isolation issues affect the patient care you provided?"

Personal Questions:

"How did this scenario make you feel?"

"What made you chose the actions/interventions/focus you chose for Jason?"

Empirical Questions:

"I would like for each of you to talk with me about the knowledge, skills, attitudes (KSA), and previous experiences that provided you the ability to provide evidence-based care to Jason."

Ethical Question:

"Talk to me about how your personal beliefs and values influenced the care provided to Jason."

Reflection:

"Will each of you tell me how you knew what to do for a CF patient with pneumonia and isolation and why?"

"If we could redo this scenario now, what would you change and why?"

"How will you use this in your professional practice?"

References

Alinier, G. (2007). A typology of educationally focused medical simulation tools. *Medical Teacher, 29*(8), e243-e250.

Beaubien, J. M., & Baker, D. P. (2004). The use of simulation for training teamwork skills in health care: How low can you go? *BMJ Quality and Safety, 13*(1), i51-i56. doi:10.1136/qshc.2004.009845

Blum, C. A., Borglund, S., & Parcells, D. (2010). High-fidelity nursing simulation: Impact on student self-confidence and clinical competence. *International Journal of Nursing Education Scholarship, 7*(1), article 18, 1-16. doi: 10.2202/1548-923X.2035

Butler, K. W., Veltre, D. E., & Brady, D. (2009). Implementation of active learning pedagogy comparing low-fidelity simulation versus high-fidelity simulation in pediatric nursing education. *Clinical Simulation in Nursing, 5*(4), e129-e136. doi: 10.1016/j.ecns.2009.03.118

Cooper, S., Cant, R., Porter, J., Bogossian, F., McKenna, L., Brady, S., & Fox-Young, S. (2012). Simulation based learning in midwifery education: A systematic review. *Women Birth, 25*(2), 64-78. doi:10.1016/j.wombi.2011.03.004

Deckers, C. M., Doyle, T. J., & Wilkinson, W. J. (2011). Effectively using instructional technologies. In B. Ulrich (Ed.), *Mastering precepting: A nurse's handbook for success* (pp. 135-157). Indianapolis, IN: Sigma Theta Tau International.

De Giovanni, D., Roberts, T., & Norman, G. (2009). Relative effectiveness of high- versus low-fidelity simulation in learning heart sounds. *Medical Education, 43*(7), 661-668.

Dieckmann, P., Gaba, D., & Rall, M. (2007). Deepening the theoretical foundations of patient simulation as social practice. *Simulation in Healthcare, 2*(3), 183-193. doi: 10.1097/SIH.0b013e3180f637f5

Farnan, J. M., Paro, J. A. M., Rodriguez, R. M. , Reddy, S. T., Horwitz, L. I., Johnson, J. K., Arora, V. M. (2010). Hand-off education and evaluation: Piloting the observed simulated hand-off experience (OSHE). *Journal of General Internal Medicine 25*(2), 129-134.

Friedman, Z., Siddiqui, N., Katznelson, R., Devito, I., Bould, M. D., & Naik, V. (2009). Clinical impact of epidural anesthesia simulation on short- and long-term learning curve: High- versus low-fidelity model training. *Anesthesia and Pain Medicine, 34*(3), 229-232.

Gates, M. G., Parr, M. B., and Hughen, J. E. (2012). Enhancing nursing knowledge using high-fidelity simulation. *Journal of Nursing Education, 51*(1), 9-15. doi: 10.3928/01484834-20111116-01

Grady, J. L., Kehrer, R. G., Trusty, C. E., Entin, E. B., Entin, E. E., & Brunye, T. T. (2008). Learning nursing procedures: The influence of simulator fidelity and student gender on teaching effectiveness. *Journal of Nursing Education, 47*(9), 403-8. doi: 10.3928/01484834-20080901-09

Howard, V., Leighton, K., & Gore, T. (2013). Simulation in healthcare education. In R. Nelson & N. Staggers (Eds.), *Informatics: An interprofessional approach for health practitioners (pp. 454-471)*. Philadelphia. PA: W.B. Saunders.

Howard, V. M., Ross, C., Mitchell, A. M., & Nelson, G. M. (2010). Human patient simulators and interactive case studies: A comparative analysis of learning outcomes and student perceptions. *Computers Informatics, and Nursing (CIN), 28*(1), 42-48.

International Nursing Association for Clinical Simulation and Learning (INASCL) Board of Directors (BOD) (2011a). Standards of best practice: Simulation. Standard I: Terminology. *Clinical Simulation in Nursing, 7*(4S), s3-s7. doi:10.1016/j.ecns.2011.05.005. Retrieved from http://download.journals.elsevierhealth.com/pdfs/journals/1876-1399/PIIS1876139911000612.pdf

International Nursing Association for Clinical Simulation and Learning (INASCL) Board of Directors (BOD) (2011b). Standards of best practice: Simulation. Standard II: Professional integrity of participant. *Clinical Simulation in Nursing, 7* (4S), s8-s9. doi:10.1016/j.ecns.2011.05.006. Retrieved from http://download.journals.elsevierhealth.com/pdfs/journals/1876-1399/PIIS1876139911000624.pdf

International Nursing Association for Clinical Simulation and Learning (INASCL) Board of Directors (BOD) (2011c). Standards of best practice: Simulation. Standard III: Participant objectives. *Clinical Simulation in Nursing, 7*(4S), s10-s11. doi:10.1016/j.ecns.2011.05.007. Retrieved from http://download.journals.elsevierhealth.com/pdfs/journals/1876-1399/PIIS1876139911000636.pdf

Jeffries, P. R., & Rizzolo, M. A. (2006). *NLN/Laerdal project summary report. Designing and implementing models for the innovative use of simulation to teach nursing care of ill adults and children: A national, multi-site, multi-method study*. New York, NY: National League for Nursing.

Kameg, K., Howard, V. M., Clochesy, J., Mitchell, A. M., & Suresky, J. (2010). Impact of high fidelity human simulation on self-efficacy of communication skills. *Issues in Mental Health Nursing, 31*(5), 315-323.

Kamp, F., Gore, T., Brown, S. C., Hoadley, T., & Smith, S. (2012). Podium Presentation: *Boots, chaps, and cowboy hats: Making simulation real*. 11th Annual Conference International Nursing Simulation and Learning Resource Centers. San Antonio, TX.

Kardong-Edgren, S., Anderson, M., & Michaels, J. (2007). Does simulation fidelity improve student test scores? *Clinical Simulation in Nursing, 3*(1), e21-e24. doi: 10.1016/j.ecns.2009.05.035

Kardong-Edgren, S., Lungstrom, N., & Bendel, R. (2009). VitalSim versus SimMan: A comparison of BSN student test scores, knowledge retention, and satisfaction. *Clinical Simulation in Nursing, 5*(3), e105-e111. doi:10.1016/j.ecns.2009.01.007

Keene, P. R. (2009). Progression from low fidelity to high fidelity simulators to provide experiential learning for nursing students. *Clinical Simulation in Nursing, 5*(3 suppl), e143. doi: 10.1016/j.ecns.2009.04.047

Keinan, G., Friedland, N., & Sarig-Naor, V. (1990). Training for task performance under stress: The effectiveness of phased training methods. *Journal of Applied Social Psychology, 20*(18), 1514-1529.

Kinney, S., & Henderson, D. (2008). Comparison of low fidelity simulation learning strategy with traditional lecture. *Clinical Simulation in Nursing, 4*(2), e15-e18. doi: 10.1016/j.ecns.2008.06.005

Lapkin, S., Levett-Jones, T., Bellchambers, H., & Fernandez, R. (2010). Effectiveness of patient simulation manikins in teaching clinical reasoning skills to undergraduate nursing students: A systematic review. *Clinical Simulation in Nursing, 6*(6), e207-e222. doi:10.1016/j.ecns.2010.05.005

Lee, K. H., Grantham, H., & Boyd, R. (2008). Comparison of high- and low-fidelity mannequins for clinical performance assessment. *Emergency Medicine Australasia, 20*(6), 508-514.

Maran, N. J., & Glavin, R. J. (2003). Low- to high-fidelity simulation-A continuum of medical education. *Medical Education, 37*(Suppl. 1), 22-28.

McGaghie, W., Issenberg, S. B., Petrusa, E., & Scalese, R. (2009). A critical review of simulation-based medical education research: 2003-2009. *Medical Education, 44*(1), 50-63.

Merriam-Webster Online Dictionary. Moulage. (2013). Springfield, MA: Merriam-Webster, Inc. Retrieved from http://www.merriam-webster.com/dictionary/moulage

Meyer, M. N., Connors, H., Hou, Q., & Gajewski, B. (2011). The effects of simulation on clinical performance: A junior nursing student clinical comparison study. *Simulation in Healthcare, 6*(5), 269-77. doi: 10.1097/SIH.0b013e318223a048

National League for Nursing Simulation Innovation Resource Center (NLNSIRC). (2010). *SIRC glossary*. New York, NY: National League for Nursing. Retrieved from http://sirc.nln.org/mod/glossary/view. php?id=183

Radhakrishnan, K., Roche, J. P., & Cunningham, H. (2007). Measuring clinical practice parameters with human patient simulation: A pilot study. *International Journal of Nursing Education Scholarship, 4*(1), 1-11.

Robinson-Smith, G., Bradley, P., & Meakim, C. (2009). Evaluating the use of standardized patients in undergraduate psychiatric nursing experiences. *Clinical Simulation in Nursing, 5*(6), e203-e211. doi:10.1016/j.ecns.2009.07.001

Rudolph, J. W., Simon, R., Raemer, D. B. (2007). Which reality matters? Questions on the path to high engagement in healthcare simulation. *Simulation in Healthcare, 2*(3), 161-163. doi: 10.1097/SIH.0b013e31813d1035

Tiffen, J., Corbridge, S., Shen, B. C., & Robinson, P. (2010). Patient simulator for teaching heart and lung assessment skills to advanced practice nursing students. *Clinical Simulation in Nursing, 7*(3), e91-e97. doi: 10.1016/j.ecns.2009.10.003

Waxman, K. T., & Telles, C. L. (2009). The use of Benner's framework in high-fidelity simulation faculty development: The Bay Area Simulation Collaborative model. *Clinical Simulation in Nursing, 5*(6), e231-e235. doi:10.1016/j.ecns.2009.06.001

Wickens, C. D. (2000). The trade-off of design for routine and unexpected performance: Implications of situation awareness. In M. R. Endsley & D. J. Garland (Eds.), *Situation awareness analysis and measurement* (pp. 211-225). Mahwah, NJ: Lawrence Erlbaum Associates.

Creating Effective, Evidence-Based Scenarios

Valerie M. Howard, EdD, MSN, RN

Simulation is one example of an experiential teaching methodology, and its use within the health care or academic setting should be guided by sound educational principles (Clapper, 2010). Because simulation offers a standardized, controlled environment for applied learning opportunities, it is an ideal environment to provide application of knowledge for low-occurrence but high-risk situations in the clinical setting. When implementing simulation either within an academic or service setting, it is beneficial to develop a scenario. A scenario is defined as "the plan of an expected and potential course of events for a simulated clinical experience. The clinical scenario provides the context for the simulation and can vary in length and complexity, depending on the objectives." (International Nursing Association for Clinical Simulation and Learning [INACSL] Board of Directors [BOD], 2011a, p. s4). Therefore, the scenario is a planned educational experience that is developed by the facilitator or educator to assist the learner with meeting the learning objectives. The scenario guides the learning opportunities for the participants.

The key to successful implementation of a simulation scenario lies in careful planning to map out the scenario details (Howard, Englert, Kameg, & Perozzi, 2011; Jeffries, 2007; Waxman, 2010).

OBJECTIVES

- Identify educational theories to guide simulation scenario development.
- Utilize the best clinical evidence when developing simulation scenarios.
- Demonstrate the critical elements of scenario development.

A clinical scenario includes "the plan of an expected and potential course of events for a simulated clinical experience" (INACSL BOD, 2011a, p. s4). When designing a scenario, the facilitator should include participant preparation, pre-briefing materials, patient information with descriptions of the situation, learning objectives, environmental conditions, related equipment and props to enhance realism, roles and expectations of participants, a progression outline for the actual simulation implementation, a standardized debriefing process, and evaluation criteria (INACSL BOD, 2011a; Jeffries, 2007).

The first step in the scenario planning process begins with choosing a topic for the simulation scenario. Topics for simulation scenarios can be generated in multiple ways (see accompanying sidebar). Scenarios can be developed in alignment with course content and objectives or to provide opportunities to practice a skill that does not often occur in a clinical situation.

Educators in the academic setting can use feedback from clinical agencies to design scenarios to enhance student performance where it may be lacking. Emerging health care trends or new policies and regulations can stimulate the need for additional training, and simulation-based educational modalities can provide these opportunities. Evaluation data from standardized tests, such as the National Council Licensure Examination (NCLEX) for registered nurses, can be used as a trigger to develop targeted scenarios to provide application of knowledge.

Scenarios can also be developed for the hospital or ambulatory care setting. For example, scenarios can be developed to evaluate ongoing competencies of clinical professionals. Simulations can also be developed to improve efficiency, assess a process for the potential for latent errors, or test the workflow design in a new hospital unit.

When designing any educational modality, educational theory and models should guide development (Kaakinan & Arwood, 2009). The same holds true for simulation. Multiple learning theories can be used to guide the educational process (see Table 4.1); however, two that uniquely align are Kolb's Experiential Learning Theory (Kolb, 1984) and the National League for Nursing (NLN)/Jeffries Simulation Framework (Jeffries, 2007).

Generating Ideas for Simulation Scenarios

Course objectives

Essential learning outcomes

High-risk, low-occurrence situations

Results of standardized tests

Student performance in the clinical setting

Health care trends

Journal articles

Policy and regulations

Competency evaluation

System assessment and improvement

Table 4.1   Educational Theories and Models Linked to Simulation

Theory	Theorist
Novice to Expert	Benner, 1984
Experiential Learning Theory	Kolb, 1984
Adult Learning Theory	Knowles, 1984
Situated Cognition	Lave & Wenger, 1991
Interactive Model of Clinical Judgment Development	Lasater, 2007
NLN/Jeffries Simulation Framework	Jeffries, 2007

The ability to transfer theoretical knowledge and apply this in a practice setting leads to the acquisition of knowledge, according to Experiential Learning Theory (Kolb, 1984). Service industry professions such as nursing and medicine have long accepted this notion by incorporating clinical experiences along with didactic lecture. The learners need to be able to apply these abstract classroom concepts during a practical learning experience in order to enhance cognitive development. According to Experiential Learning Theory, learning is enhanced when learners are actively involved in gaining knowledge through experience with problem solving and decision-making, and active reflection is integral to the learning process (Dewey, 1938; Kolb, 1984). Education is a result of experience (Dewey, 1938). The process of reflection is a cognitive process that can be enhanced through a structured learning activity. Kolb's theory has been used many times in service learning industries to explain the necessity for incorporating practice into the curriculum, such as through a nursing student's clinical experiences and simulation. The debriefing experience after the simulation experience directly mirrors the importance of reflection as an integral part of the learning process. It is during this experience that learners cognitively and purposefully think about the learning experience, and the abstract principles learned in the classroom become concrete as a result of their application.

The National League for Nursing (NLN), in partnership with the Laerdal Corporation, developed a simulation framework based upon empirical and theoretical literature (Jeffries, 2007). This framework, known as the NLN/Jeffries Simulation Framework, is useful in designing, implementing, and evaluating simulations (see Figure 4.1). The simulation framework comprises five major components: teacher (or educator) characteristics, student (or learner) characteristics, educational practices, design characteristics of the simulation (the educational or evaluation activity), and outcomes. Although the framework was initially developed for the academic setting, each component can be applied to scenario development in the service or hospital setting. For example, the *teacher* in the academic setting is equivalent to the *nurse educator* or *staff development personnel* in the hospital setting. According to the INACSL standards, the more appropriate term would be *facilitator* (see Table 4.2) (INACSL BOD, 2011a).

Table 4.2   Terms

Terms used in NLN/Jeffries Simulation Framework for Nursing Education or academic setting	Terms used in the service, hospital, or clinical setting	INACSL Standard I Terminology that can be used interchangeably in any setting
Teacher	Nurse Educator	Facilitator
	Staff Development Specialist	
Student	Learner	Participant

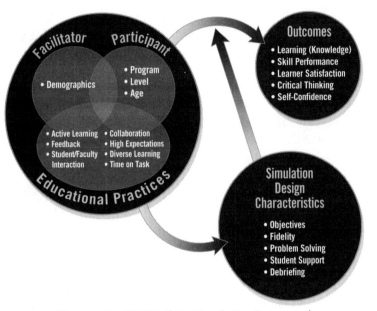

Figure 4.1 NLN/Jeffries Simulation Framework
Used with permission of the National League for Nursing

Within each component of the framework, variables exist that should be addressed when designing simulations. For example, educators need to be facilitators of learning in this learner-centered environment. In addition, educators may need support with technology and simulation design. Within the simulation environment, the roles of the learners within the scenario should be clearly defined. Learners are expected to be self-motivated and responsible for their own learning. Educational practices consist of active learning, providing appropriate feedback, facilitating student-faculty interaction (or learner-educator interaction), and fostering diverse, collaborative learning. A time frame for each scenario should be established. Objectives should be clearly defined. Learners should receive relatively little information at the start of the scenario so that the details of the scenario are not exposed prior to the scenario being run. The participants have the opportunity to analyze the situation and ask appropriate questions to gather more data during the scenario. Debriefing may be the most powerful tool used following the simulation experience, allowing participants to reflect and analyze their performance critically, and adequate time should be allotted for this activity. Finally, the outcomes of a simulated experience can be those of knowledge attainment, improved skill performance, learner satisfaction, and increased self-confidence, among others. Utilizing the NLN/Jeffries Simulation Framework can maximize the amount of learning that occurs, and it is described in more detail throughout subsequent sections of this chapter.

In addition, INACSL developed standards of best practice for simulation that can guide scenario development (INACSL BOD, 2011b). The standards were developed with input from simulation experts and address the following topics: terminology, professional integrity, participant objectives, facilitation methods, simulation facilitator, the debriefing process, and evaluation of expected outcomes. Many of these standards address elements related to scenario development and will be referenced accordingly.

Kolb's Experiential Learning Theory, the NLN/Jeffries Simulation Framework, and the INACSL standards provide a sound basis to guide simulation research and training. A conceptual framework should be utilized when designing simulation experiences and research studies (Paige & Daley, 2009). The NLN/Jeffries Simulation Framework provides the details necessary for the simulation experience to be integrated using Kolb's framework and the INACSL standards, thus maximizing the potential for learning.

Scenario Development

Proper planning is paramount to successful implementation of a simulation scenario for education and training purposes. The scenario development process can be broken down into three distinct phases:

- Phase I: Planning and Pre-Briefing
- Phase II: Scenario Implementation
- Phase III: Debriefing and Evaluation

The constructs of the NLN/Jeffries Simulation Framework can provide guidance in each phase.

Phase I: Planning and Pre-Briefing

Often called the "pre-scenario" phase, the planning phase incorporates all the activities that need to occur before the scenario is actually implemented. The facilitator needs to allot enough time to plan the scenario accordingly, and also dedicate time to pilot test the scenario prior to participation by the learners. Because of the level of detail needed to plan a scenario, a standardized planning form or template can be helpful when designing a simulation scenario (Howard, Ross, Mitchell, & Nelson, 2010; Waxman, 2010). This tool helps ensure all aspects of scenario development are considered and that the simulation experience can be replicated in the future, thus providing a standardized educational experience for all learners.

Although templates developed at several organizations are publicly available, one example of a scenario planning template is included at the end of this chapter in Table 4.12. Each element of this particular template is discussed in detail. A note about the use of scenario templates: Although the example provided in this chapter follows the NLN/Jeffries Simulation Framework and is used by the Robert Morris University (RMU) Regional RISE Center, there are many standard templates available on the Internet. You can find examples on the NLN Simulation Innovation Resource Center (SIRC) and many simulation vendor websites. It is important to find the one that applies to your situation and that can be modified to meet your own organization needs.

Initial Elements

A scenario planning template should have clear identifiable information, such as the name of the simulation course and the simulation focus, listed first. To help make sure the most up-to-date evidence is being used for development and implementation, clinical content experts should review each scenario (Waxman, 2010). This ensures scenario content closely mirrors the best practices of the clinical setting—a goal for simulation experiences. References should be included in the template and updated as standards and guidelines for clinical treatment of conditions are revised. Although there is no evidence that establishes a specific time limit for each scenario, the time limit should be specified, in addition to indicating the time needed for the debriefing experience. This is helpful for planning and scheduling in the simulation center.

A trained facilitator should conduct simulation scenarios and use different types of facilitation methods to guide the learning activities for the participants to assist them in meeting the scenario objectives (INACSL BOD, 2011d, 2011e). The methods of facilitation should be based upon the level of the learner and determined prior to implementing the scenario.

There are three types of facilitation prompting: full, partial, and none (INACSL BOD, 2011d). For example, if the scenario is being used for evaluative purposes, the facilitator would refrain from prompting in order to maintain a controlled testing environment for the participant. Alternatively, full facilitator or maximal facilitator intervention might be needed for less experienced participants in order to guide them to attain the educational objectives. Although any level may be used, identifying the level prior to implementing the scenario is important to ensure standardized conditions for learning within the simulation room (INACSL BOD, 2011d; Waxman, 2010).

To maximize successful performance, the scenario should be developed at a level appropriate for the learner (INACSL BOD, 2011c). In other words, facilitators and educators must assess the level of the learner before developing the scenario in order to effectively build upon prior learning. Prerequisite knowledge should be addressed, and any pre-scenario learning activities for the participant should be identified. This enables participants to adequately prepare to meet the challenges of the scenario and intervene effectively with the patient. The scenario description is a one- to two-paragraph summary of the scenario and can help guide future facilitators in your institution when choosing scenarios. An example of the initial elements portions of a scenario planning template is shown in Table 4.3.

Table 4.3   Scenario Planning Template: Initial Elements

Course: NURS 4031 Transition to Professional Practice

Scenario Topic/Name: Acute Alcohol Withdrawal

References Used:

Boyd, M. A. (2008). *Psychiatric nursing: Contemporary practice* (4th ed.). Philadelphia, PA: Lippincott Williams & Wilkins.

Chabria, S. (2008). Inpatient management of alcohol withdrawal: A practical approach. *SIGNA VITAE 2008, 3*(1), 24-29.

Mayo-Smith, M., Beecher, L., Fischer, T., Gorelick, D., Guillaume, J., Hill, A.,…Melbourne, J. (2004). Management of acute alcohol withdrawal delirium. *Archives of Internal Medicine, 164*(13), 1405-1412.

Estimated Scenario Time: 30 minutes

Estimated Debriefing Time: 30 minutes

Instructors of the Course:

Simulation Facilitator:

Facilitation Prompting: Partial

Student level: Senior BSN Students

Prerequisite Knowledge/Pre-scenario Learning Activity:

1. Successful completion of NURS 4020 Advanced Management of the Adult II

2. Successful completion of NURS 4025 Nursing Care of Psychiatric Clients

3. Read Chapter 25 of Boyd, M. A. (2008). *Psychiatric nursing: Contemporary practice* (4th ed.). Philadelphia, PA: Lippincott Williams & Wilkins.

Scenario Description

Helene Bender is a 70-year-old female admitted to the hospital for acute gastritis. On the second day of admission, she becomes anxious, jittery, and begins to hallucinate. Her husband, George, brings these behaviors to the attention of the nurse. During the scenario, the nursing student will have the opportunity to provide nursing care for a client experiencing symptoms of acute alcohol withdrawal.

Development of Objectives

The development of educational objectives can address the three domains of learning: cognitive, affective, and psychomotor. Educational objectives should be written as clearly and concisely as possible. These objectives guide the experience and provide assistance in determining the outcomes from the experience. Objectives should be measureable and use verbs based upon Bloom's Taxonomy of Learning (Bloom, Krathwohl, Englehart, Furst, & Hill, 1956). Because simulation requires application of knowledge, the objectives should be written at Bloom's Taxonomy level of "Application" or higher. Participant objectives should address the domains of learning, be congruent with the program outcomes and learner level, incorporate evidence-based practice, and be achievable within the recommended time frame (INACSL BOD, 2011c). Childs and Sepples (2006) suggest using the nursing process to design scenario objectives. An example of objectives that align with the nursing process and address the three domains of learning is shown in Table 4.4.

Table 4.4   Scenario Planning Template: Objectives

Learning Objectives

Upon completion of this scenario, the participant will be able to:

1. Assess the client who is experiencing signs and symptoms of alcohol withdrawal (Psychomotor Domain).
   - Tremors, diaphoresis, hypertension, tachycardia, hallucinations
   - CAGE (Cutting down, Annoyance by criticism, Guilty feelings, Eye openers) Questionnaire—four clinical questions for detection of alcoholism (O'Brien, 2008)
   - The Clinical Institute Withdrawal Assessment (CIWA) for alcohol scale score

2. Utilize therapeutic communication while caring for the client who is experiencing signs and symptoms of alcohol withdrawal (Affective Domain).
   - Establish rapport with the patient and husband
   - Use open-ended questions, empathy, clarification, etc.

3. Utilize appropriate nursing diagnoses to plan care for the client who is experiencing signs and symptoms of alcohol withdrawal (Cognitive Domain)
   - Deficient knowledge
   - Ineffective individual coping
   - Ineffective health maintenance
   - Risk for injury

4. Intervene effectively for the client who is experiencing signs and symptoms of alcohol withdrawal (Psychomotor Domain).
   - Quiet, well-lit room with environmental cues
   - IVF: NSS at 100 mL/hour
   - Thiamine 100mg IV prior to giving any IV fluid containing glucose
   - Folate 1mg
   - Multivitamin with B12
   - CIWA Score: 18–Lorazepam 0.5-1 mg IV q 15 min prn withdrawal symptoms

5. Evaluate the effectiveness of interventions for the client who is experiencing signs and symptoms of alcohol withdrawal (Cognitive and Psychomotor Domains).
   - Vital signs
   - Level of agitation/anxiety
   - Sedation scale
   - Absence of seizure activity
   - Absence of falls
   - Absence of hallucinations

Table 4.4   Scenario Planning Template: Objectives   *(cont.)*
6. Reflect upon the learning that occurred during the simulation scenario (Affective Domain) <ul><li>Journal</li><li>Discussions during debriefing</li><li>Administer postsimulation evaluation survey upon conclusion of experience</li></ul>

Fidelity and Supplies

Adequate planning also includes matching the appropriate level of fidelity with the objectives, and this leads to the identification of necessary supplies. Situated Cognition Theory stresses the importance of learning within social situations and a social context (Lave & Wenger, 1991), which is why the experience in the simulation lab should closely mimic the reality of the clinical setting. Simulation facilitators should try to replicate the clinical setting as much as possible. Fidelity refers to the level of realism in the scenario (INACSL BOD, 2011a). Depending upon the objectives, it may be realistic to use a standardized patient rather than a high fidelity full-body simulator. For example, many scenarios with objectives primarily focusing on therapeutic communication may be best developed using standardized patient simulation techniques. However, a programmable mannequin might be best suited for objectives related to care of a patient experiencing a cardiac arrest due to the invasive nature of the psychomotor skills that need to be performed. Therefore, the type of mannequin, task trainer, or standardized patient should be predetermined using the scenario template (Jeffries, 2007; Waxman, 2010). In addition, any supplies related to the implementation of the scenario should be identified, such as medications, health care supplies, and those moulage materials meant to enhance the fidelity or realism of the environment (see Table 4.5). Detailed information on creating effective simulation environments can be found in Chapter 3.

Table 4.5	Scenario Planning Template: Supplies

Identify Type of Mannequin, Task Trainer, or Standardized Patient

High-fidelity mannequin for patient
Standardized patient or actor to play the role of spouse

Equipment Needed

	PPE gloves		Mask		Goggles
	Isolation Gown		Stethoscope		
X	SpO$_2$	X	ECG Monitor		Defibrillator/Pacer
	Lab Reports	X	MD Orders	X	Medical Records
	EMR— SLS#_____	X	iPod touch/PDA		Reference Material (book)
	Oxygen NC		Oxygen FM		Oxygen Non-Rebreather
X	Suction		Tracheostomy		Foley
X	IV in Place		IV Start Kit		Crash Cart
X	Glucometer		X-rays		12 Lead Type, i.e. NSR
	ECG Machine (12 lead)		Blood		Baby Bottle
	Ventilator		Vaginal Bleeding		Pediatric Supplies
	Diaphoresis		Bloody wound	X	ID/Allergy Band
	Nasal Secretions		Mouth Secretions		Urine
	Other:		Other:		Other:

Medications and IV Fluids: Dosage, Diluents Used, Methods of Delivery

1. NSS 1 liter bag

2. Thiamine 100mg IV

3. Folate IV

4. Multivitamin/B12 for IV bag

5. Lorazepam 1mg IV q15 minutes for symptoms of alcohol withdrawal—Monitor sedation scale

The Use of Standardized Patients

A standardized patient is a person trained to consistently portray a patient or other individual in a scripted scenario for the purposes of instruction, practice, or evaluation (INACSL BOD, 2011a, s6; Robinson-Smith, Bradley, & Meakim, 2009). Standardized patients are particularly valuable when implementing scenarios focusing upon development of communication skills. When using standardized patients in a simulation scenario, many experts suggest a detailed process to follow when developing the scripts, training the actor, and allowing the standardized patient to participate in the debriefing process (Bosek, Li, & Hicks, 2007).

Patient Information

Just as in the clinical setting, the simulated patient's history and physiologic vital signs play an important part in clinical decision-making. Therefore, when planning the scenario, it is helpful to provide as much information as possible about the patient's history to guide the participant in meeting the objectives. Although some simulation experts may prefer to fully develop a simulated patient's medical record in order to enhance realism, many suggest that just the important details be included in the patient's history in order to guide the decision-making process during the scenario. The facilitator must make a conscious decision to determine which elements of a simulated patient's history are necessary to include to enable the participant to meet the objectives of the scenario. The facilitator must also provide the initial simulator settings for the presenting patient condition. The settings are dependent upon the simulator chosen and the functions provided. An example of the patient information portion of a scenario template is shown in Table 4.6.

Table 4.6   Scenario Planning Template: Patient Information
Simulated Patient History

Name: Helene Bender

Age: 70

Weight: 140 lb.

Height: 5'6"

Gender: Female

Past Medical History: Gastritis

Medications: Pepcid 20mg qd

Allergies: Penicillin

MD: Dr. Molnar

Simulation Setting: Inpatient Unit—Medical Surgical Floor

Background of presenting illness: Mrs. Bender was admitted 2 days ago for severe epigastric distress and heme positive emesis while at home. Her hemoglobin/hematocrit (H/H) were 10.9 gr/dL / 35%. An endoscopy performed yesterday revealed gastritis, and she was placed on IV Protonix. She was admitted to monitor H/H and epigastric symptoms.

Initial Vital Signs for Mannequin	
Temperature	99.0° F
SpO$_2$	94%
Heart Rate	120
NIBP	150/90
ABP	
CVP/PA	
ECG Rhythm	Sinus Tachycardia
Sweating	Yes
Pulses normal, weak, or absent Pedal, dorsal, femoral, carotid, brachial	Pulses normal
Respirations shallow, labored, or normal	30—labored

Embedded Actors and Roles

An embedded actor or confederate is a person assigned a specific role within a simulation scenario. This individual is used to guide the participant to meet the objectives (INACSL BOD, 2011b). Embedded actors can play the roles of family members, neighbors, or health care providers. In order for the embedded actor to function effectively, the role must be described and a script for potential responses to questions provided (see Table 4.7). The embedded actor can ask critical-thinking questions, such as "How does that medication work?" or "Why is my loved one acting so funny?" Although it is impossible to anticipate every action of a scenario, the preparation of a script to provide answers to potential questions or situations can assist all involved in the simulation scenario (Waxman, 2010). Often, the facilitator plays the role of the patient via the simulator voice function and the voice of other members of the health care team via telephone. Because the facilitator might be playing different roles based upon the resources available in the simulation lab, a script is especially helpful to guide the conversations. Trained actors can be used to play the additional roles in the scenario, but this requires additional cost for payment of services. Therefore, many simulation facilities use retired health care professionals, students, or faculty members to play these roles. Keep in mind that the use of embedded actors works best when the participant does not know the real identity of the person, because this can create role confusion. For example, using a faculty member to play the role of an embedded actor may create additional performance anxiety for the student in a simulation scenario because of the fear of unintended evaluation or judgment on the part of the faculty member.

Table 4.7   Scenario Planning Template: Roles, Embedded Actors, and Scripts

Scenario Roles and Embedded Actors		
XX	Primary Nurse	
	Secondary Nurse	
XX	Family Member: George (husband)	
	Family Member	
XX	MD or NP	
	Ancillary Personnel (type)	

Table 4.7   Scenario Planning Template: Roles, Embedded Actors, and Scripts   *(cont.)*
Scripts
Helene Bender

Initially:

What is climbing on the wall?

Why am I shaking?

Where am I?

Where's my purse? I need to leave to go to the bingo.

Helene Bender's Responses to Alcohol Withdrawal Assessment Scoring Guidelines (CIWA-Ar)

Nausea/Vomiting: 0

Anxiety: 4

Paroxysmal Sweats: 1

Tactile Disturbance: 0

Visual Disturbance: 4

Tremors: 2

Agitation: 3

Orientation and Clouding of Sensorium: 2

Auditory Disturbances: 3

Headache: 1

Helene Bender's Responses to CAGE Questionnaire:

Following Lorazepam administration:

Helene: I'm feeling much more relaxed. What happened? Why am I in the hospital?

RN: *Helene, I am concerned about your drinking. When was your last drink and how much did you drink?*

Helene: Oh, honey, I'm not sure. I think I had a few drinks with my friends at lunch the day before I came in. Then my stomach started to bother me. I thought it was from the crab cakes.

RN: *Have you ever experienced something similar to this before?*

Helene: No.

RN: *C: Have you ever felt you should cut down on your drinking?*

Helene: Well, sometimes George tells me this, but he is so conservative and straight-laced. All my friends drink like I do. I have to have drinks with them when we go out to lunch.

George: I am concerned about her. I just see her drinking more and more.

RN: *A: Have people annoyed you by criticizing your drinking?*

Helene: George is always the first to get on my nerves about my drinking. And, sometimes, my friends agree with him. Do you believe it? What kinds of friends are these?

RN: *G: Have you ever felt bad or guilty about your drinking?*

Helene: Well…only when my friends make a comment. But I've tried to quit several times.

RN: *E: Have you ever had an eye-opener, a drink first thing in the morning to steady your nerves or get rid of a hangover?*

Helene: I usually have a shot of whiskey in my coffee. It calms my nerves in the morning and helps me to think clearly. Then, my luncheons usually start around 12 noon, so I will have whatever is on the menu…spiked, of course.

RN expected actions:

Educate on complications of alcohol abuse/dependence

Utilize therapeutic communication

Contact MD with repeat CIWA score

MD Script

"What are the vital signs and CIWA-Ar score for Mrs. Bender?"

"I'm giving you a verbal order for Lorazepam 0.5-1 mg IV q15 minutes X 4 prn symptoms of agitation and hallucinations. Give her Thiamine 100mg IV X 1. Also, start IVF NSS at 100mL/hour and add MVI, B12, Folate 100mg. Call me after she has received these medications. Perform the CAGE assessment when you can."

After CAGE Questionnaire:

"Okay. Continue the CIWA protocol and the Ativan order. I will order a psychiatric consultation to discuss substance abuse."

Table 4.7	Scenario Planning Template: Roles, Embedded Actors, and Scripts *(cont.)*
	George Bender (Helene's husband)

George has been the loving and enabling husband of Helene for 50 years. He is aware of her alcohol use, but has not made the determination that it is detrimental to her health. He is caring and very concerned and scared about her initial state of withdrawal. He asks many questions of the primary nurse and does everything within his power to calm Helene down, yet his over-attentiveness begins to contribute to the anxiety of the situation. He tries to respond to the questions asked of Helene during the CIWA and CAGE assessments. The primary nurse should reinforce that Helene should be the one responding to the questions.

During the course of the scenario, George can ask or state:

"Why is she acting so funny?"

"Why are you giving her those medications? Do they have any side effects?"

"She usually has a drink around noontime each day."

"She is quite a socialite and attends many functions during the week."

Patient Report

Just prior to scenario implementation, the simulation facilitator may read a patient report to provide the framework and background history for the impending scenario (see Table 4.8). This report sets the context for the participant and is the beginning of the scenario implementation phase. It is best to mirror the patient report to that which the learner may receive in the real-life clinical situation.

Table 4.8	Scenario Planning Template: Patient Report

Helene Bender is a 70-year-old female admitted with acute epigastric distress and heme-positive emesis (coffee ground) 2 days ago. Her admitting hemoglobin and hematocrit (H/H) was 10.9 gm/dL / 35%. She had an EGD yesterday that revealed a small gastric ulcer, and she was placed on IV Protonix. She continues to be monitored for her H/H and signs of epigastric pain. VS have been stable with trends: Temp 98.4°; BP 120/76; Pulse 90; RR 16. It is admission day 3 at 10 a.m. Her husband, George, is at the bedside today and has just called for the nurse. As you enter the room, George states that his wife is "acting funny."

Phase II: Planning for Scenario Implementation

The next step in the scenario development process is to design the actual scenario implementation phase. During this phase, the learners actually participate in the scenario and provide care for the simulated patient (which could be a mannequin or a standardized patient). However, this process should be documented in advance via the scenario template so that the simulator can be programmed and the response to interventions from participants can be anticipated. As with the planning phase, the objectives guide the simulator programming and implementation phase. Note in Table 4.9 how the objectives for the scenario are then placed in the planning template to serve as a further guide for the simulation facilitator.

When developing the scenario implementation phase, the facilitator tries to anticipate the participant's actions and plan accordingly. However, as previously mentioned, it is impossible to predict every action that might occur during a live simulation scenario. Therefore, the facilitator must maintain a high level of flexibility and use the proper facilitation methods in order to cue the participant toward meeting the objectives. Cueing is used during full and partial facilitation methods, but should be minimized during sessions where simulation is used for summative evaluation, as this could give one participant an unfair advantage over another. The implementation is outlined in Table 4.9.

Table 4.9   Scenario Planning Template: Implementation

Scenario Implementation Phase

Opening State and Objectives

Assess the client who is experiencing signs and symptoms of alcohol withdrawal
- Tremors, diaphoresis, hypertension, tachycardia, hallucinations
- CAGE Questionnaire
- CIWA Score

Utilize therapeutic communication while caring for the client who is experiencing signs and symptoms of alcohol withdrawal.
- Establish rapport with the patient
- Use of open-ended questions, empathy, clarification, etc.

Table 4.9   Scenario Planning Template: Implementation   *(cont.)*

Initial VS/Physiologic Parameters:

BP: 150/90; Temp: 99.0° F; Pulse 120; RR 30; Patient states: "I feel so nervous. Please get that crawly thing off the wall now! Where's my purse? I need to leave to go to the bingo."

Anticipated Interventions:

Upon entering the room, the student acting in the role of the primary nurse notes that Mrs. Bender's vital signs are abnormal and that she is having hallucinations. The student should explore the patient's alcohol use and should utilize the CIWA tool and calculate a score. During this period, the student must utilize therapeutic communication techniques to develop a therapeutic environment of trust.

Next State and Objectives

Intervene effectively for the client who is experiencing signs and symptoms of alcohol withdrawal.

- Quiet, well-lit room with environmental cues
- IV fluid: NSS at 100 mL/hour
- Thiamine 100mg IV prior to giving any glucose-containing IV fluid
- Folate 1mg
- Multivitamin with B12
- CIWA Score: 18–Lorazepam 0.5-1 mg IV q 15 min prn withdrawal symptoms

Vital Signs / Physiologic Parameters: No change

Anticipated Interventions:

After calculating the CIWA score (18), the student telephones the MD on call to obtain orders to treat the acute alcohol withdrawal symptoms. The MD orders IV fluid, Thiamine, Folate, Multivitamin, and Lorazepam as listed above. The student should provide a quiet, well-lit room and ensure that the environmental cues (clock, calendar) are within the patient's view in order to provide frequent reorientation. The student will then initiate the IV fluid and medication regimen, assuring appropriate nursing considerations and assessments are in place prior to initiation. The student must continue to provide therapeutic communication techniques with both the patient and the husband, George. The student provides brief and concise patient education regarding the signs and symptoms of acute alcohol withdrawal and the need for immediate intervention.

Final State and Objectives

Evaluate the effectiveness of interventions for the client who is experiencing signs and symptoms of alcohol withdrawal.

- VS
- Level of agitation/anxiety
- Sedation scale
- Absence of seizure activity
- Absence of falls
- Absence of hallucinations

Vital Signs/Physiologic Parameters:

Following Medication Administration: VS: 98.6°, 92, 14, 130/80; CIWA = 2

Patient's diaphoresis resolves and patient states, "I'm starting to feel sleepy. What just happened?"

Anticipated Interventions:

Following medication and IV fluid administration, the student nurse reevaluates the VS and patient's level of sedation. The student nurse must continue to educate both Helene and George about side effects of the medications, and the need for frequent reorientation and assessment for seizure activity. The student nurse also explores the patient's alcohol use and administers the CAGE questionnaire.

Phase III: Planning for Debriefing and Evaluation

The period immediately following the simulation experience is commonly referred to as the debriefing phase; it has been cited as one of the most important aspects of the scenario and is where the majority of the learning occurs (Decker, Gore, & Feken, 2011; Jeffries, 2007). During this phase, the participant reflects upon his or her performance, and the facilitator can pose evidence-based clinical questions to the participants to stimulate critical thinking. All simulation experiences should be followed by a debriefing sessions conducted by a trained individual in a psychologically safe environment (INACSL BOD, 2011f). Particular debriefing methods are discussed in Chapter 5. A debriefing session can begin with a set of standard questions to be used in all scenarios, followed by specific questions that pertain to the actual scenario and reflect evidence-based clinical practice. The questions should be developed in advance per the scenario planning template so that the learning experience is standardized for all participants (see Table 4.10).

Simulation can be used for summative or formative evaluation purposes, and the concept of simulation evaluation is discussed in detail in Chapter 6. However, when developing a scenario and using a template, facilitators and educators need to indicate if the participants will be evaluated, and what type of instrument will be used. The participants should also be informed if summative evaluation is planned, and reliable and valid instruments should be used (INACSL BOD, 2011g). In addition, learners should evaluate the simulation experience to ensure continuous quality improvement of the scenarios (Howard et al., 2010). Regardless, if the participants or the experience is to be evaluated, facilitators and educators should designate it on the scenario planning template in order to ensure standardization of the experience from beginning to end (see Table 4.10).

Table 4.10   Scenario Planning Template: Debriefing and Evaluation
Objective 6: Reflect upon the learning that occurred during the simulation scenario (Affective Domain)
<ul><li>Journal</li><li>Discussions during debriefing</li><li>Administer post-simulation evaluation survey upon conclusion of experience</li></ul>
Debriefing Questions
1. What worked well during the scenario? 2. If you had the opportunity to participate in the same scenario again, what would you do differently? 3. What was the primary problem? 4. What were your priorities of care? 5. Please provide the rationales for the interventions you performed. 6. How will you use this information in the real-life clinical setting?
Evidence-Based Clinical Questions
Question   What are the signs and symptoms of acute alcohol withdrawal (AWD)?
Answer   "Current diagnostic criteria for AWD include disturbance of consciousness, change in cognition or perceptual disturbance developing in a short period, and the emergence of symptoms during or shortly after withdrawal from heavy alcohol intake.... The classic clinical presentation of AWD includes hyperpyrexia, tachycardia, hypertension, and diaphoresis" (Mayo-Smith et al., 2004, p. 1405).

Rationale and Reference	"Neurotransmitters are thought to play an important role in the manifestations of alcohol withdrawal. The gamma amino butyric acid (GABA) receptor is down regulated and its neuronal activity decreased in alcohol withdrawal, resulting in hyperarousal. Elevated levels of norepinephrine are found in the cerebrospinal fluid of patients in alcohol withdrawal. This is believed to be due to a decrease in the alpha-2 receptor-mediated inhibition of presynaptic norepinephrine release. Dysfunctional serotonergic neurotransmission has been linked to an increased propensity toward ethanol addiction" (Chabria, 2008, p. 24).
Question	When do symptoms of AWD appear?
Answer	Clinical features of alcohol withdrawal syndrome can appear within hours of the last drink, but delirium typically does not develop until 2 to 3 days after cessation of drinking. Alcohol withdrawal delirium usually lasts 48 to 72 hours, but there have been case reports of much longer duration (Mayo-Smith et al., 2004).
Rationale and Reference	Alcohol is a CNS depressant. Upon abrupt cessation of alcohol intake, an individual may experience CNS activation causing the symptoms of alcohol withdrawal.
Question	What is the purpose for administering nutritional supplements (MVI, Folate, Thiamine) for the treatment of AWD? Why must the Thiamine be given prior to any glucose-containing fluids?
Answer	Patients with alcohol dependence are often Thiamine deficient. Thiamine deficiency is associated with Wernicke encephalopathy and Wernicke-Korsakoff syndrome.
Rationale and Reference	Thiamine administration has a low risk of adverse effects and can prevent the development of these conditions. In particular, Thiamine should be given before administration of IV fluids containing glucose, as the IV administration of glucose may precipitate acute Thiamine deficiency (Mayo-Smith et al., 2004). Multivitamins containing or supplemented with folate should be given routinely, and deficiencies of potassium, magnesium, glucose, and phosphate should be corrected as needed (Chabria, 2008).
Question	What is the purpose of the CAGE Questionnaire?
Answer	The CAGE Questionnaire is used to assess your patient's drinking pattern and determine your patient's dependence upon alcohol.

Table 4.10	Scenario Planning Template: Debriefing and Evaluation *(cont.)*
Rationale and Reference	The CAGE questionnaire was first published in *JAMA* 25 years ago and has been validated in numerous studies as a good, quick primary indicator of the need for further investigation of alcohol use (O'Brien, 2008).
Question	What is the CIWA-Ar tool and why is this used?
Answer	The CIWA-Ar scale (The Clinical Institute Withdrawal Assessment for alcohol scale) is used widely as a means to gauge the severity of alcohol withdrawal. The CIWA-Ar is a numeric scale with numbers being assigned to severity of symptoms such as anxiety, nausea, headache, and several other parameters.
Rationale and Reference	The CIWA-Ar score is used to guide treatment parameters with benzodiazapines (Chabria, 2008).
Question	What are common side effects of benzodiazepines and why are they used for treatment of alcohol withdrawal?
Answer	Common side effects include an exacerbation of the therapeutic effects of sedation and somnolence. Benzodiazepines are most commonly used and recommended by addiction specialists because of a favorable therapeutic/toxic effect index.
Rationale and Reference	The initial therapeutic goal in patients with AWD is control of agitation, the symptom that should trigger use of the medication regimens described in this guideline. Rapid and adequate control of agitation reduces the incidence of clinically important adverse events. Sedative hypnotic drugs are recommended as the primary agents for managing AWD. Current evidence does not clearly indicate that a specific sedative-hypnotic agent is superior to others or that switching from one to another is helpful. Careful monitoring of sedation scale is key following administration (Mayo-Smith et al., 2004).

Pilot Testing and Periodic Review

Now that the scenario has been developed, it is important to pilot test it prior to actually implementing it with the learners. Do not underestimate the importance of this practice session and allow an adequate amount of time. The simulation center staff can play the different roles in the scenario to determine if all of the equipment needed is listed, if the objectives are clear, and if any other changes need to be made prior to introducing the experience with the learners. Just as in the real-life clinical setting, scenarios need to be updated periodically as practice standards change, with most simulation experts suggesting at least an annual review of all scenario content within your facility. The scenario review process can be one part of the quality improvement plan for your simulation program or facility.

Conclusion

Developing an effective, evidence-based scenario takes significant planning on the part of the simulation facilitator, and adequate time should be allotted to this activity. Proper planning ensures that all of the details related to the scenario have been addressed and can assist the facilitator in a smooth scenario implementation for learners. In response to the lack of time and limited resources many simulation facilitators have, many corporations and organizations have developed preplanned scenarios for purchase (see Table 4.11). Although these scenarios can save simulation educators time and resources, you need to ensure that the preplanned scenario objectives do indeed correlate with your own particular program objectives and the educational level of the participant. Ultimately, with adequate time, planning, clinical evidence, practice, and mentoring, the most novice simulation educators can develop the skills necessary to develop and implement a successful simulation scenario.

Table 4.11   Preplanned Simulation Scenarios for Purchase

Program	Developer
Simulation Learning System	Elsevier Publishing Company
Program for Nursing Curriculum Integration	CAE Healthcare
Real Nursing Simulations	Pearson Publishing Company
Lippincott's Clinical Simulations	Lippincott Publishing Company
Simulation Innovation Resource Center	National League for Nursing
Nursing Scenarios	Laerdal Corporation and NLN

Table 4.12   Complete Acute Alcohol Withdrawal Scenario

Developed by Kameg, K., Howard, V., Perozzi, K., & Englert, N.
Robert Morris University
School of Nursing & Health Sciences
Template adapted from J. Sarasnick, MSN, RN

Course: NURS 4031 Transition to Professional Practice

Scenario Topic/Name: Acute Alcohol Withdrawal

References Used:

Boyd, M. A. (2008). *Psychiatric nursing: Contemporary practice* (4th ed.). Philadelphia, PA: Lippincott Williams & Wilkins.

Chabria, S. (2008). Inpatient management of alcohol withdrawal: A practical approach. *SIGNA VITAE 2008, 3*(1), 24-29.

Mayo-Smith, M., Beecher, L., Fischer, T., Gorelick, D., Guillaume, J., Hill, A.,... Melbourne, J. (2004). Management of acute alcohol withdrawal delirium. *Archives of Internal Medicine, 164*(13), 1405-1412.

Estimated Scenario Time: 30 minutes

Estimated Debriefing Time: 30 minutes

Instructors of the Course:

Simulation Facilitator:

Facilitation Prompting: Partial

Student level: Senior BSN Students

Prerequisite Knowledge/Pre-scenario Learning Activity:

1. Successful completion of NURS 4020 Advanced Management of the Adult II

2. Successful completion of NURS 4025 Nursing Care of Psychiatric Clients

3. Read Chapter 25 of Boyd, M. A. (2008). *Psychiatric nursing: Contemporary practice* (4th ed.). Philadelphia, PA: Lippincott Williams & Wilkins.

Scenario Description

Helene is a 70-year-old female admitted to the hospital for acute gastritis. On the second day of admission, she becomes anxious, jittery, and begins to hallucinate. Her husband, George, brings these behaviors to the attention of the nurse. During the scenario, the nursing student will have the opportunity to provide nursing care for a client experiencing symptoms of acute alcohol withdrawal.

Learning Objectives

Upon completion of this scenario, the participant will be able to:

1. Assess the client who is experiencing signs and symptoms of alcohol withdrawal (Psychomotor Domain).
    - Tremors, diaphoresis, hypertension, tachycardia, hallucinations
    - CAGE (Cutting down, Annoyance by criticism, Guilty feelings, Eye openers) Questionnaire—four clinical questions for detection of alcoholism (O'Brien, 2008)
    - The Clinical Institute Withdrawal Assessment (CIWA) for alcohol scale score

2. Utilize therapeutic communication while caring for the client who is experiencing signs and symptoms of alcohol withdrawal (Affective Domain).
    - Establish rapport with the patient and husband
    - Use open-ended questions, empathy, clarification, etc.

3. Utilize appropriate Nursing Diagnoses to plan care for the client who is experiencing signs and symptoms of alcohol withdrawal (Cognitive Domain).
    - Deficient knowledge
    - Ineffective individual coping
    - Ineffective health maintenance
    - Risk for injury

4. Intervene effectively for the client who is experiencing signs and symptoms of alcohol withdrawal (Psychomotor Domain).
    - Quiet, well-lit room with environmental cues
    - IVF: NSS at 100 ml/hour
    - Thiamine 100mg IV prior to giving any glucose-containing IVF
    - Folate 1mg
    - Multivitamin with B-12
    - CIWA Score: 18–Lorazepam 0.5-1 mg IV q 15 min prn withdrawal symptoms

5. Evaluate the effectiveness of interventions for the client who is experiencing signs and symptoms of alcohol withdrawal (Cognitive and Psychomotor Domains).
    - Vital signs
    - Level of agitation/anxiety
    - Sedation scale
    - Absence of seizure activity
    - Absence of falls
    - Absence of hallucinations

Table 4.12   Complete Acute Alcohol Withdrawal Scenario   *(cont.)*

6. Reflect upon the learning that occurred during the simulation scenario (Affective Domain).

- Journal
- Discussions during debriefing
- Administer post-simulation evaluation survey upon conclusion of experience

Identify Type of Mannequin, Task Trainer, or Standardized Patient

High-fidelity mannequin for patient
Standardized patient or actor to play the role of spouse

Equipment Needed

	PPE gloves		Mask		Goggles
	Isolation Gown		Stethoscope		
X	SpO$_2$	X	ECG Monitor		Defibrillator/Pacer
	Lab Reports	X	MD Orders	X	Medical Records
	EMR—SLS#_____	X	iPod touch/PDA		Reference Material (book)
	Oxygen NC		Oxygen FM		Oxygen Non-Rebreather
X	Suction		Tracheostomy		Foley
X	IV in Place		IV Start Kit		Crash Cart
X	Glucometer		X-rays		12 Lead Type, i.e. NSR
	ECG Machine (12 lead)		Blood		Baby Bottle
	Ventilator		Vaginal Bleeding		Pediatric Supplies
	Diaphoresis		Bloody wound	X	ID/Allergy Band
	Nasal Secretions		Mouth Secretions		Urine
	Other:		Other:		Other:

Medications and IV Fluids: Dosage, Diluents Used, Methods of Delivery

1. NSS 1 liter bag
2. Thiamine 100mg IV
3. Folate IV
4. Multivitamin/B12 for IV bag
5. Lorazepam 1mg IV q15 minutes for symptoms of Alcohol Withdrawal—Monitor Sedation Scale

Simulated Patient History

Name:	Helene Bender
Age:	70
Weight:	140 lb.
Height:	5'6"
Gender:	Female
Past Medical History:	Gastritis
Medications:	Pepcid 20mg qd
Allergies:	PCN
MD:	Dr. Molnar

Simulation Setting: Inpatient Unit—Medical Surgical Floor

Background of presenting illness: Mrs. Bender was admitted 2 days ago for severe epigastric distress and heme positive emesis while at home. Her hemoglobin/hematocrit (H/H) were 10.9 gr/dL / 35%. An endoscopy performed yesterday revealed gastritis and she was placed on IV Protonix. She was admitted to monitor H/H and epigastric symptoms.

Initial Vital Signs for Mannequin

Temperature	99.0 F
SpO$_2$	94%
Heart Rate	120
NIBP	150/90
ABP	
CVP/PA	
ECG Rhythm	Sinus Tachycardia
Sweating	Yes
Pulses normal, weak, or absent.	Pulses normal
Pedal, dorsal, femoral, carotid, brachial	
Respirations shallow, labored, or normal	30—labored

Table 4.12 Complete Acute Alcohol Withdrawal Scenario *(cont.)*		
Scenario Roles and Embedded Actors		
XX	Primary Nurse	
	Secondary Nurse	
XX	Family Member: George (husband)	
	Family Member	
XX	MD or NP	
	Ancillary Personnel (type)	

Scripts
Helene Bender

Initially:

What is climbing on the wall?

Why am I shaking?

Where am I?

Where's my purse? I need to leave to go to the bingo.

Helene Bender's Responses to Alcohol Withdrawal Assessment Scoring Guidelines (CIWA-Ar)

Nausea/Vomiting: 0

Anxiety: 4

Paroxysmal Sweats: 1

Tactile Disturbance: 0

Visual Disturbance: 4

Tremors: 2

Agitation: 3

Orientation and Clouding of Sensorium: 2

Auditory Disturbances: 3

Headache: 1

Helene Bender's Responses to CAGE Questionnaire:

Following Lorazepam administration:

Helene: I'm feeling much more relaxed. What happened? Why am I in the hospital?

RN: *Helene, I am concerned about your drinking. When was your last drink and how much did you drink?*

Helene: Oh, honey, I'm not sure. I think I had a few drinks with my friends at lunch the day before I came in. Then my stomach started to bother me. I thought it was from the crab cakes.

RN: *Have you ever experienced something similar to this before?*

Helene: No.

RN*: C: Have you ever felt you should cut down on your drinking?*

Helene: Well, sometimes George tells me this, but he is so conservative and straight-laced. All my friends drink like I do. I have to have drinks with them when we go out to lunch.

George: I am concerned about her. I just see her drinking more and more.

RN: *A: Have people annoyed you by criticizing your drinking?*

Helene: George is always the first to get on my nerves about my drinking. And, sometimes, my friends agree with him. Do you believe it? What kinds of friends are these?

RN: *G: Have you ever felt bad or guilty about your drinking?*

Helene: Well…only when my friends make a comment. But I've tried to quit several times.

RN: *E: Have you ever had an eye-opener, a drink first thing in the morning to steady your nerves or get rid of a hangover?*

Helene: I usually have a shot of whiskey in my coffee. It calms my nerves in the morning and helps me to think clearly. Then, my luncheons usually start around 12 noon, so I will have whatever is on the menu…spiked, of course.

RN expected actions:

Educate on complications of alcohol abuse/dependence

Utilize therapeutic communication

Contact MD with repeat CIWA score

MD Script

"What are the vital signs and CIWA-Ar score for Mrs. Bender?"

"I'm giving you a verbal order for Lorazepam 0.5-1 mg IV q15 minutes X 4 prn symptoms of agitation and hallucinations. Give her Thiamine 100mg IV X 1. Also, start IVF NSS at 100mL/hour and add MVI, B12, Folate 100mg. Call me after she has received these medications. Perform the CAGE assessment when you can."

Table 4.12   Complete Acute Alcohol Withdrawal Scenario   *(cont.)*

After CAGE Questionnaire:

"Okay. Continue the CIWA protocol and the Ativan order. I will order a psychiatric consultation to discuss substance abuse."

George Bender (Helene's husband)

George has been the loving and enabling husband of Helene for 50 years. He is aware of her alcohol use, but has not made the determination that it is detrimental to her health. He is caring and very concerned and scared about her initial state of withdrawal. He asks many questions of the primary nurse and does everything within his power to calm Helene down, yet his over-attentiveness begins to contribute to the anxiety of the situation. He tries to respond to the questions asked of Helene during the CIWA and CAGE assessments. The primary nurse should reinforce that Helene should be the one responding to the questions.

During the course of the scenario, George can ask or state:

"Why is she acting so funny?"

"Why are you giving her those medications? Do they have any side effects?"

"She usually has a drink around noontime each day."

"She is quite a socialite and attends many functions during the week."

RN Report

Mrs. Bender is a 70-year-old female admitted with acute epigastric distress and Heme positive emesis (coffee ground) 2 days ago. Her admitting hemoglobin and hematocrit (H/H) was 10.9 gm/dL / 35%. She had an EGD yesterday that revealed a small gastric ulcer and she was placed on IV Protonix. She continues to be monitored for her H/H and signs of epigastric pain. VS have been stable with trends: Temp 98.4°; BP 120/76; Pulse 90; RR 16. It is admission day 3 at 10 a.m. Her husband, George, is at the bedside today and has just called for the nurse. As you enter the room, George states that his wife is "acting funny."

Scenario Implementation Phase

Opening State and Objectives:

Assess the client who is experiencing signs and symptoms of alcohol withdrawal.

- Tremors, diaphoresis, hypertension, tachycardia, hallucinations
- CAGE Questionnaire
- CIWA Score

Utilize therapeutic communication while caring for the client who is experiencing signs and symptoms of alcohol withdrawal.

- Establish rapport with the patient
- Use of open-ended questions, empathy, clarification, etc.

Initial VS/Physiologic Parameters:

BP: 150/90; Temp: 99.0 F; Pulse 120; RR 30; Patient states: "I feel so nervous. Please get that crawly thing off the wall now! Where's my purse? I need to leave to go to the bingo."

Anticipated Interventions:

Upon entering the room, the student acting in the role of the primary nurse notes that Mrs. Bender's vital signs are abnormal and that she is having hallucinations. The student should explore the patient's alcohol use and should utilize the CIWA tool and calculate a score. During this period, the student must utilize therapeutic communication techniques to develop a therapeutic environment of trust.

Next State and Objectives

Intervene effectively for the client who is experiencing signs and symptoms of alcohol withdrawal.

- Quiet, well-lit room with environmental cues
- IVF: NSS at 100 mL/hour
- Thiamine 100mg IV prior to giving any glucose-containing IV fluid
- Folate 1mg
- Multivitamin with B-12
- CIWA Score: 18–Lorazepam 0.5-1 mg IV q 15 min prn withdrawal symptoms

Vital Signs/Physiologic Parameters: No change

Anticipated Interventions:

After calculating the CIWA score (18), the student telephones the MD on call to obtain orders to treat the acute alcohol withdrawal symptoms. The MD orders IVF, Thiamine, Folate, Multivitamin, and Lorazepam as listed above. The student should provide a quiet, well-lit

Table 4.12   Complete Acute Alcohol Withdrawal Scenario   *(cont.)*

room and ensure that the environmental cues (clock, calendar) are within the patient's view in order to provide frequent reorientation. The student will then initiate the IVF and medication regimen, assuring appropriate nursing considerations and assessments are in place prior to initiation. The student must continue to provide therapeutic communication techniques with both the patient and the husband, George. The student nurse provides brief and concise patient education regarding the signs and symptoms of acute alcohol withdrawal, and the need for immediate intervention.

Final State and Objectives

Evaluate the effectiveness of interventions for the client who is experiencing signs and symptoms of alcohol withdrawal.

- VS
- Level of agitation/anxiety
- Sedation scale
- Absence of seizure activity
- Absence of falls
- Absence of hallucinations

Vital Signs/Physiologic Parameters:

Following Medication Administration: VS: 98.6, 92, 14, 130/80; CIWA = 2

Patient's diaphoresis resolves and patient states, "I'm starting to feel sleepy. What just happened?"

Anticipated Interventions:

Following medication and IVF administration, the student nurse reevaluates the VS and patient's level of sedation. The student nurse must continue to educate both Helene and George about side effects of the medications, and the need for frequent reorientation and assessment for seizure activity. The student nurse also explores the patient's alcohol use and administers the CAGE questionnaire.

Objective 6: Reflect upon the learning that occurred during the simulation scenario (Affective Domain)

- Journal
- Discussions during debriefing
- Administer post-simulation evaluation survey upon conclusion of experience

1. What worked well during the scenario?
2. If you had the opportunity to participate in the same scenario again, what would you do differently?
3. What was the primary problem?
4. What were your priorities of care?
5. Please provide the rationales for the interventions you performed.
6. How will you use this information in the real-life clinical setting?

Question	What are the signs and symptoms of acute alcohol withdrawal (AWD)?
Answer	"Current diagnostic criteria for AWD include disturbance of consciousness, change in cognition or perceptual disturbance developing in a short period, and the emergence of symptoms during or shortly after withdrawal from heavy alcohol intake…. The classic clinical presentation of AWD includes hyperpyrexia, tachycardia, hypertension, and diaphoresis" (Mayo-Smith et al., 2004 p. 1405).
Rationale and Reference	"Neurotransmitters are thought to play an important role in the manifestations of alcohol withdrawal. The gamma amino butyric acid (GABA) receptor is down regulated and its neuronal activity decreased in alcohol withdrawal, resulting in hyperarousal. Elevated levels of norepinephrine are found in the cerebrospinal fluid of patients in alcohol withdrawal. This is believed to be due to a decrease in the alpha-2 receptor-mediated inhibition of presynaptic norepinephrine release. Dysfunctional serotonergic neurotransmission has been linked to an increased propensity toward ethanol addiction" (Chabria, S., 2008, p. 24).
Question	When do symptoms of AWD appear?
Answer	Clinical features of alcohol withdrawal syndrome can appear within hours of the last drink, but delirium typically does not develop until 2 to 3 days after cessation of drinking. Alcohol withdrawal delirium usually lasts 48 to 72 hours, but there have been case reports of much longer duration (Mayo-Smith et al., 2004).
Rationale and Reference	Alcohol is a CNS depressant. Upon abrupt cessation of alcohol intake, an individual may experience CNS activation causing the symptoms of alcohol withdrawal.

Table 4.12	Complete Acute Alcohol Withdrawal Scenario *(cont.)*
Question	What is the purpose for administering nutritional supplements (MVI, Folate, Thiamine) for the treatment of AWD? Why must the Thiamine be given prior to any glucose-containing fluids?
Answer	Patients with alcohol dependence are often Thiamine deficient. Thiamine deficiency is associated with Wernicke encephalopathy and Wernicke-Korsakoff syndrome.
Rationale and Reference	Thiamine administration has a low risk of adverse effects and can prevent the development of these conditions. In particular, Thiamine should be given before administration of IV fluids containing glucose, as the IV administration of glucose may precipitate acute Thiamine deficiency (Mayo-Smith et al., 2004).
Question	What is the purpose of the CAGE Questionnaire?
Answer	The CAGE Questionnaire is used to assess your patient's drinking pattern and determine your patient's dependence upon alcohol.
Rationale and Reference	The CAGE questionnaire was first published in *JAMA* 25 years ago and has been validated in numerous studies as a good, quick primary indicator of the need for further investigation of alcohol use (O'Brien, 2008).
Question	What is the CIWA-Ar tool and why is this used?
Answer	The CIWA-Ar scale (The Clinical Institute Withdrawal Assessment for alcohol scale) is used widely as a means to gauge the severity of alcohol withdrawal. The CIWA-Ar is a numeric scale with numbers being assigned to severity of symptoms such as anxiety, nausea, headache, and several other parameters.
Rationale and Reference	The CIWA-Ar score is used to guide treatment parameters with benzodiazapines (Chabria, 2008).
Question	What are common side effects of benzodiazepines and why are they used for treatment of alcohol withdrawal?
Answer	Common side effects include an exacerbation of the therapeutic effects of sedation and somnolence. Benzodiazepines are most commonly used and recommended by addiction specialists because of a favorable therapeutic/toxic effect index.

Rationale and Reference	The initial therapeutic goal in patients with AWD is control of agitation, the symptom that should trigger use of the medication regimens described in this guideline. Rapid and adequate control of agitation reduces the incidence of clinically important adverse events. Sedative hypnotic drugs are recommended as the primary agents for managing AWD. Current evidence does not clearly indicate that a specific sedative-hypnotic agent is superior to others or that switching from one to another is helpful. Careful monitoring of sedation scale is key following administration (Mayo-Smith, M. et al., 2004).

References

Benner, P. (1984). *From novice to expert: Excellence and power in clinical nursing practice.* Menlo Park, CA: Addison-Wesley.

Bloom, B. S., Krathwohl, D. R., Englehart, M., Furst, E., & Hill, W. (1956). *Taxonomy of educational objectives: The classification of educational goals, by a Committee of College and University Examiners.* Handbook I: Cognitive domain. New York, NY: Longmans Green.

Bosek, M., Li, S., & Hicks, F. D. (2007). Working with standardized patients: A primer. *International Journal of Nursing Education Scholarship, 4*(1), Article 16 Epub.

Boyd, M. A. (2008). *Psychiatric nursing: Contemporary practice* (4th ed.). Philadelphia, PA: Lippincott Williams & Wilkins.

Chabila, 3. (2008). Inpatient management of alcohol withdrawal. A practical approach. *SIGNA VITAE 2008, 3*(1), 24-29.

Childs, J. C., & Sepples, S. (2006). Clinical teaching by simulation: Lessons learned from a complex patient care scenario. *Nursing Education Perspectives, 27*(3), 154-158.

Clapper, T. C. (2010). Beyond Knowles: What those conducting simulation need to know about adult learning theory. *Clinical Simulation in Nursing, 6*(1), e7-e14.

Decker, S., Gore, T., & Feken, C. (2011). Simulation. In T. Bristol, & J. Zerwehk (Eds.), *Essentials of e-learning for nurse educators* (pp.277-294). Philadelphia, PA: F. A. Davis.

Dewey, J. (1938). *Experience and Education.* New York, NY: Macmillan.

Howard, V. M., Englert, N., Kameg, K., & Perozzi, K. (2011). Integration of simulation across the undergraduate curriculum: Student and faculty perspectives. *Clinical Simulation in Nursing, 7*(1), e1-e10.

Howard, V., Ross, C., Mitchell, A. M., & Nelson, G. M. (2010). Human patient simulators and interactive case studies—A comparative analysis of learning outcomes and student perceptions. *Computers, Informatics, and Nursing (CIN), 28*(1), 42-48.

International Nursing Association for Clinical Simulation and Learning (INASCL) Board of Directors (BOD) (2011a). Standards of best practice: Simulation. Standard I: Terminology. *Clinical Simulation in Nursing, 7*(4S), s3-s7. doi:10.1016/j.ecns.2011.05.005 Retrieved from http://download.journals.elsevierhealth.com/pdfs/journals/1876-1399/PIIS1876139911000612.pdf

International Nursing Association for Clinical Simulation and Learning (INASCL) Board of Directors (BOD) (2011b). Standards of best practice: Simulation. Introduction. *Clinical Simulation in Nursing, 7*(4S), s1. doi: 10.1016/j.ccns.2011.05.003 Retrieved from download.journals.elsevierhealth.com/pdfs/journals/1876-1399/PIIS1876139911000594.pdf

International Nursing Association for Clinical Simulation and Learning (INASCL) Board of Directors (BOD) (2011c). Standards of best practice: Simulation. Standard III: Participant objectives. *Clinical Simulation in Nursing, 7*(4S), s10-s11. doi:10.1016/j.ecns.2011.05.007 Retrieved from http://download.journals.elsevierhealth.com/pdfs/journals/1876-1399/PIIS1876139911000636.pdf

International Nursing Association for Clinical Simulation and Learning (INASCL) Board of Directors (BOD) (2011d). Standards of best practice: Simulation. Standard IV: Facilitation methods. *Clinical Simulation in Nursing, 7*(4S), s12-s13. doi:10.1016/j.ecns.2011.05.008 Retrieved from http://download.journals.elsevierhealth.com/pdfs/journals/1876-1399/PIIS1876139911000648.pdf

International Nursing Association for Clinical Simulation and Learning (INASCL) Board of Directors (BOD) (2011e). Standards of best practice: Simulation. Standard V: Simulation facilitator. *Clinical Simulation in Nursing, 7*(4S), s14-s15. doi:10.1016/j.ecns.2011.05.009 Retrieved from http://download.journals.elsevierhealth.com/pdfs/journals/1876-1399/PIIS187613991100065X.pdf

International Nursing Association for Clinical Simulation and Learning (INASCL) Board of Directors (BOD) (2011f). Standards of best practice: Simulation. Standard VI: The debriefing process. *Clinical Simulation in Nursing, 7*(4S), s16-s17. doi:10.1016/j.ecns.2011.05.010 Retrieved from http://download.journals.elsevierhealth.com/pdfs/journals/1876-1399/PIIS1876139911000661.pdf

International Nursing Association for Clinical Simulation and Learning (INASCL) Board of Directors (BOD) (2011g). Standards of best practice: Simulation. Standard VII: Evaluation of expected outcomes. *Clinical Simulation in Nursing, 7*(4S), s18-s19. doi:10.1016/j.ecns.2011.05.011 Retrieved from http://download.journals.elsevierhealth.com/pdfs/journals/1876-1399/PIIS1876139911000673.pdf

Jeffries, P. R. (2007). *Simulations in nursing education: From conceptualization to evaluation.* New York, New York: The National League for Nursing.

Kaakinen, J., & Arwood, E. (2009). Systematic review of nursing simulation literature for use of learning theory. *International Journal of Nursing Education Scholarship, 6*(1), 1-20.

Knowles, M. S. (1984). *The adult learner: A neglected species* (3rd ed.). Houston, TX: Gulf.

Kolb, D. A. (1984). *Experiential learning.* Englewood Cliffs, NJF: Prentice Hall.

Lasater, K. (2007). High-fidelity simulation and the development of clinical judgment: Students' experience. *Journal of Nursing Education, 46*(6), 269-276.

Lave, J., & Wenger, E. (1991). *Situated learning: Legitimate peripheral participation.* Cambridge: Cambridge University Press.

Mayo-Smith, M., Beecher, L., Fischer, T., Gorelick, D., Guillaume, J., Hill, A.,…Melbourne, J. (2004). Management of acute alcohol withdrawal delirium. *Archives of Internal Medicine, 164*(13), 1405-1412.

O'Brien, C. P. (2008). The CAGE questionnaire for detection of alcoholism: A remarkably useful but simple tool. *Journal of the American Medical Association, 300*(17), 2054-2056.

Paige, J. B., & Daley, B. J. (2009). Situated cognition: A learning framework to support and guide high-fidelity simulation. *Clinical Simulation in Nursing, 5*(3), e97-e103.

Robinson-Smith, G., Bradley, P., & Meakim, C. (2009). Evaluating the use of standardized patients in undergraduate psychiatric nursing experiences. *Clinical Simulation in Nursing, 5*(6), e203-e211.

Waxman, K. T. (2010). The development of evidence-based clinical simulation scenarios: Guidelines for nurse educators. *Journal of Nursing Education, 49*(1), 29-35.

"Without reflection, we go blindly on our way, creating more unintended consequences, and failing to achieve anything useful."

–Margaret J. Wheatley

Debriefing and Reflective Practice

Shelly J. Reed, DNP, FNP, CPNP

Reflection upon experiences is a powerful way to promote learning. For health care providers, reflecting, critically reviewing, and trying to make sense of personal experiences helps them to learn and develop new insights and perspectives about their practice. Reflection is an active process. During reflection, cognitive thought processes come into play, helping make a plan for improvement with future similar experiences. Thus, through reflection, learning occurs, as well as changes in one's approach to practice (Ausselin, 2011; Bulman, Lathlean, & Gobbi, 2011).

Kolb's Experiential Learning Theory explains learning as a continuous process, where reflection on experiences creates learning, changing how a person thinks and behaves (Kolb, 1984). Kolb's learning cycle explains the learning process as continuous learning in four related parts: reflective observation, abstract conceptualization, active experimentation, and concrete experience (DeCoux, 1990; Fanning & Gaba, 2007; Kolb, 1984; Sewchuk, 2005). Experiential learning has been used as a framework in many educational areas to guide and define the learning experience. Experiential learning is useful in areas in which theory and practice merge. Experiential methods are commonly accepted in health professions education, although limited research exists exploring the nature and extent of use (Brackenreg, 2004).

OBJECTIVES

- Understand the importance of the reflective practice of debriefing as a part of simulation.
- Identify debriefing techniques that promote participant learning.
- Differentiate among various debriefing methods and identify situations where each might be implemented.
- Gain a basic understanding of available evaluation tools for debriefing.

Simulation and debriefing fit well with Kolb's Experiential Learning Theory. Simulation is usually preceded by learner preparation, including familiarization of the learner with objectives for the simulation, the scenario, and related content. This fits into the abstract conceptualization, or thinking, component of Kolb's theory. The simulation itself provides the active experimentation, or doing, component of the learning cycle, and debriefing provides the concrete experience, or reflection, component of Kolb's learning cycle. The reflective observation component occurs through observation during both simulation and debriefing. Experiential learning such as simulation hinges on the solidification of learning (concrete learning) through reflection (Kolb, 1984; Reed, 2009).

Debriefing has been described as the most important feature of simulation-based education (Dreifuerst, 2009; Fanning & Gaba, 2007; Grant, Moss, Epps & Watts, 2010; Mayville, 2011; Shinnick, Woo, Horwich, & Steadman, 2011). During debriefing, session participants are guided by a facilitator through reflection on what occurred during the simulation. The goal of reflection is to allow participants to incorporate prior learning with learning that occurred during the simulation for the purpose of transferring learning to future situations (Neill & Wotton, 2011; International Nursing Association for Clinical Simulation and Learning [INACSL] Board of Directors [BOD], 2011a).

In an effective debriefing, session participants reflect on their simulation performance, clarify their thought processes and actions, explore their emotions, and question themselves, others, and/or the facilitator. The outcomes for debriefing developed by INACSL are shown in the accompanying sidebar. Constructive, nonjudgmental feedback is provided by the facilitator and from other debriefing group participants (INACSL BOD, 2011a; Mayville, 2011). Debriefing is most successful when it is structured, providing a reference point for the participants to frame their own learning. In nursing, a common structure to use is the nursing process. Dreifuerst (2009) suggests that integration of the nursing process into debriefing is helpful for learners to be able to apply their learning in future nursing experiences.

> ## International Nursing Association for Clinical Simulation and Learning (INACSL) Debriefing Outcomes
>
> The integration of the process of debriefing into simulation:
>
> - Enhances learning
> - Heightens self-confidence for the learner
> - Increases understanding
> - Promotes knowledge transfer
> - Identifies best practices
> - Promotes safe, quality patient care
> - Promotes lifelong learning
>
> *Source: INACSL BOD, 2011b*

Setting the Stage for Debriefing

Effective debriefing requires preparation. Educators and facilitators need to have an understanding of the learning objectives as well as control of the environment and the process.

Learning Objectives

A well-planned simulation should include learning objectives that cover the simulation and subsequent debriefing (Arafeh, Hansen, & Nichols, 2010). The objectives are used to guide the processes and provide a template of what will be covered during the simulation and debriefing. For example, objectives for debriefing a team training simulation might differ from debriefing an instructional simulation for individual learners. An appropriate objective for team training simulation would be to improve team performance; therefore during debriefing, facilitators would want to examine the performance of the team.

Examples of team training debriefing questions include the following:

- "I noticed that you seemed frustrated when Tim did not have the medication ready when you put your hand out for it. What might help to improve that process?"

- "There are five team members in this code, yet no one thought to check to see if the oxygen had been turned on. How do you think this could have gone better?"

In contrast, during an instructional simulation, an appropriate objective may be to learn skills to care for patients with a particular diagnosis, without focusing on team care.

Examples of individual debriefing questions include the following:

- "At what point did you think it would be best to ask for additional help?"
- "What symptoms led you to notice that the baby was becoming more ill?"

Learning objectives should also vary based on the learning level of the participants. For example, the objectives for a simulation involving beginning nursing students should differ from the objectives for the same students when they have had more advanced clinical experiences and are familiar with learning in a simulation environment. In the same way, simulations for experienced health care providers should have different objectives than those with limited clinical experience. Cantrell (2008) noted that when debriefing follows an instructional simulation, well-planned learning objectives are crucial to facilitating the teaching-learning process. The objectives provide the individual doing the debriefing with a blueprint to use to facilitate the learning.

Environment

Debriefing typically takes place in a separate room from the simulation. The space required for debriefing is dependent on the number of participants. The space should allow for privacy and, if video review is included, appropriate equipment. Seating the participants and facilitator around a table or arranging chairs in a circle helps establish an environment of equality (Mayville, 2011; Wickers, 2010).

The debriefing session should begin by clarifying expectations, including the length of the debriefing and the debriefing format (McDonnell, Jobe, & Dismukes, 1997). One of the expectations to be established is an environment of trust (Fanning & Gaba, 2007). Participants might feel vulnerable discussing mistakes made in a simulation. Impressing upon them that the debriefing discussion should not leave the room helps them to feel safe (Wickers, 2010). Although data related to the required characteristics of a safe environment is not found in the literature, Ganley & Linnard-Palmer (2012) reported nursing students participating in simulations identified the characteristics of such an environment as one in which they were not ridiculed or embarrassed by their mistakes. Establishing rules for open communication and providing a supportive environment are highly recommended by simulation experts (Arafeh et al., 2010).

Sharing objectives and expectations for the debriefing helps participants identify their roles during debriefing. Generally, objectives for the debriefing are the same as for the simulation, or they are an extension of the simulation objectives. Participants might watch a video of their performance and be expected to complete a checklist during the review (Wickers, 2010). The debriefing may involve a discussion in which the participants are asked to identify what they have learned during the simulation. Facilitators might explain other activities that enrich the debriefing, such as journaling. Through this introductory discussion, participants can clarify their roles during debriefing.

Length and Timing

Debriefing is generally held immediately after a simulation. This allows for better recall of scenario performance. However, because of logistics or an intentional desire to have the learner spend time in individual reflection before coming together as a group for debriefing, the debriefing may occur at a later point in time. Available evidence shows nursing students prefer debriefing immediately after the simulation as the experience is in the forefront of their minds (Cantrell, 2008; Neill & Wotton, 2011; Reed, 2009; Wotton, Davis, Button, & Kelton, 2010). The Center for Advanced Pediatric Education (CAPE) recommends starting the debriefing within 5 to 10 minutes, helping to reduce anxiety of waiting for the video-recorded performance to be viewed (American Academy of Pediatrics [AAP] and American Heart Association [AHA], 2011).

One study compared post-simulation debriefing with "in-simulation" debriefing, in which the simulation was temporarily suspended for a period of instruction and then restarted. An advantage of in-simulation debriefing is avoiding negative learning as errors are corrected as they occur in the simulation. Advantages of post-simulation debriefing include allowing learning from mistakes made during the simulation, as well as having more time to comprehensively review the case. Medical students stated they learned from both types, although post-simulation debriefing was rated as more effective overall (Van Heukelom, Begaz, & Treat, 2010).

Adequate time is needed to debrief thoroughly (Reed, 2012a), although the amount of time has not been established by research. A general rule of thumb for establishing a targeted length of time for debriefing is to spend as much time (or more) debriefing as was spent performing the scenario (Flanagan, 2008). Students participating in two different research studies identified that debriefing sessions lasting 10 and 20 minutes did not provide adequate time to debrief (Childs & Sepples, 2006; Wotton et al., 2010). Brackenreg (2004) emphasized allowing enough time to explore the implications and consequences of the facilitated experience.

Group Size

No evidence is available on an optimal size for a debriefing group. The participants in the simulation, including the facilitators, should all be present for the debriefing. Flanagan (2008) recommended limiting observers in debriefing, as they may distract participants and provide unsolicited comments.

Facilitator

The facilitator, the person who conducts the debriefing, guides the learners to interpret the simulation and put it into an accurate perspective (Lasater, 2007). The facilitation of a debriefing, particularly facilitator behaviors during debriefing, has received the most attention in the debriefing literature. It is generally agreed that the facilitator should not dominate the conversation with questions or lecture; the goal is for participants to analyze and evaluate the simulation through discussion. To achieve this goal, McDonnell et al. identify several desirable facilitator behaviors:

- Asking questions that identify issues
- Active listening
- Pausing at least 3 to 4 seconds rather than immediately answering
- Promoting group participants to answer first (McDonnell et al., 1997)

Examples of the type of questions a facilitator might use to promote discussion include:

- "I noticed that you hesitated when Mr. Smith's mother asked you what was happening. What were you thinking at that point in time?"

- "There were three medications available to you to help manage postpartum hemorrhage. Why did you decide to choose Pitocin?"
- "Mary, I think I am hearing that you were afraid to call the doctor about this because of a negative experience you have had in the past. Is there anyone in the group that has a suggestion for Mary as to how to help decrease her anxiety when calling the doctor?"

Research has identified certain facilitator behaviors as being helpful for debriefing (see accompanying sidebar). For example, student nurses identified that they value a facilitator who is an expert in the content area (Reed, 2012a). However, there are times when an expert facilitator is not a content expert. In this case, the facilitator can involve the content expert in the simulation experience, including the debriefing. As noted earlier, facilitators should not dominate the conversation. They should allow participants time to talk about their feelings before making comments (Reed, 2012a). Cantrell (2008) found that nursing students also felt the demeanor of the facilitator was important—for example, whether the facilitator used humor, provided instructions, and offered helpful evaluation.

Components Contributing to an Effective Debriefing Process

Being facilitated by an individual competent in the process of debriefing

Being facilitated by an individual who has observed the simulated experience

Use of evidence-based debriefing methodologies

Being based on a structured framework for debriefing

Being based on the objectives, the learners, and the outcome of the simulated experience

Being conducted in an environment that supports confidentiality, trust, open communication, self-analysis, and reflection (INACSL BOD, 2011b)

Debriefing Types

Every debriefing should involve a discussion; the difference is whether this discussion should include a review of all or parts of the video-recorded simulation performance or include written reflective techniques such as journaling.

Discussion Alone

When debriefing simulations for educational purposes, Chronister & Brown (2011) and Reed (2012b) found discussion without video review had a positive effect on learning and knowledge retention. On the other hand, Salvodelli et al. (2006) found no benefit to adding video review to discussion debriefing of nontechnical skills performance. Discussion-only debriefing can be easily accomplished in multiple environments, whereas the use of video to aid the discussion requires a video system that can be expensive, prone to failure, and anxiety provoking (Flanagan, 2008). In addition, technical support may be needed to locate video clips or to run the video system, adding to the number of nonparticipant observers in the room. Facilitators who debrief using a video system need training on its use as inability to view video segments smoothly can be disruptive to the group discussion.

Discussion of a Video Recording

The use of a video recording in debriefing can provide an accurate account of events and stimulate learning and discussion in an organized way. The debriefing facilitator chooses portions of the video-recorded simulation that are pertinent to the objectives to view during debriefing and centers the discussion on these viewings. Facilitators can also use checklists during video-recorded debriefings to identify key behaviors or performance quality (Grant et al., 2010; Lasater, 2007).

Skill-improvement and team-based simulations may benefit from video review. Chronister & Brown (2011) found that reviewing parts or all of the video-recorded simulation improved skill performance and response times. Scherer, Chang, Meredith, & Battistella (2003) showed that video review of trauma code behaviors improved performance of medical residents. Viewing a video may also help transfer knowledge to real-world settings (Reed, Andrews, & Ravert, 2013, in press). In contrast, in a study on skills-based training, 30 residents showed no difference between debriefing with discussion only and debriefing with video-assisted discussion except for time to achieve tasks in the discussion-only group (Sawyer et al., 2012). Another comparison study of video-facilitated feedback (n=20) and oral feedback alone (n=20) showed no significant improvement on the overall targeted performance between the two groups, although the members of the video-facilitated feedback group were significantly more likely to perform three individual behaviors (Grant et al., 2010).

Facilitators need to make the decision to use video during debriefing judiciously, after consideration of the learning objectives. In a study of undergraduate nursing students, the students reported they did not feel safe when being videotaped for the purpose of review and debriefing (Ganley & Linnard-Palmer, 2010). Also, playing lengthy or unrelated video segments may distract from discussing key issues and accomplishing the objectives of the debriefing session (Fanning and Gaba, 2007).

Written Debriefing

Petranek (2000) proposed that learning could be extended with the addition of written debriefing after discussion debriefing. He based this recommendation about journaling on debriefing of simulated gaming experiences. In nursing, Reed (2009) conducted a debriefing study comparing discussion-only debriefing with written debriefing in the form of journaling or blogging. Nursing students definitely preferred their experience with discussion debriefing over the written debriefing types. Another study compared discussion-only debriefing with discussion followed by journaling or discussion followed by blogging. Nursing students again preferred their experience with discussion-only debriefing, and identified no learning benefit from adding written debriefing after discussion. In fact, students expressed annoyance at having to complete a debriefing blog (Reed, 2012b). Additional research is needed to determine whether written debriefing can extend learning or whether it provides a distraction to learners.

No debriefing type has been established as better than another. Therefore, the selection of a debriefing type should be made based on learning objectives for the simulation/debriefing, facilitator expertise, and the debriefing structure used.

Debriefing Structures

A crucial part of experiential learning is a systematic debriefing process that enables participants to discover and evaluate their own solutions (Brackenreg, 2004). Some have suggested structured debriefing as a means to provide a positive learning environment (Dreifuerst, 2009; Neill & Wotton, 2011). Structured reflection can promote learning and provide opportunities to develop critical thinking, clinical decision-making, clinical reasoning, and clinical judgment skills (Dreifuerst, 2009). The following are some debriefing models and structures used for debriefing simulations, with available research results. All of these structures require training for effective use.

Debriefing for Meaningful Learning

Debriefing for Meaningful Learning (DML) uses a consistent structure to guide nursing students to develop clinical reasoning and to "think like a nurse." Debriefing for Meaningful Learning uses six components—engage, evaluate, explore, explain, elaborate, and extend—to structure the debriefing process and promote active reflection. The debriefing facilitator uses Socratic questioning to examine student actions and thinking that occurred during the simulation. Wickers (2010) provides several examples of Socratic-type questions, including the following:

- "What other assessment data would have been helpful to have before phoning the doctor?"
- "How did you prioritize your nursing care and why?"
- "Where could you have found information concerning _____?"

Debriefing for Meaningful Learning worksheets and a written record of the simulation experience enhance learning opportunities. Using these tools, participants are supported to translate their thinking into knowledgeable decision-making, with the goal of applying the knowledge gained to subsequent clinical encounters (Dreifuerst, 2012; Dreifuerst & Decker, 2012; Mariani, Cantrell, Meakim, Prieto, & Dreifuerst, 2012).

In a comparison study (n=238), Debriefing for Meaningful Learning participants scored statistically higher on the Health Sciences Reasoning Test, on the Debriefing Assessment of Simulation in Healthcare (DASH) (student version), and on supplemental questions (Dreifuerst, 2012). In another study (n=86), students participating in the Debriefing for Meaningful Learning model and students receiving "unstructured" debriefing had no significant differences when scored with Lasater Clinical Judgment Rubric (Mariani et al., 2012).

Debriefing with Good Judgment

Debriefing with good judgment is an approach that enables the debriefer to deliver important feedback while avoiding a negative experience for those being debriefed. When maintaining the "good judgment" approach, debriefers supply their interpretation of the simulation actions (advocacy), and pair it with a "curious" desire to understand those actions (inquiry). In this approach, the debriefing is designed to increase what the participant hears and internalizes without the participant becoming defensive or humiliated.

Examples of advocacy/inquiry questioning include the following:

- "It looked to me like it was confusing. How did you feel?"
- "So, it looked to me as if confusion may have prevented you from effectively executing respiratory resuscitation and, later, the ACLS algorithm. How did you all see it?" (Rudolph, Simon, Rivard, Dufresne, & Raemer, 2007).

Outcome, Present State, Test Model Debriefing

The Outcome, Present State, Test (OPT) Model of Clinical Reasoning is a structured debriefing used to frame client situations and focus on outcomes (Pesut & Herman, 1999). During debriefing, students complete OPT model worksheets following interactions associated with the identified nursing diagnosis. A priority focus, called a "keystone issue," is identified and serves as the basis for defining a present state. This is described and compared to the desired outcome state, with participants identifying interventions to fill the gaps between present and desired states.

In a study using OPT model worksheets for debriefing simulations, Kuiper and colleagues found that worksheet scores were comparable to authentic clinical experiences, with the authors concluding that clinical reasoning was supported by OPT worksheet use (Kuiper, Heinrich, Matthias, Graham, & Bell-Kotwall, 2008). Mariani et al. (2012) noted no significant difference on the OPT worksheet mean scores for the two methods.

Other Debriefing Structures

Flanagan (2008) recommends a general structure for debriefing in which debriefers promote discussion of the events, experience, and participant concerns about the simulation during the body of the debriefing. Following are some suggested questions to encourage this discussion:

- "What did you do to manage the situation and why?"
- "What went well? Why did it go well?"
- "What was difficult?"
- "What would you do differently next time?"
- "What have you learned?"

A method described in an aviation debriefing manual by McDonnell, Jobe, and Dismukes (1997) spawned many of the health care debriefing practices that exist today. This method focuses on crew resource management (CRM), or, in other words, teamwork. A suggestion for debriefing from this manual is to use video to set the scene for debriefing. Simple questions such as "What went well?" start the debriefing conversation. The "crew" (team) is led to topics by asking questions requiring an explanation rather than a yes/no answer. The discussion is deepened by asking more in-depth questions, such as "Was there anything that made you uncomfortable when you…?" Finally, importance is placed on following up on topics raised by participants, with full exploration of those topics using "what," "how," and "why" questions.

Evaluating Debriefing

Evaluating debriefings helps to provide evidence about how to maximize the learning that occurs during these sessions. Often, developing the skill of debriefing is forgotten with the excitement of learning how to use new simulation technologies. At present, two evaluation tools have been identified as useful when evaluating debriefings as well as those who debrief.

Debriefing Experience Scale (DES)

The Debriefing Experience Scale (DES) was designed to evaluate the participant experience during debriefing (Reed, 2012a). It comprises 20 items, rated in the scale areas of "experience" and "importance." Four of the scale items are related to processing the experience, five items are related to learning, and 11 items are related to the session facilitator (Reed, 2012a).

The scale was created from a review of simulation literature and feedback from three nursing simulation experts. It was refined, with redundant items removed, through a two-step factor analysis process. Cronbach's alpha on the experience and importance portion of the dual 20-item scales is high, with 0.93 for the experience portion and 0.91 for the importance portion (Reed, 2012a). Although use of the tool thus far has involved only nursing students, indications are that its use could be expanded as the reliability and validity of the scale were established using nursing simulation experts as well as nursing students.

Suggested areas for comparative investigation include length of debriefing, debriefing types, and facilitator training (Reed, 2012a), as well as any other factors that might influence the debriefing experience.

Debriefing Assessment for Simulation in Healthcare (DASH)

The Debriefing Assessment for Simulation in Healthcare (DASH) tool is designed for evaluating debriefing session facilitators on the quality they deliver in debriefings for the purpose of providing feedback to the facilitators to allow improvement on DASH-established comportments (Simon, Raemer, & Rudolph, 2009).

The DASH tool is a behaviorally anchored rating scale that requires a training course for its use. Six facilitator behaviors are rated on the tool, including the following:

- Establishing an engaging learning environment
- Maintaining an engaging learning environment
- Structuring the debriefing in an organized way
- Provoking engaging discussions
- Identifying and exploring performance gaps
- Helping trainees achieve or sustain good future performance

These behaviors are rated from 1 (extremely ineffective/abysmal) to 7 (extremely effective/outstanding; Brett-Fleegler et al., 2012).

The scale was developed by a consensus of eight emergency medicine physicians with experience in simulation and debriefing. The reliability and validity of the scale was established through webinar by physicians, nurses, and other highly educated professionals who were debriefing a team-based critical-care simulation with the objectives of management, role establishment, and team leadership. Statistical significance was achieved by rating the three different videos. Intraclass correlation for the DASH overall was 0.74, and the Cronbach alpha for the average video was 0.89 across the entire webinar-rater data set. The DASH evaluation tool has been established as useful to rate expert facilitator behaviors for critical-care, medical, and team-based simulation debriefings (Brett-Fleegler et al., 2012).

Debriefing Training

Many facilitator training programs are available to help individuals learn best debriefing practices. Some training programs are associated with simulation centers, whereas other programs are available in connection with simulation and education conferences. In one study, participants were found to be more satisfied with educators who had been through a debriefing training course; however, there was no significant relationship found between cognitive student outcomes and faculty training (Hallmark, 2010). Examples of the resources available are shown in Table 5.1.

Table 5.1   Examples of Debriefing Training Resources

Educational Activity	Sponsor
Debriefing and Guided Reflection Course Beyond Basic Debriefing Course	Simulation and Resource Center, (SIRC), National League of Nursing, http://sirc.nln.org/
Structured and Supported Debriefing Course	American Heart Association, http://www.heart.org/HEARTORG/CPRAndECC/InstructorNetwork/InstructorResources/Structured-and-Supported-Debriefing-Course_UCM_304285_Article.jsp
DASH—Debriefing Assessment for Simulation in Healthcare	Center for Medical Simulation, http://www.harvardmedsim.org/debriefing-assesment-simulation-healthcare.php
Advancing Crisis Management Training in Health Care (Includes debriefing training)	Stanford School of Medicine VA PA Sim Center, http://med.stanford.edu/VAsimulator/
Sim 104: Briefing and Debriefing—The Key to Learning with Simulation	University of Washington Center for Health Science Interprofessional Education, Research and Practice, http://collaborate.uw.edu/faculty-development/teaching-with-simulation/teaching-with-simulation.html-0

Conclusion

Debriefing is an essential component of the simulation experience, helping participants to integrate and create meaning of their simulation learning experiences (Lasater, 2007). The goal of providing feedback in a nonthreatening manner during debriefing is to improve actions in future events. Although evidence for best practices in debriefing is still incomplete, it is considered so important for learning that it has become an essential component of every simulation experience (Shinnick et al., 2011).

References

American Academy of Pediatrics (AAP) and American Heart Association (AHA). (Producer). (2011). *An interactive tool for facilitation of simulation-based learning.* [DVD]. United States: Producer.

Arafeh, J. M. R., Hansen, S. S., & Nichols, A. (2010). Debriefing in simulated-based learning: Facilitating a reflective discussion. *Journal of Perinatal & Neonatal Nursing, 24*(4), 302-309.

Ausselin, M. E. (2011). Using reflection strategies to link course knowledge to clinical practice: The RN-to-BSN student experience. *Journal of Nursing Education, 50*(3), 125-133.

Brackenreg, J. (2004). Issues in reflection and debriefing: How nurse educators structure experiential activities. *Nurse Education in Practice, 4*(4), 264-270. doi:10.1016/j.neph.2004.01.005

Brett-Fleegler, M., Rudolf, J., Eppich, W., Monuteaux, M., Fleegler, E., Cheng, A., & Simon, R. (2012). Debriefing assessment for simulation in healthcare: Development and psychometric properties. *Simulation in Healthcare, 7*(5), 288-291.

Bulman, C., Lathlean, J., & Gobbi, M. (2011). The concept of reflection in nursing: Qualitative findings on student and teacher perspectives. *Nurse Education Today, 32*(5), e8-e13.

Cantrell, M. A. (2008). The importance of debriefing in clinical simulations. *Clinical Simulation in Nursing, 4*(2), e19-e23. doi:10.1016/j.ecns.2008.06.006

Childs, J. C., & Sepples, S. (2006). Clinical teaching by simulation: Lessons learned from a complex patient care scenario. *Nursing Education Perspectives, 27*(3), 154-158.

Chronister, C., & Brown, D. (2012). Comparison of simulation debriefing methods. *Clinical Simulation in Nursing, (8)*7, e281-e288. doi:10.1016/j.ecns.2010.12.005

DeCoux, V. M. (1990). Kolb's Learning Style Inventory: A review of its applications in nursing research. *Journal of Nursing Education, 29*(5), 202-207.

Dreifuerst, K. T. (2009). The essentials of debriefing in simulation learning: A concept analysis. *Nursing Education Perspectives, 30*(2), 109-114.

Dreifuerst, K. T. (2012). Using debriefing for meaningful learning to foster development of clinical reasoning in simulation. *Journal of Nursing Education, 51*(6), 326-333.

Dreifuerst, K. T., & Decker, S. I. (2012). Debriefing: An essential component for learning in simulation pedagogy. In P. Jeffries (Ed.), *Simulation in nursing education: From conceptualization to evaluation* (2nd ed.) (pp. 105-129). New York, NY: National League for Nursing.

Fanning, R. M., & Gaba, D. M. (2007). The role of debriefing in simulation-based education. *Simulation in Healthcare 2*(2), 115-125. doi:10.1097/SIH.0b013e3180315539

Flanagan, B. (2008). Debriefing: Theory and techniques. In R. Riley (Ed.), *Manual of simulation in healthcare* (pp. 155-170). Oxford: Oxford University Press.

Ganley, B. J., & Linnard-Palmer, L. (2012). Academic safety during nursing simulation: Perceptions of nursing students and faculty. *Clinical Simulation in Nursing, 8*(2), e49-e57.

Grant, J. S., Moss, J., Epps, C., & Watts, P. (2010). Using video-facilitated feedback to improve student performance following high-fidelity simulation. *Clinical Simulation in Nursing, 6*(5), e177-e184.

Hallmark, E. F. (2010). *The effect of faculty debriefing training on the achievement and satisfaction of pre-licensure nursing students participating in simulation.* (Doctoral dissertation). Retrieved from ProQuest Dissertations and Theses database (815829062).

International Nursing Association for Clinical Simulation and Learning (INASCL) Board of Directors (BOD). (2011a). Standards of Best Practice: Simulation. Standard I: Terminology. *Clinical Simulation in Nursing, 7*(4S), s3-s7. doi:10.1016/j.ecns.2011.05.005. Retrieved from http://download.journals. elsevierhealth.com/pdfs/journals/1876-1399/PIIS1876139911000612.pdf

International Nursing Association for Clinical Simulation and Learning (INASCL) Board of Directors (2011b). Standards of Best Practice: Simulation. Standard VI: The debriefing process. *Clinical Simulation in Nursing, 7* (4S), s16-s17. doi:10.1016/j.ecns.2011.05.010. Retrieved from http://download.journals. elsevierhealth.com/pdfs/journals/1876-1399/PIIS1876139911000661.pdf

Kolb, D., (1984). *Experiential learning: Experience as a source of learning and development.* Upper Saddle River, NJ: Prentice-Hall.

Kuiper, R., Heinrich, C., Matthias, A., Graham, M. J., & Bell-Kotwall, L. (2008). Debriefing with the OPT model of clinical reasoning during high fidelity patient simulation. *International Journal of Nursing Education Scholarship, 5*(1), 1-14, doi:10.2202/1548-923X.1466

Lasater, K. (2007). High-fidelity simulation and the development of clinical judgment: Students' experiences. *Journal of Nursing Education, 46*(6), 269-276.

Mariani, B., Cantrell, M.A., Meakim, C., Prieto, P., & Dreifuerst, K. (2012). Structured debriefing and student's clinical judgment abilities in simulation. *Clinical Simulation in Nursing,* e1-e9. doi: 10.1016/j. ecns.2011.11.009

Mayville, M. L. (2011). Debriefing: The essential step in simulation. *Newborn and Infant Nursing Reviews, 11*(1), 35-39.

McDonnell, L. K., Jobe, K. K., & Dismukes, R. K. (1997). Facilitating LOS debriefings: A training manual. *Flight Safety Digest, 16*(11), 1-24.

Neill, M. A., & Wotton, K. (2011). High-fidelity simulation debriefing in nursing education: A literature review. *Clinical Simulation in Nursing, 7*(5), e161-e168. doi:10.1016/j.ecns.2011.02.001

Pesut, D. J., & Herman, J. (1999). *Clinical reasoning: The art & science of critical & creative thinking.* Albany, NY: Delmar.

Petranek, C. F. (2000). Written debriefing: The next vital step in learning with simulations. *Simulation & Gaming, 31*(1), 108-118.

Reed, S. J. (2009). *Comparison of debriefing methods following simulation: Development of pilot instrument* (Doctoral thesis). Case Western Reserve University.

Reed, S. J. (2012a). Debriefing experience scale: Development of a tool to evaluate the student learning experience in debriefing. *Clinical Simulation in Nursing, 8*(6), e211-e217. doi:10.1016/j.ecns.2011.11.002

Reed, S. J. (2012b, November). *Written debriefing: Comparison study of debriefing with and without a written component.* Paper presented at the American Association of Colleges of Nursing Baccalaureate Education Conference, San Antonio, TX.

Reed, S. J., Andrews, C., & Ravert, P. (2013, in press). Debriefing simulation: Comparison of debriefing with video and debriefing alone. *Clinical Simulation in Nursing*. doi: 10.1016/j.ecns.2013.05.007

Rudolph, J. W., Simon, R., Rivard, P., Dufresne, R. L., & Raemer, D. B. (2007). Debriefing with good judgment: Combining rigorous feedback with genuine inquiry. *Anesthesiology Clinics, 25*(2), 361-376.

Salvodelli, G. L., Naik, V. R., Park, J., Joo, H. S., Chow, R., & Hamstra, S. J. (2006). Value of debriefing during simulated crisis management: Oral versus video-assisted oral feedback. *Anesthesiology, 105*(2), 279-85.

Sawyer, T., Sierocka-Castaneda, A., Chan, D., Berg, B., Lustik, M., & Thompson, M. (2012). The effectiveness of video-assisted debriefing versus oral debriefing alone at improving neonatal resuscitation performance. *Simulation in Healthcare, 7*(4), 213-221.

Scherer, L. A., Chang, M. C., Meredith, J. W., & Battistella, F. D. (2003). Videotape review leads to rapid and sustained learning. *The American Journal of Surgery, 185*(6), 516-520.

Sewchuk, D. (2005). Experiential learning—A theoretical framework for perioperative education. *AORN Journal, 81*(6), 1311-1318.

Shinnick, M. A., Woo, M., Horwich, T. B., & Steadman, R. (2011). Debriefing: The most important component in simulation? *Clinical Simulation in Nursing, 7*(3), e105-e111.

Simon, R., Raemer, D. B., & Rudolph, J. W. (2009). *Debriefing assessment for simulation in healthcare—Rater version*. Cambridge, MA: Center for Medical Simulation.

Van Heukelom, J. N., Begaz, T., & Treat, R. (2010). Comparison of postsimulation debriefing versus in-simulation debriefing in medical simulation. *Simulation in Healthcare, 5*(2), 91-97.

Wickers, M. P. (2010). Establishing a climate for a successful debriefing. *Clinical Simulation in Nursing, 6*(3), e83-e86. doi:10.1016/j.ecns.2009.06.003

Wotton, K., Davis, J., Button, D., & Kelton, M. (2010). Third-year undergraduate nursing students' perceptions of high fidelity simulation. *Journal of Nursing Education, 19*(11), 632-639.

"The most elegant design of a study will not overcome the damage caused by unreliable or imprecise measurements."

–Joseph L. Fleiss

Evaluating Simulation Effectiveness

Katie Anne Adamson, PhD, RN

Health profession educators have long used various forms of simulation for teaching and learning. However, they have historically given little attention to evaluating the effectiveness of simulation endeavors. This chapter focuses on the culminating step in planning and implementing a successful simulation program: evaluation. For many charged with the responsibility of managing or running a simulation program, even those who have established competence and confidence in teaching with simulation, evaluating the effectiveness of simulation endeavors might seem like a daunting task. This chapter seeks to make it less intimidating by:

1. Answering the essential question of why we evaluate

2. Describing a framework for categorizing simulation evaluation strategies

3. Suggesting guidelines and instruments from practice and the literature that may be used for each type of evaluation

4. Providing exemplars of simulation evaluation

OBJECTIVES

- Describe the rationale for evaluating simulation endeavors.

- List the four levels of evaluation, including characteristics and guidelines for completing evaluations at each level.

- Identify resources for finding evaluation instruments to suit various evaluation objectives.

Why Evaluate?

The first and most important question to answer before attempting to evaluate the effectiveness of simulation endeavors is, "Why?" Why should we be interested in learning about the efficacy of simulation? Bourke and Ihrke (2005) identify five purposes of evaluation (see the accompanying sidebar). Essentially, evaluation is a form of reflection. It allows simulation participants to reflect on their performance and how it may be improved. It allows simulation facilitators to reflect on how the program is doing and how it may be improved. Finally, it allows the outside world (administrators, funders, and so on) an opportunity to see how simulation endeavors are contributing to the mission of the organization (Kellogg Foundation, 1998).

Purposes of Evaluation

Help participants learn and identify what they have learned (or not learned)

Identify actual or potential problems, including shortfalls in participant learning or gaps in a specific simulation activity or program

Assign participant scores

Improve current practices

Identify how well or efficiently intended outcomes were achieved

Source: Bourke & Ihrke, 2005

In health care education, simulation is called upon to address several challenges, including expanding enrollments, faculty shortages, graduates who are underprepared for the workforce, limited clinical placement sites, and reduced opportunities for patient care in existing clinical placement sites due to patient acuity and regulatory constraints. In hospitals and health care systems, simulation is used to validate and develop competencies, improve quality of care, decrease risks, and optimize resources. Inadequate evidence exists, however, about whether simulation is successful in addressing these challenges. Therefore, we need to increase efforts to document the efficacy of simulation activities.

From a universal perspective, the evidence supporting the efficacy of simulation is growing; however, many evaluations about the efficacy of simulation endeavors will be done to meet immediate, local needs. For example, after the purchase of simulation equipment and the early implementation of a simulation program, administrators will likely ask the question, "How do we know simulation is working?" This question can have several meanings, but, in general, people want to know how the implementation of simulation activities affects the outcomes they care about, including patient care and the bottom line.

To that end, the focus of a simulation evaluation may range from an individual simulation participant to an entire simulation program or strategy. Likewise, the purpose of a simulation evaluation may range from gathering formative data about an individual participant's satisfaction with a particular activity to gathering summative data about the results of an entire simulation training program in order to guide future research, practice, and policy (Kellogg Foundation, 1998).

> ## Formative and Summative Evaluations
>
> Formative evaluations answer the question, "Is this working?" and illuminate opportunities for immediate remediation or improvement.
>
> Summative evaluations answer the question, "Did this work?" and illuminate opportunities for future changes.

Kirkpatrick's Framework

Kirkpatrick (1998) suggested the following framework to categorize evaluation strategies. This framework is helpful for identifying the scope and purpose of an evaluation. Kirkpatrick's (1998) four levels of evaluation are reaction, learning, behavior, and results. These levels can be used to categorize different types of simulation evaluations. Table 6.1 shows each of the levels, what questions are answered at each level of evaluation, and examples of strategies that may be used to complete evaluations at each level.

Table 6.1	Questions and Strategy Examples for Levels of Evaluation	
Level	*Questions*	*Strategy Example*
1. Reaction	What were the participants' reactions to the simulation activity? Were they satisfied with the simulation experience? Did the simulation activity improve their confidence?	Surveying participants about their level of satisfaction with the simulation experience
2. Learning	What did the participants learn from the simulation activity? What domains of learning did the simulation activity contribute to: cognitive, affective, psychomotor?	Evaluating participants' demonstrations of critical thinking or technical skills in simulation, or pre- and posttesting participants' knowledge and attitudes
3. Behavior	How did the simulation activity affect the participants' behavior in the actual clinical environment? Did learning that occurred in simulation transfer to actual patient care?	Evaluating the competency of new graduates or residents who were educated using simulation
4. Results	What were the longer term results of the simulation activity? How were patient or organizational-level outcomes affected?	Calculating cost-savings (Cohen et al., 2010) or improved patient outcomes (Draycott et al., 2008) that result from simulation-based training

Guidelines for Evaluations at Each Level

Kirkpatrick (1998) identified guidelines for completing evaluations at each level. Similarities between evaluations at every level include starting with the end in mind (Wiggins & McTighe, 2005) to determine what information you want to gather and identifying a standard or benchmark against which you will compare your results. A strategy for evaluation should be included in the early simulation planning process and not tacked on at the end. It is also important, regardless of the types of evaluation you will be doing, to establish whether the evaluations will be formative, summative, or whether you will use both types of evaluations.

Regardless of what level of evaluation you are doing and whether it is formative or summative, after you have collected your data, you need to communicate your results to stakeholders and to make any necessary changes based on these results.

The following describes the unique characteristics of each level of evaluation:

- **Reaction:** In addition to standardized response questions, encourage participants to provide written comments. Design the evaluation form and participant experience to encourage maximum participation and honesty.

- **Learning:** Consider using a control group so that you can make objective comparisons. Evaluate multiple domains of learning: cognitive, affective, and psychomotor. This may be accomplished using measures such as a multiple-choice exam (cognitive); an observation-based performance evaluation (psychomotor); and a written reflection about attitudes or beliefs (affective).

- **Behavior:** Allow adequate time for behavior change to take place and consider identifying a control group for comparison. Get a 360-degree view of participants' practice behaviors by seeking input from multiple sources: clinical instructors, preceptors, staff, peers, patients, and the participant. Repeat the evaluation of behavior as appropriate.

- **Results:** Allow adequate time for results to occur. Consider what you will use for your comparison. This may mean taking measurements before and after implementation of a simulation program. Consider doing a cost-benefit analysis and repeat the evaluation of results as appropriate in the form of periodic monitoring or tracking.

Highlights and Challenges of Evaluations at Each Level

Evaluations become increasingly more challenging and increasingly more meaningful as you move from Level 1 (Reaction) to Level 4 (Results; see Figure 6.1). Although it might be easy to ask simulation participants about their satisfaction with a simulation activity, it is much more difficult to measure how simulation-based training affects a participant's behavior and ultimately affects patient and organizational outcomes (Results). In parallel, it also might be interesting to know how well participants enjoyed a simulation activity, but it is much more important to know the answer to the large question, "Is simulation working?"

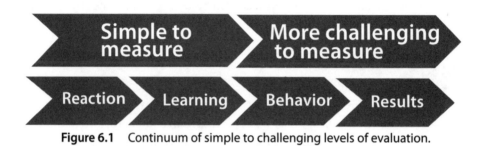

Figure 6.1   Continuum of simple to challenging levels of evaluation.

Measuring Progress

Evaluations often involve measuring progress over time. For example, a staff education department faced with complacent or unmotivated learners may be very interested in measuring changes in participant satisfaction with the department's educational offerings. In this case, it may be important to evaluate participants' reactions to simulation activities. Educators are interested in students' development and learning in the cognitive, affective, and psychomotor domains. Patient safety advocates are interested in practitioners' behaviors (hand washing, for instance) and the results of these behaviors. Data about these behaviors and results are most valuable when they are presented in a context in which change over time may be observed. In these cases, it is valuable to repeat the same evaluation at multiple points in time in order to document progress.

Instruments and Methods for Evaluation at Each Level

Table 6.2 shows examples of instruments from the literature that may be used to facilitate evaluations at each level. While it may be tempting to develop unique evaluation instruments for specific evaluation needs, consider using an instrument that has already been assessed for validity and reliability that meets your needs.

Table 6.2 Examples of Measurement Instruments	
Level	*Instrument Examples*
1. Reaction	Satisfaction and self-confidence in learning scale (NLN, 2005)
	Emergency Response Confidence tool (Arnold et al., 2009)
2. Learning	
Cognitive	Multiple-choice exam questions such as ATI
Psychomotor	Skills checklists—(Elkin, Perry, & Potter, 2007)
Multiple domains	Lasater Clinical Judgment Rubric (Lasater, 2007)
	Sweeny-Clark Simulation Evaluation Rubric (Clark, 2006)
	Clinical Simulation Evaluation Tool (Radhakrishnan, Roche, & Cunningham, 2007)
3. Behavior	Creighton Simulation Evaluation Instrument (Todd, Manz, Hawkins, Parsons, & Hercinger, 2008)
4. Results	Cost/benefit analysis
	Cost savings (Cohen et al., 2010) or improved patient outcomes (Draycott et al., 2008) that result from simulation-based training

Additional Resources for Identifying Existing Instruments

You might find certain recent review articles helpful for identifying possible evaluation instruments.

- Bray, Schwartz, Odegard, Hammer, and Seybert (2011) review simulation evaluation strategies used in pharmacy education.

- Davis and Kimble (2011) review evaluation instruments using the American Association of Colleges of Nursing Baccalaureate Essentials.

- Kardong-Edgren, Adamson, and Fitzgerald (2010) review evaluation instruments from the health sciences literature designed to evaluate cognitive, affective, and psychomotor learning, as well as team performance.

- Kogan, Holmboe, and Hauer (2009) review 55 evaluation instruments used with medical trainees.

- Yuan, Williams, and Fang (2012) review simulation studies from medical and nursing education and include listings of instruments used in each study.

Methods for Evaluating Participants in Simulation Endeavors

In addition to specific evaluation instruments, it may be helpful to consider general methods for evaluating participants in simulation endeavors. Table 6.3 includes examples of strategies that may be used to reflect participants' experiences, performances, and learning.

Table 6.3   Examples of Strategies

Method	Uses
360-degree survey of performance	Feedback from multiple sources can provide a more complete picture of participants' performance and/or learning.
Anecdotal faculty notes	Consistent and well-organized notes may reflect participant progress and provide documentation for formative and summative evaluation.
Attitude scales	Frick, Chadha, Watson, Wang, and Green (2009) suggest that participants' perceptions influence their learning. Gathering data about participants' attitudes toward and satisfaction with simulation activities may reflect the efficacy of the activities.
Observation-based evaluations including short checklists	These evaluations enable educators to observe and rate participant performance systematically.
Reflection papers, blogs, or journals	These types of reflections provide self-reported data about participants' experience in and learning from a simulation activity. Examples from the literature include Marchigiano, Eduljee, and Harvey (2010), who used journaling for the development of critical thinking skills, and Weller (2004) and McElhinney (2011), who employed unique reflective practices in simulation.
Typical course clinical evaluation tools	These instruments are likely familiar to educators and are typically designed to reflect course or program objectives.

Considerations When Selecting an Instrument

You need to consider several important questions when selecting an evaluation instrument (Bourke & Ihrke, 2005):

- Does the instrument measure what you are interested in measuring?
- Does it measure everything you are interested in measuring or will you need to add questions or use more than one instrument?
- Is the instrument accessible and understandable to those who will be using it?
- What type of training will you need to provide to those who will be using it?
- What evidence is there to support the validity and reliability of the results and how you plan to use them?

If you are not satisfied with the answers to these questions, you might consider modifying an existing instrument or designing your own. Be warned, however, that designing and validating a new evaluation instrument requires a significant investment of time, effort, and expertise in tool development.

> One of the key considerations when selecting an evaluation strategy or instrument is deciding what you want to measure. Should the evaluation reflect the performance of an individual or a team? If you are working with an interprofessional team, are the expectations for each member of the team similar or different? How should this be accounted for in the evaluation?

Observation-based evaluation instruments are powerful in that they have the potential to capture what the person being rated is actually doing—not just what they report they know or how they would act in a hypothetical situation. However, they also have several weaknesses. A key weakness of observation-based evaluation instruments is that the data they produce is influenced not only by the performance of the person being observed, but by variables associated with the person doing the observing and scoring. Rater bias (intentional or not) is a factor that must be considered when selecting an instrument and evaluation strategy. Rater training and careful consideration of how rater characteristics might influence the ratings they assign will help ensure a more valid and reliable evaluation process.

Evaluation Exemplar—Academic Setting

One exemplar of a multiple-level evaluation of simulation effectiveness is the National Council of State Boards of Nursing (NCSBN) National Simulation Study (Hayden, 2012; NCSBN, 2013). In this study, nursing students were randomized into three study groups, with each group using simulation to replace a percentage of their traditional clinical hours. One group has up to 10% of their traditional clinical hours substituted with simulation experiences; one group has 25% of their traditional clinical hours substituted with simulation experiences; and one group has 50% of their traditional clinical hours substituted with simulation experiences. Students were evaluated throughout their nursing education and will continue to be evaluated into the first year of practice. This study seeks to answer the following research questions (Hayden, 2012; NCSBN, 2013):

- Are there differences in clinical competency among graduating nursing students in the three study groups?
- Are there differences in knowledge among graduating nursing students in the three study groups?
- Are there perceived differences in how well learning needs are met in the clinical and simulation environments among the three study groups?
- Are there differences in clinical competency among the three study groups in each of the core clinical courses?

Table 6.4 shows a description of how each of these questions corresponds with different levels of evaluation and the instruments used.

Table 6.4	Levels of Questions Asked in Phase I and Phase II of the NCSBN National Simulation Study	
Question	*Evaluation Level*	*Instruments*
Are there perceived differences in how well learning needs are met in the clinical and simulation environments among the three study groups?	Reaction—Level 1	Clinical Learning Environment Comparison Survey
Are there differences in knowledge among graduating nursing students in the three study groups?	Learning—Level 2	ATI Comprehensive Assessment and Review Program
Are there differences in clinical competency among graduating nursing students in the three study groups?	Behavior—Level 3	Creighton Competency Evaluation Instrument
Are there differences in clinical competency among the three study groups in each of the core clinical courses?		

In Phase III after graduation, data will be collected from the graduates' National Council Licensure Examination (NCLEX) results and the graduates will be followed for their first year of practice. During that year, the NCSBN will evaluate the graduates' translational outcomes of simulation into the workforce (Results–Level 4). The longitudinal follow up of graduates will focus on clinical competency, safety competency, job satisfaction, retention, and stress. Data collection for the study will be completed in December 2014.

Evaluation Exemplar—Practice Setting

A hypothetical exemplar of a multilevel simulation evaluation in a hospital setting involves an effort to reduce catheter-associated urinary tract infections (CAUTIs) through a simulation-based CAUTI Prevention Training Program. In this exemplar, staff education has been tasked with implementing the hospital-wide training program for nurses and support staff and to then evaluate the efficacy of the program.

Staff educators are interested in the quality of their programs and might have several questions related to evaluation:

- Are staff satisfied with the training they received as part of the CAUTI Prevention Training Program?
- Did staff demonstrate improved knowledge and skill related to CAUTI prevention after participating in the training program?
- How did the CAUTI Prevention Training Program affect participants' behavior in the actual clinical environment?
- How did the CAUTI Prevention Training Program affect hospital CAUTI rates?

Table 6.5 describes how each of these questions corresponds with different levels of evaluation and ideas for instruments that may be used.

Table 6.5   Levels of Questions Asked in the Hypothetical Study

Question	Evaluation Level	Instruments
Are staff satisfied with the training they received as part of the CAUTI Prevention Training Program?	Reaction—Level 1	Satisfaction survey distributed to participating staff after completion of the program
Did staff demonstrate improved knowledge and skill related to CAUTI prevention after participating in the training program?	Learning—Level 2	Pre- and post-knowledge exam about CAUTI prevention Lab-based skills check-off for catheter insertion, care, and removal.

Question	Evaluation Level	Instruments
How did the CAUTI Prevention Training Program affect participants' behavior in the actual clinical environment?	Behavior—Level 3	Peer observation of catheter insertion, care, and removal Self-report survey of behavior in clinical environment
How did the CAUTI Prevention Training Program affect hospital CAUTI rates?	Results—Level 4	Comparing CAUTI rates before and after the CAUTI Prevention Training Program or comparing CAUTI rates between units where the program has been implemented and those where it has yet to be implemented

Take a moment to consider education and training needs in your facility. How are these needs being addressed and is there a formal evaluation process in place to measure their efficacy? This exemplar may be used as a template for evaluating reactions, learning, behavior, and results from education and training programs covering topics ranging from hand washing to complex invasive procedures.

Conclusion

Evaluating the efficacy of simulation endeavors is a complex, but necessary, step in the process of planning, implementing, and continuously improving a successful simulation program. This chapter has described the reasons to evaluate simulation endeavors, described a system for categorizing simulation evaluation strategies, and provided guidelines and examples from the literature for completing different types of evaluations. Using these resources and the exemplars will help you and your simulation team take on the challenge of evaluating your simulation endeavors.

References

Arnold, J. J., Johnson, L. M., Tucker, S. J., Malec, J. F., Henrickson, S. E., & Dunn, W. F. (2009). Evaluation tools in simulation learning: Performance and self-efficacy in emergency response. *Clinical Simulation in Nursing, 5*(1), e35-e43. doi:10.1016/j.ecns.2008.10.003

Bourke, M., & Ihrke, B. (2005). The evaluation process. In D. Billings & J. Halstead (Eds.), *Teaching in nursing: A guide for faculty* (2nd ed.) (pp. 443-464). Philadelphia: W. B. Saunders.

Bray, B. S., Schwartz, C. R., Odegard, P. S., Hammer, D. P., & Seybert, A. L. (2011). Assessment of human patient simulation-based learning. *American Journal of Pharmaceutical Education, 75*(10), Article 208. doi: 10.5688/ajpe7510208

Clark, M. (2006). Evaluating an obstetric trauma scenario. *Clinical Simulation in Nursing, 2*(2), e75-e77. doi:10.1016/j.ecns.2009.05.028

Cohen, E. R., Feinglass, J., Barsuk, J. H., Barnard, C., O'Donnell, A., McGaghie, W. C., & Wayne, D. B. (2010). Cost savings from reduced catheter-related bloodstream infection after simulation-based education for residents in a medical intensive care unit. *Simulation in Healthcare, 5*(2), 98-102.

Davis, A. H., & Kimble, L. P. (2011). Human patient simulation evaluation rubrics for nursing education: Measuring the essentials of baccalaureate education for professional nursing practice. *Journal of Nursing Education, 50*(11), 605-611.

Draycott, T. J, Crofts, J. F., Ash, J. P., Wilson, L. V., Yard, E., Sibanda, T. & Whitelaw, A. (2008). Improving neonatal outcome through practical shoulder dystocia training. *Obstetrics and Gynecology, 112*(1), 14-20.

Elkin, M. K., Perry, A. G., & Potter, P. A. (2007). *Nursing interventions & clinical skills* (4th ed.). St. Louis, MO: Mosby.

Frick, T. W., Chadha, R., Watson, C., Wang, Y., & Green, P. (2009). College students perceptions of teaching and learning quality. *Educational Technology Research and Development, 57*(5), 705-720.

Hayden, J. (2012, September 11). *The National Council of State Boards of Nursing National Simulation Study: Results from year 1.* Presented at 2012 NCSBN Scientific Symposium, Arlington, VA. Retrieved from www.ncsbn.org/3309.htm

Kardong-Edgren, S., Adamson, K., & Fitzgerald, C. (2010). A review of currently published evaluation instruments for human patient simulation. *Clinical Simulation in Nursing, 6*(1), e25-e35. doi:10.1016/jecns.2009.08.004

Kellogg Foundation. (1998). *Evaluation handbook.* Battle Creek, MI: Author. Retrieved from http://www.epa.gov/evaluate/pdf/eval-guides/evaluation-handbook.pdf

Kirkpatrick, D. L. (1998). *Evaluating training programs: The four levels* (2nd ed.). San Francisco, CA: Berrett-Koehler.

Kogan, J. R., Holmboe, E. S., & Hauer, K. E. (2009). Tools for direct observation and assessment of clinical skills of medical trainees. *Journal of the American Medical Association, 302*(12), 1316-1326.

Lasater, K. (2007). Clinical judgment development: Using simulation to create an assessment rubric. *Journal of Nursing Education, 46*(11), 496-503.

Marchigiano, G., Eduljee, N., & Harvey, K. (2010). Developing critical thinking skills from clinical assignments: A pilot study on nursing students' self-reported perceptions. *Journal of Nursing Management, 19*(1), 143-152. doi:10.1111/j.1365-2834.2010.01191.x

McElhinney, E. (2011). An evaluation of clinical simulation in a virtual world and its impact on practice—An action research project. *Clinical Simulation in Nursing, 7*(6), e258, doi:10.1016/j.ecns.2011.09.050

National Council of State Boards of Nursing (NCSBN). (2013). *National simulation study.* Chicago, IL: Author. Retrieved from www.ncsbn.org/2094.htm

National League for Nursing (NLN). (2005). *The student satisfaction and self confidence in learning scale.* Retrieved from http://www.nln.org/researchgrants/nln_laerdal/instruments.htm

Radhakrishnan, K., Roche, J., & Cunningham, H. (2007). Measuring clinical practice parameters with human patient simulation: A pilot study. *International Journal of Nursing Education Scholarship*, 4(1), Article 8, 1-11.

Todd, M., Manz, J., Hawkins, K. S., Parsons, M. E., & Hercinger, M. (2008). The development of a quantitative evaluation tool for simulation in nursing education. *International Journal of Nursing Education Scholarship*, 5(1), Article 41, 1-17.

Weller, J. M. (2004). Simulation in undergraduate medical education: Bridging the gap between theory and practice. *Medical Education*, 38(1), 32-38.

Wiggins, G., & McTighe, J. (2005). *Understanding by design.* Alexandria, VA: Association for Supervision and Curriculum Development.

Yuan, H. B., Williams, B. A., & Fang, J. B. (2012). The contribution of high-fidelity simulation to nursing students' confidence and competence: A systematic review. *International Nursing Review, 59*(1), 26-33.

"I hear and I forget. I see and I remember. I do and I understand."

–Confucius

Using Simulation With Specific Learner Populations

Carol Cheney, MS, CCC-SLP, CHSE

Karen Josey, MEd, BSN, RN, CHSE

Linda Tinker, MSN, RN, CHSE

OBJECTIVES

- Know the basic differences and similarities in simulation with different levels of learners.

- Identify foundational issues that unify all levels of learners.

- Understand pragmatic elements of simulation that might inadvertently affect learner populations and outcomes.

- Understand how simulation can be used to bridge the gap between all different types of clinicians from academia to practice.

Simulation foundations and theories largely remain constant. But simulation should be managed and utilized based on the different types and levels of learners. Simulation is an instructional methodology used to provide learning with patient safety in mind. It is simply no longer acceptable to attempt something for the first time on someone's loved one when there is a means to practice repeatedly before performing on a patient (Finkelman & Kenner, 2009). The targeted population of learners will drive the type of simulation needed and used. Simulation debriefing methodologies, scenario types, and outcomes may vary depending on whether the learner is a new graduate nurse, a team, or an experienced physician. It also depends on the objective for the simulation. Typically with new graduates, the environment is one in which more learning occurs in the moment. With an experienced team of clinicians, learning is most robust during periods of reflected self-discovery. Many simulation activities, regardless of the type or level of the learner, begin with motor skills acquisition or evaluation. According to Fitts and Posner's theory of motor skill acquisition, new learners have to think through and perform step by step, methodologically, before they are able to perform in a more rote and fluid fashion, and certainly before increased complexity can be added to the situation (Fitts & Posner, 1967). In order to ensure a new graduate has the simple steps of motor skills down, those tasks have to be repeated over and over, often following a checklist or procedural guideline such as the example shown in Figure 7.1.

Critical Behavior Reference for Competency Tool
Complete for Employee File ONLY with action plans, RCA's, or other special circumstances

Employee Name: _____ Employee Number: _____ Date: _____

TITLE	Foley Catheter Insertion				
EFFECTIVE DATE	2/2009	DATE REVISED:		REVIEWED	
SKILL LEVEL:				DEPARTMENT	Clinical Education/Simulation
Associated Policy & Procedure					
Target Populations:	AGE POPULATION: ☐ All Populations ☐ Neonate ☐ Infant ☐ 2Toddler ☐ Child ☐ Adolescent ☑ Adult ☐ Geriatric				

Skill Validation Methods: D-Demonstration   O-Observation of Daily Work   SP-Simulated Practice

	CRITICAL BEHAVIORS Verify physician order, verify patient using two identifiers, explain procedure, and perform hand hygiene before and after procedure.	Weight	Initial Validation	Remediation
1.	Do perineal care and position pt. Apply sterile gloves. Organize sterile supplies: pour solution over cotton balls, open lubricant and lubricate catheter. P CK	10		
2.	Place sterile drape over the perineal area exposing the labia/penis. Place catheter tray on sterile field. Use saturated cotton ball to cleanse. Male: Retract foreskin on uncircumcised patients – cleanse from urethral meatus to base of glans; Female: Retract labia to expose urethral meatus and cleanse. P, CK	20		
3.	Insert catheter until urine appears. Advance catheter another 2-5cm. Do not force catheter. Inflate catheter balloon. Allow bladder to empty 800-1000ml. Clamp tubing for 15minutes. Unclamp. P DM,CK	10		
4.	Anchor the catheter securely allowing slack for pt movement. Make sure tubing is not looped, kinked, clamped, or position above the level of the bladder. Position collection bag on bed frame. DM P CK	10		
5.	Provide perineal care after each bowel movement and at least once per shift assessing urethral meatus and surrounding tissue for inflammation, swelling, discharge, and if any discomfort is being experienced. Empty collection bag once per shift. P,DM,CP	15		
6.	Discontinues catheter by attaching syringe to inflation valve and removes fluid from balloon. Pulls catheter out smoothly and slowly. P,CK	20		
7.	Document D	15		

Validated By:_____Date: _____
(Signature and Credentials)

Figure 7.1   Example of a weighted checklist.
Used with permission of Banner Health.

With learners who have relevant experience, often the simulation team needs to validate the learner's ability to perform skills independently and competently. Assessment using task trainers is an excellent way of achieving this goal. After this occurs over a variety of skills and tasks, those tasks can be superimposed and the learner placed in a more complex environment in which a simulated patient or family receives education simultaneously with the care or has other complex medical issues. This superimposition of tasks and objectives, using a mannequin to teach and assess, occurs through the scenario development process. Scenarios can be designed and, in the case of new graduates, should be designed to progressively increase in complexity with the addition of distractors (such as noises, interruptions, and so on) found in the natural or live environment. Regardless of the level of learner, factors such as generational differences with technology utilization, vulnerability of the learner in the environment, and group versus individual learning styles must be considered as well.

All Learners

With all learners, pre-briefing and orientation to the simulator is often a good place to equilibrate all participants in a simulated event.

Pre-Briefing

The pre-briefing prepares the learner and sets the expectations of the simulation event. It lets the learner know if the event is an assessment of learning needs, a practical learning application, or even a high stakes assessment of performance. In an assessment of learning needs or practical application, learners should realize that simulation is about learning from their mistakes and practicing the events that lead to better patient care. Simulation allows one to practice without harming patients. In a high stakes simulation, the learner is held accountable for knowing how to perform at a certain level. High stakes testing is a summative evaluation or a competency that has consequences—such as moving to the next level in a residency program. Pre-briefing should be performed regardless of the type or level of learner in the simulation experience or the objective of the experience.

Suspension of disbelief is important to discuss in the pre-briefing to let learners know that the situation is to be treated as they would in actual practice. It is not always about the high technology of the mannequins or the realistic smells and textures of daily patient care, but the immersion into the simulation. Whether it's plastic vomit or real vomit, something is occurring with the patient that needs to be addressed. Explaining to learners the importance of assessing, communicating, diagnosing, and treating the patient as they would in the real environment enables the scenario to move forward in order to meet the intended objectives. Disbelief can halt or make ineffective the scenario or a part of the scenario. If you were not able to suspend disbelief when watching a movie, for example, you would not cry or laugh when watching it. A great example of suspended disbelief occurred in our simulation center during a scenario when one of our emergency residents had to perform an emergency C-section on an obstetric mannequin. His hands were shaking as he was cutting, as they might if he was cutting on a real patient, yet he was "cutting" a plastic mannequin.

Orientation

Orientation to the environment, equipment, and mannequin occurs before the simulation with all levels of learners. This gives them information they need to participate as they would with a typical patient. For example, if the mannequin normally does not have a pulse on one arm and learners are not informed of this, they may take the wrong path and make the wrong assumptions, taking away from the real purpose of the experience or impeding the flow of learning.

Vulnerability

Facilitators also need to consider and account for vulnerability with all learner types. Just as a new graduate or student may be unsure and feel uncomfortable being watched while performing alone for others to see, experts who are unaccustomed to the simulation environment may hesitate to perform in front of subordinates for fear the simulation event and their own performance might undermine their credibility. Truog and Meyer (2013) speak to the potential of the simulation being "stressful and shameful as well as stimulating and empowering" (p. 3). They also discuss building trust and being honest in delivering simulations. Simulation can be the ideal environment to teach and assess challenging an authority or even questioning a plan of action with the purpose of preventing patient harm (Gaba, 2013).

Death and Dying

Allowing the patient/mannequin to die is a controversial issue. If death isn't part of the learning objective, novices who might never have experienced death in the real environment may be focused on the death and emotional aspect, especially if they are not sure if actions taken in the scenario led to the demise. Experienced learners might know their actions did not cause the death and realize that death happens even when appropriate actions are taken, or they might feel comfortable that they will learn from their mistakes and not repeat them when caring for patients. End-of-life care, communication about death, and working through feelings about a patient death are valuable simulation experiences. If it is a planned objective of the scenario and covered in the pre-briefing, the acceptance of death can be less stressful and more accepted by the learners, especially the novice or inexperienced learner (Corvetto & Taekman, 2013).

Learning Objectives

The learning objectives need to drive the simulation scenario. Distraction from the learning objectives might be related to experience. Learners' previous experiences with simulation may also affect how they perform in future scenarios. It might take time and effort to change negative experiences. Those who value and embrace simulation learning can benefit tremendously in getting "experience" that they might not otherwise get to help prepare them for the real environment.

Students

Student simulations in academic programs are as varied as the number and types of clinical students. It is in the academic setting that many of our newer workforce members experience simulation for the first time. Simulation is now widely used in a variety of academic environments from nursing to dentistry to social work. Simulation experiences in academia often start with basic skills acquisition and practice. This might occur in a classroom setting with learning to place an intravenous (IV) line, with students sitting behind counters with latex limbs on display ready to receive their IV lines. As the students master each subsequent skill, the learning advances to interaction in the simulation environment where they may experience a patient history or head-to-toe assessment. Often the objectives with students are to learn and master the foundational skills and sequentially introduce or stack new skills/principles.

Simulation with students might not initially include recorded playback debriefing; instead the educator might pause the simulation experience to provide a clarification or solicit a learning opportunity in the moment. Debriefing in the moment might provide a greater benefit to students because the students might not yet have gained a deep enough cognitive awareness of what they should or should not do to be able to reflect and have that "aha" moment upon watching a recorded playback, as you might expect from an experienced practicing clinician. Issues such as whether the mannequin should deteriorate and/or die in a scenario if steps are missed or errors occur might not be relevant to the learning objective and, in fact, might distract a student learner from the objective at hand. For example, if the scenario's focus is on communication with a hysterical family member during a tense event such as a sudden onset pediatric respiratory event, the administration of the proper dose of Albuterol or the initiation of the pediatric asthma protocol might be a nonissue and serve to detract from the objective of communication because the learner is focused on the death aspect. A death and dying scenario, whether the outcome may or may not have been prevented, might be a more appropriate situation to address these sorts of issues with students. It is important to note that these death and dying issues should be addressed in some manner so as not to overprotect students from the reality of the roles in which they are seeking educational foundations.

Bridging the Gap

In the academic environment, the student is learning the basics of the concepts and competencies. Students get some opportunities in simulation and clinical rotations to practice a few of these concepts firsthand. Mastery of these skills and concepts is not likely to occur as the student might have only performed the skill once and that might have been in a simulation environment rather than with a live patient. There is a difference between practice, demonstration of learning, and competency. Bridging the gap between education and service has been an ongoing challenge.

Many state boards of nursing and academic programs are working to incorporate the IOM Future of Nursing recommendations, including the recommendation on the use of simulation in pre-licensure clinical education (IOM, 2011). In Arizona, for example, this work is lead by the Arizona Action Coalition Education-Practice Collaborative, a collaboration between education and service, which is sponsored by the Arizona Action Coalition. This group has been working on bridging the education-service gap for new graduates and has adopted the Massachusetts Nurse of the Future Competency Model (Massachusetts Department of Higher Education [MDHE], 2010).

The Arizona Education-Practice Collaborative Simulation Sub-group of academic and practice experts used the Massachusetts Nurse of the Future core competencies as a guide and identified the common topics covered in both academic and practice settings in simulation. For example, in both settings the safety competencies of infection control, patient identifiers, and medication administration are included in simulation content, as are the communication competencies of SBAR (Situation-Background-Assessment-Recommendation), therapeutic communication, and handoffs. By identifying common topics, this collaboration between education and nursing is essential to improving new graduate RN practice readiness to meet the quality and safety needs of patients and families (Arizona Action Coalition, 2013).

Massachusetts Nurse of the Future Core Competencies

Safety

Communication

Patient-Centered Care

Professionalism

Teamwork and Collaboration

Informatics and Technology

Leadership

Systems-Based Practice

Quality Improvement

Evidence-Based Practice

Source: MDHE, 2010

New Graduate Registered Nurses

New graduates tend to benefit from well-designed and structured training programs that give them access to learn both the things they need to understand and perform routinely and those that they might experience only rarely. Simulation can be a valuable tool to help weave the combination of theoretical knowledge; skills and tasks; and communication with patients, caregivers, and colleagues. Integrating and perfecting clinical reasoning, problem solving, deductive and inductive reasoning, sequencing, pragmatics, and timing into a practice environment in which no harm can be done on multiple simulated patients is quite powerful and shows tremendous benefit to the new graduate learner. Simulation opportunities might also reduce the length of precepted time on the units and allow unit-based educators and preceptors to focus on the opportunities and greatest learning needs. Although everyone benefits from debriefing, new graduates, much like students, do not always need to see themselves perform in order to benefit from a debriefing. However, unlike students, the debriefing may be much more structured and in a more traditional format focusing on what went well and what did not go well and identifying key strengths and opportunities.

To bridge the gap, the new graduates will need opportunities to practice and master what they have learned and learn to identify what may yet be opportunities for learning and improvement. Simulation provides the opportunity to review what they might have only experienced a few times before or not at all. It also provides a safe environment to remediate and practice to specific needs, problems, cases, and errors, as well as regulatory requirements.

Physicians graduate from medical schools and then go into residency programs to bridge the gap between academia and practice. Physical therapists and pharmacists also have residencies. Paramedics and emergency medical technicians (EMTs) have had extensive clinical experiences in emergency departments to practice skills they will perform in the field. Until recently, residencies have not routinely existed in nursing. Historically, hospital-based nursing programs allowed more time in the clinical setting for learning and practicing nursing skills and making nursing judgments. In the past, skills were practiced on real people first, whether it was a peer student or a real patient. Today, nurse residency programs exist, but there is much variation in these programs. They run the gamut of a few weeks' duration to up to a year or more. They may be a facility-based program or a formal standardized program. Regardless of the form of the residency program, simulation can play an important part in preparing new graduates to translate the knowledge and skills they acquired in their academic programs into the actual clinical setting.

Our organization, Banner Health, onboards new graduate nurses by validating basic practice skills. The skills have critical actions, and those steps are weighted to assist the validator in assessment. If the learner does not demonstrate the correct actions and steps to receive a score of 80% or more or misses a critical step, remediation occurs. After skills, the new graduate is immersed into 3 days of 4- to 5-hour scenarios. These scenarios are intended to replicate a "typical" day on the unit and target the domains of time management, communication with the patient and team, procedures, decision-making, and clinical knowledge. A report is generated that is specific for each learner's opportunities and strengths and sent to the learner's manager who shares it with the learner's preceptor. The preceptor then adapts the clinical orientation period to include needed learning. For example, if the learner struggles with communication with the physician but is great with time management, the orientation would focus on the communication component. A sample Simulation Summary Report Form is shown in Figure 7.2.

Banner Health's version of a new graduate registered nurse residency program is the On-Boarding Across the Continuum program, which includes clinical orientation, electronic medical record (EMR) documentation training, specialty academy, professional development courses, preceptor training, and other necessary training such as Basic Life Support, Advanced Life Support, Basic ECG, and so on. The specialty academies come after clinical orientation and EMR training. The purpose of the academies is to help prepare newly graduated and new to service RNs with more advanced knowledge and skills. Simulation is an integral part of these programs. The Banner Health ED New Graduate On-Boarding Pathway is depicted in Figure 7.3.

Practicing on actual people, such as has traditionally been done in the apprenticeship model in medicine, is no longer an accepted mechanism for learning new skills (Finkelman & Kenner, 2009). Simulation allows a means to train and practice in a safe and repetitive "pretend" environment versus practicing and learning on patients. Would average consumers feel comforted in having a nurse who has never even practiced IV insertion try to put an IV in their elderly mother or father or child? It is much better to have a nurse who has practiced on a skill trainer that actually has veins that can also accept an infusion of fluids or medicines instead of performing that same skill on someone's parent or child, for the first time. Patient consumer advocates (such as the Agency for Healthcare Research and Quality [AHRQ]) encourage us to ask our physicians how many times they have performed a procedure before we decide if we want that physician to perform the procedure on us.

Banner Simulation
Medical Center

**Simulation
Summary Report**

Name
Employee ID
Facility
Unit

Attended On:
02/11/13 - 02/20/13

Skill Summary

Skill	First Attempt	Second Attempt	Third Attempt
Safe Medication Administration	100%	Completed	Completed
Urinary Catheters: Indwelling Catheter Insertion, Maintenance, & Removal	80%	100%	Completed
Initially Remediated on:			
•Open insertion kit maintaining sterility. Apply sterile gloves. Organize sterile supplies: pour solution over cotton balls, open lubricant and lubricate catheter			
Blood Component Administration	85%	100%	Completed
Initially Remediated on:			
•Verify Transfusion record against the blood product label by two licensed personal utilizing:			
Blood component type, Unit number, Unit ABO/Rh type, Patient ABO/Rh type (on transfusion record), Expiration date			
CVC Site Care	85%	100%	Completed
Initially Remediated on:			
•Change Caps			
Comment: Remediated to Nursing Skill			
Suctioning: Nasotracheal & Tracheostomy	55%	100%	Completed
Initially Remediated on:			
•Maintains sterility throughout entire procedure			
•Retracts 1-2cm before applies suction			
Comment: Remediated to Nursing Skill			
Peripheral Intravenous Catheter: Starting Maintenance, & Discontinuation	100%	Completed	Completed
IV Smart Pump	100%	Completed	Completed
Chest Drainage Unit Set Up: Atrium Oaisis	0%	100%	Completed
Initially Remediated on:			
•Demonstrate where to fill water seal chamber			
•Demonstrate where to adjust dry suction control regulator			
•Connect chest drain unit to patient			
•Secure patient connection site with tape to facilitate complete visualization of entire length of tube			
•Connect wall suction to chest drain unit			
•Place chest tube to "water seal" or "gravity" drainage			
Comment: Remediated to Nursing Skill; watched dvd.			
CVC Removal	100%	Completed	Completed
Nasogastric Tube Insertion, Maintenance, & Removal	90%	100%	Completed
Initially Remediated on:			
•Tape tube to nose and secure to gown to prevent dislodgement.			
Specimen Labeling	100%	Completed	Completed

Scenario Summary

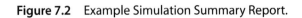

Overall SBAR Breakdown				
Situation	Background	Assessment	Recommendation	Readback
5/5	4/5	1/5	3/5	3/4

Overall Documentation Breakdown				
MAR	Handoff	Procedure	Assessment	MD Notification
0/3	0/3	0/3	2/3	1/3

Chart legend:
—■— Prioritization
—▲— Timely Intervention
—▲— SBAR
—●— Med Administration
—+— Procedural
—×— Documentation

Scenario	Scenario Facilitator: Name Here	Percent Completion
MedSurg Post-Op Ileus Day 1		57%

Patient with nausea/vomitting, and an NG tube
Steps: (Missed steps denoted by *)

Delivering NG or Zofran within 30 minutes
*NG Placement within 30 minutes of order
*IS teaching or turn/cough/deep breath prior to end of shift

SBAR Seeking NG
NG connected to suction
NG to Nare
NPO signage on/near door
*Identify and replace infiltrated IV

Fall band on wrist
*Fall signage on/near door

Figure 7.2   Example Simulation Summary Report.

MedSurg PLE Day 1   58%
  patient requiring heparin
  Steps: (Missed steps denoted by *)
    *Start Heparin within 60 minutes of report end
    *Heparin @ 18 u/k/hr

    IVF @ 100 ml/hr
    Nicotine patch on patient
    Dressing on Wound
    Consult wound RN order on chart
    *SCD's on left leg

    HoB up
    10am Meds
    PRN Meds

MedSurg Post-Op Ileus Day 2   92%
  Patient with nausea/vomitting, and an NG tube
  Steps: (Missed steps denoted by *)
    Obtain blood sugar within 10 minutes of hypoglycemic episode
    Obtain blood sugar between 10-15 minutes after D50 push
    Start KCl within 90 minutes of scenario start
    SBAR Updating physician for hypoglycemic episode (Situation; Background; *Assessment; Recommendation; Readback)

    Foley D/C'd
    NG to suction
    NG to nare
    *Incision open to Air

    IVF @ 125ml/hour
    10am Meds
    11am Meds
    PRN Meds

MedSurg PLE Day 2   90%
  patient requiring heparin
  Steps: (Missed steps denoted by *)
    Stop Heparin within 60 minutes of report end
    Resume heparin within 75 minutes of stopping
    Call for RT within 10 minutes of SoB episode start
    Heparin @ 17 ml/kg/hr
    *IVF @ 100 ml/hr

    Moist to dry dressing
    10am Meds
    PRN Meds

MedSurg POA   87%
  Post-Op Appy who complains for nicotine
  Steps: (Missed steps denoted by *)
    Provide nicotine patch within 1 hour of initial complaint
    Hang blood within 30 minutes of arrival on the unit
    SBAR Abnormal Labs (Situation; *Background; *Assessment; Recommendation; Readback)

    Nicotine patch on patient
    IVF programmed @ 100 ml/hr using guardrails & Maint IV
    SCD's on both legs
    IS at bedside
    Correctly hung and running blood
    *Krames transfusion education at bedside
    *Smoking cessation education at bedside

    10am Meds
    11am Med
    PRN Meds

MedSurg Sepsis   81%
  Patient requiring lab assessment and multiple tasks
  Steps: (Missed steps denoted by *)
    Conduct assessment within 1 hour of report end
    Hang IVF within 15 minutes of order
    SBAR Unstable Vitals (Situation; Background; *Assessment; *Recommendation; *Readback)
    SBAR Handoff report to ICU RN (Situation; Background; *Assessment; *Recommendation)
    *NC on patient and @ 2-6L

    IVF Bolus @ 999 or 100 ml/hr
    Foley in place
    Pt transferred off unit
    10am Meds
    11am Meds
    PRN Meds

| Additional Topics Covered in Scenarios or Debriefing: |

  Infection Control Measures
  Hand Hygiene

Figure 7.2   Example Simulation Summary Report.   (cont.)

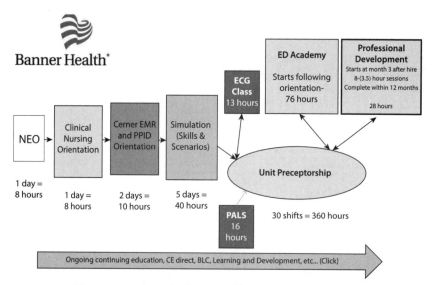

Figure 7.3   Sample New Graduate On-Boarding Pathway.

Simulation can be used to enforce advanced skills and decision-making; however, with new graduates, it is used more as the development opportunity, that is, as an education and action planning strategy to build up to those advanced skills and clinical reasoning moments. Simulations can also help new graduates move from didactic concepts and theories to practical application modality. For new graduate clinicians and health care employees, simulation might be the first introduction to the transference of theory and foundational principles into practice. Less is often more, and the scenarios and skills need not be designed with "intentional" errors, as most new graduates will make unintentional errors on their own. A novice differs from an expert in the ability to identify and rectify an error quickly.

Experienced Clinical Staff

As much as new graduates benefit from structure, experienced individuals might learn more about themselves and what they have or have not mastered in a more chaotic environment, that is, in large teams, with complex issues, noise, and adrenaline. Sometimes, it is not just the complexity of the simulated event that progresses with experience but also the location in which the simulations occur. Mock codes address a low-frequency, high-risk event. Most practitioners do not have much experience participating in codes. However, all need to be able to perform at optimal level when a code occurs. In situ simulations such as unit-based mock codes are ideal, in that the team that normally performs together practices together in the actual environment where the event would occur. In situ simulations can identify deficiencies in an individual, the team, the environment, or a process.

Banner Health has a system-wide postpartum hemorrhage scenario rollout, in which in situ simulations are done at every facility throughout seven states. This is a multidisciplinary effort in which blood bank, transport, administrative assistants, nurses, physicians, and anyone who would be involved at that facility if an actual event occurred are part of this simulated process. In 2012, at almost every facility in which the in situ simulations were performed, within a day or two, an actual postpartum hemorrhage occurred. The feedback was overwhelmingly positive that the communication between groups was efficient and the process ran more smoothly than ever. Everyone knew what they had to do and knew how to respond to a request from another group because they had practiced it.

Simulation is used for team training, new initiatives, skills, regulatory requirements, annual education, and rollouts that include a change in processes for practice. Basic courses can be available for those who have not performed the skills recently, such as airway management, chest tube care or insertion, lumbar puncture, paracentesis, and thoracentesis to name a few procedures. Annual deep sedation training and malignant hyperthermia training (regulatory) or sepsis and pediatric asthma scenarios (initiatives) are examples of simulation scenarios that the experienced practitioner needs. The patient experience is an example of the practitioner demonstrating effective communication, questioning, and responsiveness with the patient based on evidence. This communication assures that the patient's concerns, needs, and questions are addressed. For the experienced learner, the patient experience is something that might be beneficial to perform in a simulation environment. The recorded playback enables practitioners to view their own responses and interactions. Remediation occurs if the behaviors do not meet the simulation objectives and the scenario can be repeated.

High stakes testing is another important use of simulation for all types and levels of learners. Normally, simulation is touted as a safe environment in which learners can make errors without retribution. High stakes testing is an exception as the results may determine whether the learner passes or fails or whether the test-taker can acquire or keep a job or remain in a program. High stakes testing is not new and has been used very extensively to demonstrate knowledge attainment. What is relatively new is that high stakes testing is now being used with simulation to demonstrate whether the learner or test-taker can perform. A few examples of high stakes testing in simulation are as follows:

- Emergency residents who must pass a number of emergency scenarios in order to remain or advance in the program
- Critical-care nurses who must demonstrate competence in advanced cardiac life support (ACLS) scenarios to receive the ACLS certification to continue in their current positions
- Physicians who have had complaints about their practice or skills and are evaluated using simulation scenarios or task trainers

Naturally, there are limitations, and, as the name implies, the stakes can be high. There are some questions to consider when using simulation in this manner:

- Is the learner a good test-taker or a good gamer?
- Is the simulation well written?
- Is there consistency of evaluators?
- What is the validity of the simulation as a test?
- How is it scored?

Community

Simulation is not only used in the medical, aeronautical, or business arenas but also in the community setting. Cardiopulmonary resuscitation (CPR) is a well-known simulated event that has a huge effect on saving lives. The American Heart Association (AHA) (2013) says that CPR provided immediately after sudden cardiac arrest can double or triple a victim's chance of survival, yet only 32% of cardiac arrest victims get CPR from a bystander. The motivation for performing bystander CPR is that it is usually performed on someone known to the bystander. Fire departments, community organizations, and medical organizations deliver CPR classes to those in the community. There are training kits from American Heart Association that can be used in the community, school, home, or wherever convenient; the kits include a mannequin and video that multiple people can use. Simulation has also been successfully used in disaster preparedness drills.

The community offers many opportunities for simulation, especially in the home care arena, that can lead to better and safer patient care. Caregivers, including family members, need to know how to give insulin shots, administer tracheotomy care, and manage pediatric asthma, to name a few skills. Just as nurses learned to inject a needle into an orange, a patient or caregiver can do so to get the feel and confidence to perform in the real setting. Return demonstration ensures learning and safe patient care. Ideally those in the community could be taught how to deal with worst-case scenarios such as a mucous plug in a tracheotomy.

Current simulation centers can also be a source of education for other venues that do not have access to simulation support. Banner Health supports physicians who take trauma education and airway management to rural communities In addition, school children and high school students can whet their interest in health care careers in the safe environment of a local simulation center.

Conclusion

Simulation is a valuable learning modality for all types and levels of learners. It is important to know how to use simulation for these different groups in order to maximize learning and meet intended objectives. Foundations of simulation cross all learner levels, although the manner in which simulation is used and the complexity of the scenarios might be different depending on the level of learner. Novices will be focused more on acquiring skills and applying basics, such as time management and procedural knowledge, to the scenarios. Advanced learners will be able to handle much more depth and complexity in the scenarios as well as have a deeper level of self-reflection; learners might even attain the level of high-stakes simulations for testing competencies. Technology utilization and vulnerability of the learner and group versus individual learning environments are foundational elements to contemplate when building simulation scenarios.

Practical elements such as pre-briefing, orientation to the simulator, and suspending disbelief are important in ensuring the simulation objectives are met versus situations in which the learner is focused on matters that are not related to the learning exercise. The mannequin/patient dying in the scenario can become the focus when it wasn't the main objective, or it can be a valued learning objective. Therefore, an important question to be discussed by the team developing the simulation is, "What will happen when a learner makes a mistake or error that could result in death?" Should the natural consequences of the action (that is, death) be allowed to occur, or should the scenario be stopped for an instructional moment? The level of the learner should be a major consideration in making this decision.

Using simulation to bridge the gap from academia to practice can help to get the learner ready to practice in a complex fast-paced environment more quickly and efficiently than previous apprenticeship models. From the perspective of the practitioner and the organization, quick assimilation into the workforce is a desirable outcome. More research is needed on the transfer of learning in simulation to actual skills, knowledge, and attitudes in the work environment. Simulation allows practice, demonstration, and application of learning as well as assessment and validation. Simulation is a safe place to make errors, to learn from mistakes, and to avoid patient harm.

References

American Heart Association (AHA) (2013). *CPR & sudden cardiac arrest (SCA)*. Retrieved from http://www.heart.org/HEARTORG/CPRAndECC/WhatisCPR/CPRFactsandStats/CPR-Statistics_UCM_307542_Article.jsp

Arizona Action Coalition. (2013, May 24). *Education practice collaborative*. Retrieved from http://www.futureofnursingaz.com/

Corvetto, M. A., & Taekman, J. M. (2013). To die or not to die? A review of simulated death. *Society for Simulation in Healthcare.8(1), 8-12.*

Finkelman, A., & Kenner, C. (2009). *Teaching IOM: Implications of the Institute of Medicine Reports for nursing education*. Silver Spring, Maryland: ANA.

Fitts, P. M., & Posner, M. I. (1967). *Human performance (Basic concepts in psychology series)*. Belmont, CA: Brooks/Cole.

Gaba, D. M. (2013). Simulations that are challenging to the psyche of participants. *Simulation in Healthcare, 8*(1), 4-7.

Institute of Medicine (IOM). (2011). *The future of nursing: Leading change, advancing health*. Washington, DC: The National Academies Press. Retrieved from www.thefutureofnursing.org/IOM-Report

Massachusetts Department of Higher Education (MDHE) (2010). *Nurse of the future— Nursing core competencies (2000-2013)*. Retrieved fromhttp://www.mass.edu/currentinit/currentinitNursingNurseFutureComp.asp

Truog, R., & Meyer, E. (2013). Deception and death in medical simulation. *Society for Simulation in Healthcare, 8*(1), 1-3.

*"Coming together is a beginning.
Keeping together is progress.
Working together is success."*

–Henry Ford

Using Health Care Simulation for Interprofessional Education and Practice

Janice C. Palaganas, PhD, RN, NP

8

With its experiential and boundless features, health care simulation is naturally evolving as a platform for interprofessional education (IPE) as the need for IPE becomes increasingly evident in patient safety and is recognized by professional, accrediting, and certifying bodies (Commission on Collegiate Nursing Education [CCNE], 2009; Institute of Medicine [IOM], 2007, 2010; Interprofessional Education and Healthcare Simulation Collaborative [IPEHCS-C], 2012; National League for Nursing Accrediting Commission [NLNAC], 2012; see Figure 8.1). Many challenges have evolved in the health care system that support the need for IPE. Over time, separate specialties and professions have been created to focus on specific aspects of patients' health and care such that a single profession today cannot adequately meet all the complex needs of patients. To keep patients safe, health care professionals are tasked to work together as a team; however, it is clear through medical error rates, root cause analyses, and patient outcome research that breaches in quality health care are often due to poor communication within health care professional teams (The Joint Commission [TJC], 2013; The Joint

OBJECTIVES

- Review the evolution of health care simulation as a platform for interprofessional education.
- Discuss the benefits and challenges of using simulation for interprofessional education.
- Inform implementation of simulation-enhanced interprofessional education within an organization using recommendations established for simulation-enhanced interprofessional education.
- Provide a framework to achieve successful simulation-enhanced interprofessional education.

Commission on Accreditation of Healthcare Organizations [JCAHO], 2005). Just as the significance of interprofessional practice has become apparent, the evidence that health care teams generally cannot figure out how to effectively work together has emerged as a major issue.

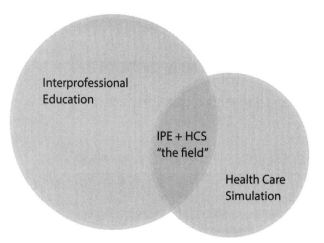

Interprofessional Education

IPE + HCS
"the field"

Health Care Simulation

Figure 8.1   The overlapping combined science of the fields of interprofessional education and health care simulation.

Teamwork failures stem from a variety of systemic gaps in our health care processes as well as fundamental human factors. Many systemic gaps have been revealed in the current education of health care professionals (Benner, Sutphen, Leonard, & Day, 2010). Interprofessional practice (IPP) opportunities are not guaranteed in pre-licensure curricula or post-licensure continuing education. Even when interprofessional conflict does occur, rather than allowing the student or junior clinician to work through the situation and gain the skills needed for effective collaboration, preceptors or experienced clinicians often step in and resolve the conflict. Students are typically educated in a silo track, graduate, and go to work in a health care setting; then they are expected to know how to work with colleagues from other disciplines. In assessing situations involving compromised patient care, it has become evident that without effective IPE, professions have difficulty figuring out how to work together as a team (Hean, Craddock, & Hammick, 2012). Educators also tend to teach the way they were taught and can be hesitant to try more effective ways (Bradshaw & Lowenstein, 2007). This becomes problematic because most clinicians learn what they do best on the job (for example, during apprenticeship) and through traditional teaching styles (for example, through unidirectional education such as a PowerPoint lecture). This style of learning does not match the style of younger, more technologically advanced students (Billings & Halstead, 2009). Accrediting, certifying, and professional bodies have recognized this need for IPP and have strongly recommended implementation of IPE. The need is clear; however, figuring out how to operationalize IPE has not been obvious.

The time for IPE is long overdue, and health care education is, therefore, shifting gears and moving in the direction of IPE to achieve safe patient care. IPE can occur using a variety of methods, including simulation. Educational modalities are continually examined for effectiveness in IPE. Team issues and interactions can be engineered through simulation-enhanced IPE, exposing future health care providers to relevant encounters that can grow effective teamwork. Simulation activities can occur in an array of settings (for example, simulation centers, in situ, virtual worlds) using varied modalities including mannequin-based simulations, standardized patients, embedded simulated persons, task training, team-based games, and serious games.

Health care simulation is increasingly recognized as an ideal vehicle for IPE. Educators and organizational leaders have become fascinated with the benefits of simulation and many simulation programs have sprouted in the last decade. Many of them purchase simulators, but they do not have the adequate resources or knowledge to use them appropriately or effectively. Other programs have discovered the science of effective simulation but have not had the resources to be able to share their knowledge with others. The result is that many organizations and educators are performing IPE using simulation without the requisite knowledge and skills. Educators look to published literature to assist in covering these gaps; however, the existing literature lacks the research evidence needed to guide educators on how to best structure and successfully implement simulation-based IPE (McGaghie, Issenberg, Petrusa, & Scalese, 2010; Palaganas, 2012; Reeves, Abramovich, Rice, & Goldman, 2012; Zhang, Thompson, & Miller, 2011). This chapter seeks to guide educators in understanding health care simulation as a platform for IPE by:

- Providing terms of reference to guide educators in simulation-enhanced IPE and to suggest a common language when sharing knowledge
- Providing thematic evidence from a synthesis of the research literature

- Providing recommendations from the 2012 Interprofessional Education and Healthcare Simulation Symposium on how to get started in simulation-enhanced IPE
- Describing challenges identified in simulation-enhanced IPE
- Providing theoretical frameworks that may serve as a foundation to simulations
- Providing a development, implementation, and practice framework for simulation-enhanced IPE that assists in overcoming the challenges in this science

Terms of Reference

Despite defined concepts in IPE and health care simulation, terminology often varies across literature, professions, geographical boundaries, and institutions. Acknowledging that a standardized language is essential, these terms of reference are listed in the nearby sidebar to create working definitions for the purposes of facilitating discussions with reduced miscommunications. Educators and researchers are encouraged to explore and refine these terms through further concept analyses and studies.

Terms Related to Interprofessional Education

Crisis resource management (CRM) is an approach to managing critical situations in a health care setting. Crisis resource management training develops communication skills. Originally developed in aviation and, as a result, also called crew resource management, crisis resource management emphasizes the role of "human factors"—the effects of fatigue and expected or predictable perceptual errors, as well as the effects of different management styles and organizational cultures in high-stress, high-risk environments (Gaba, Howard, Fish, Smith, & Sowb, 2001; Helmreich, Merritt, & Willhelm, 1999).

Interdisciplinary learning "involves integrating the perspective of professionals from two or more professions, by organizing the education around a specific discipline, where each discipline examines the basis of their knowledge" (Howkins & Bray, 2008, p. xviii).

Interprofessional education/training (IPE) describes those occasions "when two or more professions learn with, from and about each other to improve collaboration and the quality of care" (Center for Advancement of Interprofessional

Education [CAIPE], 2005, para. 1). "It is an initiative to secure *interprofessional learning* and promote gains through interprofessional collaboration in professional practice" (Freeth, Hammick, Reeves, Koppel, & Barr, 2005, p. xv). "**Formal interprofessional education** aims to promote collaboration and enhance the quality of care; therefore, it is an educational or practice development initiative that brings people from different professions together to engage in activities that promote interprofessional learning. The intention for formal interprofessional education is for curricula to achieve this aim" (Freeth et al., 2005, p. xiv). **"Informal (or 'serendipitous') interprofessional education** is unplanned learning between professional practitioners, or between students on *uniprofessional* or *multi-professional* programs, which improves interprofessional practice. At its inception, it lacks the intention of interprofessional education. At any point in time after that it may be acknowledged that learning with, from and about each other is happening between participants. However, in many such initiatives, this remains unacknowledged or is only recognized on reflection in and on the learning practice" (Freeth et al., 2005, p. xiv).

Interprofessional learning (IPL) is "learning arising from interaction between members (or students) of two or more professions. This may be a product of *interprofessional education* or happen spontaneously in the workplace or in education settings (for example, from *serendipitous interprofessional education*)" (Freeth et al., 2005, p. xv).

Interprofessionalism is "the effective integration of professionals through mutual respect, trust, and support, from various professions who share a common purpose to mold their separate skills and knowledge into collective responsibility and awareness that can be achieved through learned processes for communication, problem solving, conflict resolution, and conducting evaluation" (Palaganas & Jones, submitted for publication).

Intraprofessional involves activity between or among individuals within the same profession with similar or different specialties or levels of practice (for example, surgeon and emergency physician; clinical nurse and nurse practitioner; resident and physician).

Multidisciplinary involves bringing professionals with different perspectives together to provide a wider understanding of a particular problem (Howkins & Bray, 2008).

Multiprofessional education (MPE) is "when members (or students) of two or more professions learn alongside one another: in other words, parallel rather than interactive learning. Also referred to as **common or shared learning**" (Freeth et al., 2005, p. xv).

continues

continued

Simulation-enhanced Interprofessional Education is the use of health care simulation modalities for interprofessional education. **Simulation-based Interprofessional Education** describes simulations that were created using interprofessional learning objectives and students from two or more professions learn with, from, and about each other during the simulation; whereas **interprofessional simulations** describe simulations that were created using clinical, diagnosis-centered, or task-focused learning objectives, and students from two or more professions participate in the simulation, learning in parallel and not necessarily from and about each other during the simulation (Palaganas, 2012).

Transdisciplinary is a strategy that crosses many disciplinary boundaries to create a holistic approach to development and attempts to overcome the confines of individual disciplines to form a team that crosses and recrosses disciplinary boundaries and thereby maximizes communication, interaction, and cooperation among team members (Freeth et al., 2005).

Uniprofessional education is when members (or students) of a single profession learn together (Freeth et al., 2005; Howkins & Bray, 2008).

State of the Science

In a recent review of health care simulation and IPE research literature (Palaganas, 2012), there were 5,547 "hits" that surfaced from a general search of six literature databases from the years 1800 to 2012 using 33 single search terms for simulation and team training and multiple Boolean combinations. Most were found to be descriptive without reported or measured outcomes. A common theme throughout the literature considered for future directions included studying patient outcomes; however, few engaged in this type of patient outcome-based research. A meta-analysis of the current literature was not appropriate because the literature generally lacked adequate methodological strength, strength of findings, and similarity in research questions, variables, populations, or measures (Palaganas, 2012). Investigators generally reported positive outcomes in regard to participant satisfaction, describing verbal enthusiastic feedback from participants and faculty. Despite positive reports, a synthesis of these studies showed low rigor in research design and inadequate report of potential variables, lowering the confidence in findings.

The Benefits and Challenges of Simulation-Enhanced IPE

Recognizing the need to assess the community, Palaganas, Wilhaus, & Andersen (manuscript submitted for publication) surveyed educators in 2012 who use health care simulation for IPE and analyzed the responses. Respondents felt that simulation is an attractive method for IPE because:

- It provides a safe environment by keeping real patients safe.
- Without IPE, there is a lack of opportunities in clinical settings for skill development.
- It provides a realistic experience.
- Learners are more engaged in experiential and active learning.
- It is deliberate practice.
- It provides a standardized experience.

Those who felt that simulation was more effective than other IPE activities at achieving interprofessional learning objectives attributed this perception to realism, practice, debriefing and reflection, increased learner engagement, relevance of the experience, fostered interaction, safe environment, opportunity for feedback, immediacy of feedback, immersive experience, framework for learning communication, and the emotional experience. Those who felt it was less effective highlighted the importance of protecting the psychological safety (intrapsychological consequences on an individual from the interpersonal risks or past cognitive connections made during the simulation) of learners during the simulation and how simulation, if not done "right," may be more detrimental to positive IPL (Palaganas et al., manuscript submitted for publication).

Palaganas, Wilhaus, and Andersen (manuscript submitted for publication) found that the challenges during implementation of the simulation-based IPE reflected common challenges found in simulation-based education as well as those found in IPE. Of the common challenges found in simulation, costs and resources were a barrier for simulation-enhanced IPE (McGaghie et al., 2010). Of the common challenges found in IPE, scheduling, logistics, and organizing the different programs or professions were large barriers for simulation-enhanced IPE (Freeth et al., 2005). Table 8.1 shows simulation-specific challenges during IPE implementation and potential strategies to address these challenges.

Table 8.1   Simulation-Enhanced IPE Challenges and Potential Strategies to Resolve Them

Simulation-Enhanced IPE Challenges	Potential Strategies for Resolution
Problems with audio recording or live streaming	Dry run using audio recording, live streaming, and playback of video
Scenario development that engages all disciplines and learning levels	Include educators or content experts from all involved disciplines during scenario development
Lab scheduling and schedule conflicts	Implement an Interprofessional Curricula Cross-Matching Committee whose responsibility is to bring to the table the programmatic curricula and competencies for their programs and highlight where the curricula or content overlap and where courses or labs can be scheduled together
Mannequin electronic failure	Educator development on creative ways to overcome potential mannequin glitches during simulations
Need for simulator operator training	Schedule inservices with vendor educators or technicians to teach faculty or technicians to use simulators; dry runs with full simulator operation
Lack of faculty expertise in technology, simulation, and debriefing	Send educators to simulation educator development training or develop apprenticeship program for faculty
Interprofessional debriefing	Reflect on personal assumptions, explore a learner's frame/mental model prior to opening to discussion; use reflective practice by allowing learners to discover areas of interprofessional practice and improvements
No technology support	Find educators or students who are technologically inclined; work with IT department

Simulation-Enhanced IPE Challenges	*Potential Strategies for Resolution*
Not having enough time	Prioritize objectives and debriefing points and limit either simulation or debriefing to the points that are critical to cover
Lack of pre-briefing	Educator development on the importance of pre-briefing and its effect on learning using simulation
Fidelity/realism/accurate reflection of the phenomenon	Dry run scenario with practicing providers
Difference in objectives of each of the involved faculty (for example, one profession is looking for team training; the other is looking for skills training)	Involve educators from each profession in the curriculum and scenario development. Understand each educator's personal objectives for the course and aim for negotiation and consensus of overall course objectives. This maintains educator buy-in and success of the course.
Difficulty with assessing team performance	Educator development around assessment; research existing team performance assessment tools; contact programs that have performed team assessment

Themes in Simulation-Enhanced IPE

A distinction has been made in IPE literature between IPE and multiprofessional educa-tion. IPE describes those occasions in which two or more professionals learn with, from, and about each other to improve collaboration and the quality of care (CAIPE, 2005). Multiprofessional education occurs when learners from two or more professions learn alongside one another—in other words, parallel rather than interactive learning (Freeth et al., 2005). IPE literature offers evidence that learning is better achieved through IPE versus multiprofessional education (Canadian Interprofessional Health Collaborative [CIHC], 2010).

This distinction can also be made in health care simulation and appears in two forms that Palaganas (2012) refers to as simulation-based interprofessional education and interprofessional simulation. These methods depend on the objectives specified for the simulation. Simulation-based IPE refers to a simulation that was structured according to IPE objectives in which two or more professionals learn with, from, and about each other to improve collaboration and the quality of care. Interprofessional simulation corresponds with multiprofessional education and involves learners from two or more professions learning alongside one another in the simulation. In interprofessional simulation, the simulation is structured around a patient condition or situation that requires coordination and demonstration of skills specific to the individual professions. By nature, debriefing as a separate modality fosters simulation-based IPE. Most high-technology simulations couple debriefing with the interprofessional simulation and, therefore, provide a hybrid approach of interprofessional simulation to simulation-based IPE.

Given the complexity of the combined science of health care simulation and IPE, multiple confounding variables exist from one simulation group to the other and from one simulation program to another. Single-site studies generally serve as a limitation; however, given the variability of simulation programs, using multiple sites might contribute a multitude of unnecessary confounding variables. Details of the published studies and activities, including potential confounding variables, were limited, which, in turn, limited the ability to study characteristics that influence positive and negative outcomes. This limitation also makes generalizability and replication extremely difficult. Palaganas (2012) suggests reporting points (directly in publication or as an addendum to the publication) that could allow another site to replicate one's work and provide the ability for future literature synthesis to determine characteristics that influence outcomes. These reporting points (see Table 8.2) may also serve as a development guide for researchers looking to use simulation-enhanced IPE.

The review of literature and survey assessment reflected the complexities of health care simulation and IPE including the use of multiple teaching methods without comparison; the lack of valid and reliable measures; multiple confounding variables (reported and not reported, with many variables yet to be identified in the field); differences in learning levels, and differences in sample sizes of the involved professions. Despite the lack of strong findings presented in the literature, the literature and survey results—as a whole—hint that simulation is an excellent platform for IPE. Learners positively perceive simulation as a learning method (McGaghie et al., 2010). The literature has also shown that if an educator does not prepare well enough, is not prepared to deal with an interprofessional group, or does not use a simulation method to reach level-appropriate objectives, then the teaching platform would not be a good fit for learning (Cooper, Carlisle, Gibbs, and Watkins, 2001; Freeth et al., 2005).

Table 8.2   Suggested Reporting Points for IPE and Health Care Simulation Research

Objectives

- Aims and purpose of study (Manuscript)
- Objectives of educational activity
- Objectives of simulation activity

Background

- Terminology and definitions used by author
- Current existing literature

Learners

- Sample sizes (total and per professional group)
- Profession or program
- Grade level
- Team composition in simulation

Educators/Researchers

- Backgrounds/credentials
- Composition for development of study and educational activity
- Composition for implementation of study and educational activity

Method

- Design
- Theoretical framework
- Interventions

Simulation Modality

- Type, model, and version
- Details of scenario (consider video supplement and scenario appendix)
- Structure of debriefing if incorporated (consider video supplement and appendix if structured or semistructured)

Table 8.2   Suggested Reporting Points for IPE and Health Care Simulation Research   *(cont.)*

Measures

- Why chosen
- Validity
- Reliability

Results

Discussion

- Simulation factors that may have led to positive outcomes
- Simulation factors that may have led to negative outcomes
- Challenges encountered
- Strengths of study design
- Limitations of study design
- Areas for future study

Source: Palaganas, 2012

Getting Started

According to Tekian, McGuire, and McGaghie (1999), expert opinion is the best and most logical source when there is an absence of clear data. The field of IPE and health care simulation has advanced logically with thoughtful due processes within individual simulation programs and the development of professional societies and interest groups. These advancements may be seen through national competencies and recommendations developed by leaders of multiple professional organizations.

Competencies and Recommendations

To create a coordinated effort across health professions and provide strategies toward collaborative learning, interprofessional competencies have been developed by the Interprofessional Education Collaborative Expert Panel (IPECEP) in 2010 that developed interprofessional competency domains (IPECEP, 2011a). The group came to consensus on four domains:

1. Values/Ethics for Interprofessional Practice

2. Roles/Responsibilities

3. Interprofessional Communication

4. Teams and Teamwork

The IPECEP met again in 2011 to develop specific competencies under these domains (see Table 8.3; IPECEP, 2011b). These competencies may be used by educators to set objectives for the simulation-based IPE.

Table 8.3   Interprofessional Collaborative Practice Competencies

Domain 1: Values/Ethics for Interprofessional Practice

VE1. Place the interests of patients and populations at the center of interprofessional health care delivery.

VE2. Respect the dignity and privacy of patients while maintaining confidentiality in the delivery of team-based care.

VE3. Embrace the cultural diversity and individual differences that characterize patients, populations, and the health care team.

VE4. Respect the unique cultures, values, roles/responsibilities, and expertise of other health professions.

VE5. Work in cooperation with those who receive care, those who provide care, and others who contribute to or support the delivery of prevention and health services.

VE6. Develop a trusting relationship with patients, families, and other team members (CIHC, 2010).

VE7. Demonstrate high standards of ethical conduct and quality of care in one's contributions to team-based care.

VE8. Manage ethical dilemmas specific to interprofessional patient- or population-centered care situations.

VE9. Act with honesty and integrity in relationships with patients, families, and other team members.

VE10. Maintain competence in one's own profession appropriate to scope of practice (IPECEP, 2011b, p. 19).

Table 8.3	Interprofessional Collaborative Practice Competencies *(cont.)*

Domain 2: Roles/Responsibilities

RR1. Communicate one's roles and responsibilities clearly to patients, families, and other professionals.

RR2. Recognize one's limitations in skills, knowledge, and abilities.

RR3. Engage diverse health care professionals who complement one's own professional expertise, as well as associated resources, to develop strategies to meet specific patient care needs.

RR4. Explain the roles and responsibilities of other care providers and how the team works together to provide care.

RR5. Use the full scope of knowledge, skills, and abilities of available health professionals and health care workers to provide care that is safe, timely, efficient, effective, and equitable.

RR6. Communicate with team members to clarify each member's responsibility in executing components of a treatment plan or public health intervention.

RR7. Forge interdependent relationships with other professions to improve care and advance learning.

RR8. Engage in continuous professional and interprofessional development to enhance team performance.

RR9. Use unique and complementary abilities of all members of the team to optimize patient care (IPECEP, 2011b, p. 21).

Domain 3: Interprofessional Communication

CC1. Choose effective communication tools and techniques, including information systems and communication technologies, to facilitate discussions and interactions that enhance team function.

CC2. Organize and communicate information with patients, families, and health care team members in a form that is understandable, avoiding discipline-specific terminology when possible.

CC3. Express one's knowledge and opinions to team members involved in patient care with confidence, clarity, and respect, working to ensure common understanding of information and treatment and care decisions.

CC4. Listen actively and encourage ideas and opinions of other team members.

CC5. Give timely, sensitive, instructive feedback to others about their performance on the team, responding respectfully as a team member to feedback from others.

CC6. Use respectful language appropriate for a given difficult situation, crucial conversation, or interprofessional conflict.

CC7. Recognize how one's own uniqueness, including experience level, expertise, culture, power, and hierarchy within the health care team, contributes to effective communication, conflict resolution, and positive interprofessional working relationships (University of Toronto, 2008).

CC8. Communicate consistently the importance of teamwork in patient-centered and community-focused care (IPECEP, 2011b, p. 23).

Domain 4: Teams and Teamwork

TT1. Describe the process of team development and the roles and practices of effective teams.

TT2. Develop consensus on the ethical principles to guide all aspects of patient care and team work.

TT3. Engage other health professionals—appropriate to the specific care situation—in shared patient-centered problem solving.

TT4. Integrate the knowledge and experience of other professions—appropriate to the specific care situation—to inform care decisions while respecting patient and community values and priorities/preferences for care.

TT5. Apply leadership practices that support collaborative practice and team effectiveness.

TT6. Engage self and others to constructively manage disagreements about values, roles, goals, and actions that arise among healthcare professionals and with patients and families.

TT7. Share accountability with other professions, patients, and communities for outcomes relevant to prevention and health care.

TT8. Reflect on individual and team performance for individual, as well as team, performance improvement.

TT9. Use process improvement strategies to increase the effectiveness of interprofessional teamwork and team-based care.

TT10. Use available evidence to inform effective teamwork and team-based practices.

TT11. Perform effectively on teams and in different team roles in a variety of settings (IPECEP, 2011b, p. 25).

Source: IPECEP, 2011b

At a third national collaborative in 2012, the Society for Simulation in Healthcare (SSH) and the National League for Nursing (NLN) Symposium on Interprofessional Education and Healthcare Simulation explored the use of simulation as an instrument for advancing IPE and practice using the domains and competencies developed by IPEC (Wilhaus et al., 2013). Commonly reported gaps identified in simulation-enhanced IPE knowledge included:

- The lack of substantive and specific accreditation mandates
- Insufficient infrastructure and resources
- A paucity of research support mechanisms that demonstrate the effect of simulation-enhanced IPE on quality and safety
- Logistical challenges (for example, scheduling and coordination)
- Cultural challenges

There were consensus recommendations developed for organizations and for individuals. The recommendations for individuals were presented in ten steps (Wilhaus et al., 2013):

1. Examine personal assumptions, knowledge, and skills relative to health care simulation, IPE, and simulation-enhanced IPE.

2. Identify and engage local spheres of influence and share information about the IPEC competencies.

3. Conduct formal and informal educational offerings.

4. Promote IPE and simulation-enhanced IPE through the use of social media.

5. Participate in regional, state, and national conferences to showcase and learn more about simulation-enhanced IPE.

6. Submit manuscripts and publications about simulation-enhanced IPE.

7. Review and enhance current simulation scenarios to ensure that they align with the IPEC competencies.

8. Use research reports to provide evidence which link simulation-enhanced IPE to quality and safe patient outcomes.

9. Employ evaluation tools that focus on IPE.

10. Access and add simulation-enhanced IPE resources through the MedEdPortal or iCollaborative.

Educators and organizations can use these steps as a guideline to prepare and implement simulation-enhanced IPE.

Characteristics That Influence Outcomes in Simulation-Enhanced IPE

With the evolving technology-integrated lifestyles of today's learners, educators are obligated to change the structured didactic curricula of the past to a more conducive learning platform. The use of simulation in health care, in its highly experiential and interactive form, fosters a new culture of learning. For optimal learning using simulation, educators must acknowledge and understand characteristics in simulation-enhanced IPE so that educational opportunities can be effectively engineered into the simulation. A few foundational characteristics are presented in this section.

The Challenge of a New Science

Health care simulation and IPE continue separately in a discovery phase attempting to define and redefine language, taxonomies, characteristics, and the variables that influence outcomes. These limitations are imposed on this combined field in a two-fold fashion, requiring a collaboration of the most artistic, inventive, tolerant, and detail-oriented scientists (Schneider, 2009). Although the literature is deemed "inadequate" with educators frequently "reinventing the wheel," the state of the field is not only appropriate; it is a necessary process. According to Uhlig, Lloyd, and Raboin (personal communication, June 16, 2012), often it is the social process of working together to understand and find new ways of doing things that generates new capabilities in a health care team, rather than the specific techniques or methods that are developed or used. In other words, the "wheel" should not be the focus; instead the focus should be on the social and relational work that's necessary for replication (for example, word limits, journal requirements for methods used). Finding additional venues (such as web addendums to journals) to report details as listed in Table 8.2 is a critical key to covering gaps in this science.

Case Example

Professor Jones has developed an interest in IPE and has been asked to work with the simulation center to develop IPE for the schools of nursing, pharmacy, and medicine. In search of a model, she found a journal article that sounds like what she wants to implement and shows significant outcomes in learning teamwork. The article only has a paragraph on the simulation scenario, and she realizes that she needs to fill in details. Taking the advice of this chapter, she assembles a team of faculty from each of the schools to develop the scenario and the objectives of the IPE. The team spends three long meetings coming to agreement on the objectives alone. Although Professor Jones may have imposed the objectives and scenario from another model to facilitate the development, the process of understanding the desires of the different faculty and schools, understanding the gaps in the literature, and finding ways to work with her team to agree on objectives generated a team and increased knowledge and ownership essential to the IPE they will develop, implement, measure, and report.

Educator Characteristics

A long-standing variable in education is the expertise, quality, and "likeability" of educators by learners, colleagues, and superiors alike. Interprofessional education requires additional knowledge in:

- Interprofessional practice as applicable to the learner groups
- IPE competencies, as well as the newest research and recommendations for IPE
- IPE planning, design, implementation, and formulation of design and evaluation teams
- Spheres of influence and change theory
- Translational research
- Assessment of learners in IPE, including existing validated and reliable evaluation instruments (Hammick, Freeth, Koppel, Reeves, & Barr, 2008; Howkins & Bray, 2008)

Furthermore, as outlined in the Society for Simulation in Healthcare (SSH) Domains for Certified Healthcare Simulation Educators (2012), educators using simulation require additional knowledge in:

- Experiential teaching and learning theory
- Simulation equipment
- Simulation principles, practice, equipment, and methodology
- Assessment of learners using simulation
- Management of simulation resources and environments
- Engagement in simulation scholarly activities

The level of an educator's knowledge in these areas, along with teaching talent, professional values, and capabilities, can greatly influence a learner group's outcomes.

Preventing Adverse Learning

While creating and implementing simulation-enhanced IPE, educators have an obligation to recognize and be mindful of the possibility that negative perspectives around interprofessional practice may develop. Although adverse learning experiences might occur randomly, the likelihood for positive outcomes may depend on factors of educator knowledge, including substantial planning using an anticipatory design, awareness for and support of possible characteristics that lead to positive outcomes, and recognition of and purposeful muting of possible characteristics that lead to negative outcomes.

Case Example

An attending obstetrician who was previously an L&D nurse was leading a debriefing with residents she had mentored previously and new nursing staff. Before the debriefing began, one of the residents joked, "At least I wasn't the nurse." The attending chuckled, remembering when she was the nurse, and began the debriefing. Throughout the debriefing, the nurses were very upset at the resident's joke and were not engaging in the debriefing; they also gave the IPE low evaluation scores. The attending was not aware of her light laughter, was not transparent in her thought in the moment (her previous nursing experience), and was not aware of the negative effect it caused for the learners.

Modality Matching

The reliability of the simulation should include "modality matching." Highly realistic and complex simulations are not always appropriate (Jeffries, Clochesy, & Hovancsek, 2009). All simulators have strengths and limitations. Educators are given yet another responsibility—to know the capabilities, strengths, and limitations of available simulation equipment. These capabilities should be matched to the learning objectives set by faculty, the learning level of the learners, and the cues necessary to guide learners toward achieving the learning objectives. Although educators involved in health care simulation often focus on the realism of the environment and the simulator, the realism chosen may not be appropriate. Because simulation-enhanced IPE seeks common learning ground, the objectives are often around teamwork, communication, and resource management and require more focus around making the communication opportunities more realistic.

Case Example

The simulation staff received a scenario developed by the university interprofessional lab committee. It involved a traumatic arrest and one objective—for the learners to call the OR team. The simulation staff spent hours moulaging the mannequin and staging the simulated trauma bay, achieving a highly realistic environment. During the simulation, the physicians were so focused on the bleeding mannequin, the nurses were so focused on beeping alarms, and the respiratory therapists were so focused on the mannequin's compromised airway, that the learners spent little time speaking and did not access the OR team. The scenario focused mainly on the realism of the environment and did not build in opportunities for communication or prompts to guide the learners to meet the objective of the scenario; instead, it created opportunities for failure to achieve the learning objective. The simulation would have been more effective in reaching the objective if there were less environmental noise and more social noise, for example, an embedded simulated health care provider to facilitate communication with the team.

Equal Opportunity for Professions

Educators have ethical obligations that require them to reflect on their individual desires for the education along with their personal assumptions. Often, educators seek participants from other professions to add a more realistic experience to a simulation designed for one profession. This creates a uniprofessional design that may benefit one group of learners more than other professional groups, potentially creating negative learning and proliferating the very stereotypes that IPE strives to alleviate. When asking other professions to participate, educators should involve other content expert educators from the added profession to create equal learning opportunities.

During debriefing, many assumptions arise in conversation—from both students and educators. Educators, in this context, are often role models and should be aware of their own personal assumptions around the professions involved, the value of IPE, and their preferences related to health care simulation to prevent modeling views that may be adverse to the intended learning.

Case Example

An attending emergency physician has been running a very successful simulation course for emergency resident physicians. The Joint Commission has been encouraging IPE. The attending decided to make the simulation course interprofessional by asking her friend, a school of nursing professor, to bring her senior level BSN students. The nursing students participated as learners alongside the residents during the simulation. The attending debriefed the residents as she normally debriefs this course and then asks the nursing students to share their experience and perspectives developed from the simulation. Although the nursing students were grateful to participate in a simulation with residents, there were no specific objectives developed for the nursing students. The participation of the nursing students, however, helped the residents meet their learning objectives. This simulation might have had equal opportunity if objectives were developed for the nursing students to meet their specific learning needs and if the residents also help them meet their learning objectives.

Debriefing Facilitation Skills

Fanning and Gaba (2007) posit that debriefing, more so than the active simulation, is where learning takes place. The idea is that guided reflection or facilitator-led discussions create prolonged learning through reconstruction of the events, self-reflection, and cognitive assimilations. Whether learning occurs primarily during the simulation (by working together) or during the debriefing (reflecting on team skills using a common experience) is unclear. In debriefing, students also learn how to provide peer-to-peer and profession-to-profession feedback and, in this process, learn how to communicate their thoughts to a team of other professions. This skill is relevant to clinical practice and often lacking in the clinical setting, contributing to compromises in patient care. A focus on developing this skill of feedback and communication may be key in teaching health care providers how to work together.

Case Example

Debriefings following in situ simulation-enhanced IPE are often held in a less private area (such as a staff break room or standing at the bedside of the mannequin) in a short amount of time (for example, 15 minutes). The difficulty of IPE debriefing is to get learners in a comfort zone to be willing to share their thoughts about each other and each other's professions. A less private area and not enough time become significant barriers to creating this comfort and opportunity for deep reflection and feedback. Hence, the debriefer must possess effective facilitation skills that can either overcome these barriers or be effective within the limitations presented.

Learner Characteristics

By the definition of interprofessional education, participants are learning "with, from, and about" each other. Each participant brings unique knowledge, previous experiences, energy, attitudes and perspectives, personality, mental frames, and communication skills. The combination of these unique factors affects the co-creation of knowledge and might greatly influence the interprofessional learning. Therefore, depending on characteristics of the participants who compose a group (for example, their ages, ethnicities, genders, and clinical experiences), the learning will differ from group to group.

Group Familiarity

Group familiarity with one or more members also influences the learning outcomes. In groups that have more than one profession (for example, three nurses), the within-profession learners are typically familiar with each other. Knowing how team members work together might increase team comfort or, on the contrary, create subgroup fragmentation if there are only a few members who are familiar with each other. Whether the interprofessional learning is more efficient in working teams versus ad hoc teams has not yet been studied in simulation-enhanced IPE, but it might be a significant group characteristic affecting outcomes.

Observers Versus Active Participants

Due to larger group sizes and limitations on simulation resources, simulation often involves observers and active participants. The participants observing a simulation in which active participants are in the clinical environment often actively engage in reflection using reflecting team-structured debriefings. Observing participants may also be "activated" by using structured observational tools. Whether observation through video projection and one-way mirrors serves as a concrete experience or not is unclear. Whether debriefing serves as a concrete experience is also not clear.

Some simulation-enhanced IPE has professions participate in the simulation as another profession to gain a sense of role differences and similarities. Although this may be a valuable experience, it should only be used for activities appropriate to objectives around role clarity or other appropriate objectives. If the objectives are around communication and a nurse is participating as a physician, the realism of the simulation is compromised in that the nurse may not communicate the way a physician would, but rather the way the nurse believes a physician communicates and vice versa. This dilemma is also present when using cross-profession evaluations or observations. Health care professions are beginning to realize that each profession has a specialized language and culture that another profession might not understand; therefore, if one profession is evaluating another, gaps in the observation might occur.

Psychological Safety

A fundamental characteristic for the use of simulation methods is the establishment of psychological safety (Council for the Accreditation of Healthcare Simulation Programs (CAHSP), 2012). For learners to fully engage in a simulation, their fears or potential fears should be addressed or insecurities resolved. For example, students may be worried if their grading professor is behind the mirror or will be reviewing the video (if used). Confidentiality of their performance may affect simulation behavior and the resulting learning outcomes. Although scenarios are typically developed to fit curricular needs, a particular scenario may elicit past memories in participants that could affect the learning of the group. These memories may be personal, traumatic, or sad. Educators must be able to address such a breach in psychological safety should it arise.

Psychological safety is particularly important to clinical-based learner groups or learners who work together on a day-to-day basis. If mistakes are made during the scenario then fear, embarrassment, and judgments may carry over to the day-to-day setting, creating discomfort and mistrust amongst the clinical team, which may contribute to ineffective patient care. Thus, educators must establish safety, address team issues, and hold these as priorities during the debriefing.

Simulation-enhanced IPE often requires the use of an embedded simulated provider who is often played by a clinician familiar to the learners. If this embedded simulated provider is a clinician who interacts with the learners frequently, their scenario and real life roles must be made clear to the learners and reinforced following the simulation so that the link to the actions during the scenario are clearly broken and the thoughts associated with the actions are not associated with the clinician.

Case Example

The nurse educator of a unit was asked to be an embedded simulated provider in a simulation involving nurses and physicians on the unit. In the simulation, the nurse educator plays the role of a clinical staff nurse who creates a medical error. The next day after the simulation course, the nurse educator works on the unit. She is paranoid that the physician she is working with during the shift might think that she is at risk of medical errors.

Simulation and Evaluation Design

Characteristics identified in simulation-enhanced IPE frequently concern the logistical design of the simulation. Questions regarding simulation design include:

- What effect do required versus elected courses involving IPE have on interprofessional learning?
- What is the most effective number of members and disciplines comprising a team for simulation-enhanced IPE?
- With pre-licensure students, is it more effective for students to engage in simulation-enhanced IPE in their current role as students or in their post-licensure role?
- What effect does clinical experience have on an individual and team involved in IPE?

Overcoming Challenges

There are many challenges in simulation-enhanced IPE. Having a solid grasp of theoretical frameworks can provide options and solutions. You can find a detailed discussion of theoretical frameworks in Chapter 1. In addition, a framework specific to establishing content validity, reliability, and assessment in simulation-enhanced IPE is suggested in this section and may be helpful in the development of quality simulations.

Theoretical Frameworks

Discovering the undeveloped areas of the IPE field, educators have turned to theoretical frameworks to guide the development of a learning program and to guide facilitation of the learning. Traditionally, theory has been defined as "an abstract generalization that offers a systematic explanation about how phenomena are interrelated" (Polit & Beck, 2012, p. 126). Generally, theory connotes an abstraction (Polit & Beck, 2012). Hence, IPE or health care simulation educators are basing their methods on varied theories (from opinions, suggestions, and recommendations). Educational theories such as cognitive theory (Piaget & Inhelder, 1973), behavioral theory (Watson, 1930), constructivist theory (Vygotsky, 1978), adult learning theory (Knowles, 1980), experiential learning theory (Kolb, 1984), educational theory (Wall, 2001), contact theory (Allport, 1954), change theory (Lewin, 1946), and situated learning theory (Lave & Wenger, 1991) have been developed and have provided structure and guidance to instructional strategies and learning activities in simulation-enhanced IPE.

SimBIE RVA Framework

When used for IPE, simulation is most often used as a tool to achieve interprofessional learning. Just like any educational tool, quality education ensues from validation and reliability testing. Based on the thoughts and findings from the study by Palaganas (2012), the following framework is offered to educators and researchers in the field.

This Simulation-based IPE Reliability-Validity-Assessment (SimBIE RVA) Framework (see Figure 8.2) might fill gaps identified in this chapter and reinforce the endeavors of the field (Palaganas, 2012). It can be a resource for educators, researchers, and simulation programs intent upon building interprofessional learning through simulation-enhanced IPE. Discussions in this chapter indicate the difficulty in establishing reliability, validity, and accurate assessment due to the complexity of and uncertainties within the IPE field.

Complexity and uncertainty cause difficulties in establishing strong, valid, and reliable findings. The SimBIE RVA Framework might help educators and researchers further understand their simulation and IPE practice, clarify complex areas already studied, and build their own curriculum for interprofessional learning using existing evidence and findings as a foundation. Many educators or organizations have already developed a similar simulation-enhanced IPE. Seeking these resources may provide roadmaps that can assist in the development of new programs or improvement of existing programs.

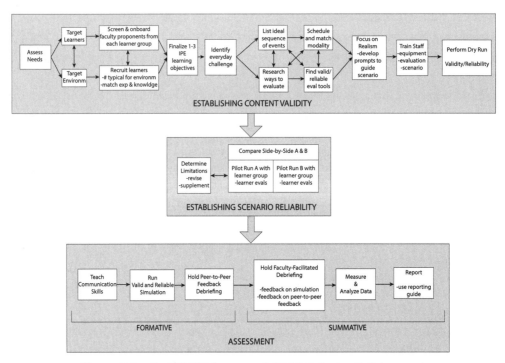

Figure 8.2   SimBIE RVA framework (2012 © Janice C. Palaganas)

Conclusion

Because the field of health care simulation and IPE has entered a discovery and exploratory stage, thoughtful reporting will be crucial to future developments. This chapter has provided information on health care simulation and IPE from the literature, national discussions and efforts, and considerable reflection of terminology and characteristics. It contributes to the growing findings around factors in IPE methods that influence positive and negative outcomes and also reveals many questions that are foundational for this science. Use of the information and tools presented in this chapter can assist in thoughtful planning for future simulation-enhanced IPE and research.

References

Allport, G. W. (1954). *The nature of prejudice.* Cambridge, MA: Perseus Books.

Benner, P., Sutphen, M., Leonard, V., & Day, L. (2010). *Educating nurses: A call for radical transformation.* San Francisco, CA: Jossey-Bass.

Billings, D. M., & Halstead, J. A. (2009). *Teaching in nursing: A guide for faculty* (3rd ed.). St. Louis, MO: Saunders Elsevier.

Bradshaw, M. J., & Lowenstein, A. J. (2007). *Innovative teaching strategies in nursing and related health professions* (4th ed.). Sudbury, MA: Jones and Bartlett.

Canadian Interprofessional Health Collaborative (CIHC). (2010). *A national interprofessional competency framework.* Vancouver, BC: Author. Retrieved from http://www.cihc.ca/resources/publications

Center for the Advancement of Interprofessional Education (CAIPE). (2005). Defining IPE. Retrieved from http://www.caipe.org.uk/about-us/defining-ipe

Commission on Collegiate Nursing Education (CCNE). (2009). *Standards for accreditation of baccalaureate and graduate degree nursing programs.* Washington, DC: Author.

Cooper, H., Carlisle, C., Gibbs, T., & Watkins, C. (2001). Developing an evidence base for interdisciplinary learning: A systematic review. *Journal of Advanced Nursing, 35*(2), 228-237.

Council for the Accreditation of Healthcare Simulation Programs (CAHSP). (2012). *Informational guide for the 2011 Society for Simulation in Healthcare Accreditation Program.* Wheaton, IL: Society for Simulation in Healthcare.

Fanning, R., & Gaba, D. (2007). The role of debriefing in simulation-based education. *Simulation in Healthcare, 2*(2), 115-125.

Freeth, D., Hammick, M., Reeves, S., Koppel, I., & Barr, H. (2005). *Effective interprofessional education: Development, delivery & evaluation.* Oxford, UK: Blackwell Publishing Ltd.

Gaba, D., Howard, S., Fish, K., Smith, B. & Sowb, Y. (2001). Simulation-based training in anesthesia crisis resource management: A decade of experience. *Simulation & Gaming, 32,* 175-193.

Hammick, M., Freeth, D., Koppel, I., Reeves, S., & Barr, H. (2008). A best evidence systematic review of interprofessional education. *Medical Teacher, 29*(8), 735-751.

Hean, S., Craddock, D., & Hammick, M. (2012). Theoretical insights into interprofessional education: AMEE guide No. 62. *Medical Teacher, 34*(2), 78-101.

Helmreich, R., Merritt, A., & Willhelm, J. (1999). The evolution of crew resource management training in commercial aviation. *International Journal of Aviation Psychology, 9*(1), 19-32.

Howkins, E., & Bray, J. (2008). *Preparing for interprofessional teaching.* Oxon, UK: Radcliffe Publishing Ltd.

Institute of Medicine (IOM). (2007). P. Aspden, J. A. Wolcott, J. Bootman, & L. R. Cronenwett (Eds.). *Preventing medication errors.* Washington, DC: The National Academies Press. Retrieved from http://www.nap.edu/catalog.php?record_id=11623

Institute of Medicine (IOM). (2010). *The future of nursing: Leading change, advancing health.* Washington, DC: The National Academies Press. Retrieved from www.thefutureofnursing.org/IOM-Report

Interprofessional Education and Healthcare Simulation Collaborative (IPEHCS-C). (2013). *A consensus report from the 2012 interprofessional education and healthcare simulation collaborative.* Wheaton, IL: Society for Simulation in Healthcare.

Interprofessional Education Collaborative Expert Panel (IPECEP). (2011a). *Team-based competencies: Building a shared foundation for education and clinical practice.* Washington, DC: Interprofessional Education Collaborative.

Interprofessional Education Collaborative Expert Panel (IPECEP). (2011b). *Core competencies for interprofessional collaborative practice: Report of an expert panel.* Washington, DC: Interprofessional Education Collaborative.

Jeffries, P. R., Clochesy, J. M.. & Hovancsek, M. T. (2009). Designing, implementing, and evaluating simulations in nursing education. In D. M. Billings & J. A. Halstead *Teaching in Nursing: A Guide for Faculty* (3rd ed.) (pp. 322-330). St. Louis, MO: Saunders Elsevier.

The Joint Commission (TJC). (2013). *Sentinel event data: Root causes by event type 2004-2012.* Chicago, IL: Author. Retrieved from www.jointcommission.org/sentinel_event.aspx

The Joint Commission on Accreditation of Healthcare Organizations (JCAHO). (2005). *Health care at the crossroads: Strategies for improving the medical liability system and preventing patient injury.* Chicago, IL: Author.

Knowles, M. (1980). *The modern practice of adult education: From pedagogy to andragogy.* Wilton, CT: Association Press.

Kolb, D. (1984). *Experiential learning: Experience as the source of learning and development.* Englewood Cliffs, NJ: Prentice-Hall.

Lave, J., & Wenger, E. (1991). *Situated learning: Legitimate peripheral participation.* Cambridge: Cambridge University Press.

Lewin, K. (1946). Action research and minority problems. *Journal of Social Issues.* 2(4), 34-46.

McGaghie, W., Issenberg, S. B., Petrusa, E., & Scalese, R. (2010). A critical review of simulation-based medical education research: 2003-2009. *Medical Education, 44*(1), 50-63.

National League for Nursing Accrediting Commission, Inc. (NLNAC). (2012). *NLNAC accreditation manual.* Atlanta, GA: Author. Retrieved from http://www.nlnac.org/manuals/NLNACManual2008.pdf

Palaganas, J. (2012). *Exploring healthcare simulation as a platform for interprofessional education* (Doctoral dissertation). Retrieved from ProQuest Dissertations and Theses database.

Palaganas, J. C., & Jones, P. *Interprofessionalism: A concept analysis.* Manuscript submitted for publication.

Palaganas, J. C., Wilhaus, J., & Andersen, J. *Results from the 2012 interprofessional education and healthcare simulation survey.* Manuscript submitted for publication.

Piaget, J., & Inhelder, B. (1973). *Memory and intelligence.* London: Routledge and Kegan Paul.

Polit, D., & Beck, C. (2012). *Nursing research: Generating and assessing evidence for nursing practice* (9th ed.). Philadelphia, PA: Wolters Kluwer Health, Lippincott Williams & Wilkins.

Reeves, S., Abramovich, I., Rice, K., & Goldman, J. (2012). *An environmental scan and literature review on interprofessional collaborative practice settings: Final report for Health Canada.* Li Ka Shing Knowledge Institute of St Michael's Hospital: University of Toronto.

Schneider, A. M. (2009). Four stages of scientific discipline; four types of scientists. *Trends in Biochemical Sciences, 34*(5), 217-223. doi: 10.1016/j.tibs.2009.02.002

Society for Simulation in Healthcare (SSH). (2012). *Certified Healthcare Simulation Educator Handbook.* Wheaton, IL: Author. Retrieved from https://ssih.org/uploads/static_pages/PDFs/Certification/CHSE_Handbook.pdf

Tekian, A., McGuire, C., & McGaghie, W. (1999). *Innovative simulations for assessing professional competence: From paper-and-pencil to virtual reality.* Chicago, IL: University of Illinois at Chicago, Dept. of Medical Education.

University of Toronto. (2008). *Advancing the interprofessional education curriculum 2009.* Curriculum overview. Competency framework. Toronto: University of Toronto, Office of Interprofessional Education.

Vygotsky, L. S. (1978). *Mind in society: The development of higher mental processes.* Cambridge, MA: Harvard University Press.

Wall, E. (Ed.). (2001). *Educational theory: Philosophical and political perspectives.* NY: Prometheus Books.

Watson, J. B. (1930). *Behaviorism* (revised edition). Chicago, IL: University of Chicago Press.

Wilhaus, J., Palaganas, J., Manos, J., Anderson, J., Cooper, A., Jeffries, P., ... Mancini, M. E. (2013). Interprofessional education and healthcare simulation symposium. IPE in healthcare simulation. Wheaton, IL: Society for Simulation in Healthcare.

Zhang, C., Thompson, S., & Miller, C. (2011). A review of simulation-based interprofessional education. *Clinical Simulation in Nursing, 7*(4), e117-e126.

Using Simulation in Academic Environments to Improve Learner Performance

Deborah Becker, PhD, ACNP, BC, CCNS

Providing education for health professions in the academic setting has changed significantly since the days of training with
the mantra "See one. Do one. Teach one." Today, in addition to
developing competent and confident health care professionals,
educators are concerned with the ethics of training with actual
patients and face the challenge of assuring consistent access
to specific clinical experiences adequate to prepare increasing
numbers of clinically competent providers confident in simple to
highly technical skills and complex reasoning (Ziv, Wolpe, Small,
& Glick, 2006).

Simulation is uniquely suited to help meet the challenges of
educating health care students in the academic environment. As
a teaching strategy, simulation has been demonstrated to provide a safe and effective approach to learning skills, developing
clinical thinking, and making critical decisions without placing
patients at risk for harm (Institute of Medicine [IOM], 2011).
Simulations can be constructed to deliver content in place of traditional lectures, to teach students how to perform specific skills,
and to teach students how to critically think through a clinical

OBJECTIVES

- Relate simulations and simulated learning strat-egies to educational theories.
- Identify a variety of ways simulation can be used for content delivery and development of psycho-motor skills.
- Describe approaches to teach early recognition and rescue situations.
- Discuss the importance of aligning technology with the objectives of the simulation.
- Compare and contrast the benefits of using various types of simula-tion approaches.
- Explain how simulation can be used for instruc-tion and evaluation.

situation. Simulations also can be designed to provide learners with a series of experiences that cannot be guaranteed to occur during their clinical practice time, as well as encourage teamwork, leadership, interprofessional practice, and communication. Learner acquisition of knowledge, skills, and abilities can be evaluated using simulation. These evaluations can be formative or summative. When properly designed, simulations can assure consistency in evaluative approach and can be used in high-stakes testing such as determining progression to the next level within a program or graduation.

Educational Theory and Simulation

The concept of learning as a function of the activity, context, and culture is based on the theory of contextual or situated learning. Active learning—in which participants are physically, mentally, and emotionally involved in the learning—is a profoundly more effective teaching strategy than more passive methods. Learners and their learning needs are at the center of active learning. Any number of teaching strategies can be employed to actively engage students in the learning process, including group discussions, problem solving, case studies, role-plays, journal writing, and structured learning groups. The benefits to using such activities are many, including improved critical-thinking skills, increased retention and transfer of new information, increased motivation, and improved interpersonal skills.

Simulation puts the learner into action, providing a contextually realistic environment in which the student is expected to demonstrate techniques, make clinically sound judgments, and respond dynamically to the situation (Bonwell & Eison, 1991). Simulation supports the educational theory of constructivism. Constructivism states that people construct their own understanding and knowledge of the world through experiencing things and reflecting on those experiences. When people encounter something new, they have to reconcile it with their previous ideas and experiences, maybe changing what they believed or maybe discarding the new information as irrelevant. In any case, learners are active creators of their own knowledge. Constructivism modifies the role of the educator to one that helps students to construct knowledge rather than recall facts. The educator provides tools such as problem-solving and inquiry-based learning activities to provide the students with the opportunities to apply their existing knowledge and real-world experience, learn to hypothesize and test their theories, and, ultimately, draw conclusions from their findings (Kolb, 1984). By actively participating in simulations, learners use their previously gained knowledge along with newly acquired abilities to work through new experiences. Afterward, learners participate in a debriefing session in which they are asked to reflect on their performances and the decision-making they exhibited during the simulation. This allows them to construct their own understanding, making changes to what they believe and either keeping or discarding the information as relevant or ir-relevant.

Adult learning principles are often employed when educating health professionals. These principles form a model of assumptions about the characteristics of adult learn-ers that are different than the traditional pedagogical assumptions made about children. Adult learning theory suggests that adults have a need to know why they should learn something; they need to be self-directed; and, because they have more experiences than youths, adults become ready to learn when they experience situations in which they de-termine a need to know or a need to be able to perform something in order to be more effective (Clapper, 2010; Knowles, 1996). Simulation provides opportunities for educators to develop reality-based situations where these principles can be applied and tested in practice almost immediately.

Achieving Objectives Through Simulation

Simulation supports educational principles, and an array of objectives can be achieved by using simulation. Basic-to-complex skill acquisition can be learned through the use of task trainers when the psychomotor components of the skill are deliberately practiced. Clinically based scenarios can be developed in which participants determine whether the patient's status warrants performance of the skill. If the learner's judgment is to proceed with the skill then the learner must prepare the patient, perform the skill, and evaluate the patient's response to the intervention. This leads to greater mastery of the skill while providing the opportunity to demonstrate the knowledge and abilities necessary to work through a dynamic situation; it also allows the learner to both develop and exhibit critical thinking and clinical judgment.

Academic institutions might have access to elaborate simulation centers with a num-ber of rooms that simulate a variety of practice settings, or they might only have access to multipurpose space. Simulation centers typically provide a contextual realism that can be important for specific educational objectives and often are equipped with technolo-gies such as a video-recording system. But just because these centers exist does not mean that all simulations have to occur there. Sometimes bringing the simulation into the classroom is appropriate, particularly when the objective is to demonstrate how to apply newly acquired information. Novices need opportunities to observe experts applying information and making clinical judgments. Bringing a simulation into the classroom can help solidify knowledge acquisition. It also demonstrates how new information and concepts are applied to situations or how this information is used to set priorities and make clinical decisions.

Content Delivery

Simulation can be an effective way to teach students in health professions programs about concepts or processes while making it an interesting and engaging experience. Bringing a mannequin into a classroom setting and demonstrating the steps of assessment or asking for volunteers and walking students through the steps is an effective way of not only delivering material but placing it in context by showing how it is done. Educators can set up the mannequin so that the signs and symptoms of a particular disease are manifested, and students can apply their newly obtained knowledge to simulated patient situations. In this way, core content is delivered along with expert modeling by the instructor. This enables students to develop a better understanding of their roles as care providers.

When delivering content in this way, educators can allow the simulation to be interrupted and can give clarification at key points. Students can ask questions about approaches demonstrated, allowing for discussions around the nuances of care provision. Simulation can be used as a means for students to demonstrate their understanding of classroom material. Educators can offer scenarios that purposely omit relevant data and include irrelevant or incomplete data that can be presented so students can engage in identifying cues and generating inferences (Su & Juestel, 2010). Educators creating the scenario must consider the background knowledge that students have on the content. By doing so, educators have the opportunity to consider where the student might get stuck and develop prompts that can redirect the student. It also provides an opportunity for the educator to consider alternative paths that students might take and determine if this will be permitted or deterred in some way. This allows educators to determine the type of pre-scenario preparation the students require and provide assignments that meet this need (Su & Juestel, 2010).

Requiring participation in simulations provides the chance for students to show their mastery of content and their ability to apply their newly acquired knowledge to a variety of clinical situations. Recently the notion of simulation replacing clinical experiences is receiving much attention. Educators can use simulation as preparation for clinical experiences by having scenarios set up around normal findings as a way to prepare students for their assigned clinical placements (Bantz, Dancer, Hodson-Carlton, & Van Hove, 2007). In contrast, scenarios demonstrating commonly encountered but abnormal findings can be used to prepare students to recognize and respond in an environment that is safe and one that allows for mistakes and corrections without doing harm.

When providing simulation experiences focused on replacing or enhancing hours traditionally spent in direct clinical experiences, the educator must consider the level of the learner, the numbers of students, the allotted time and space, and the desired clinical objectives for the experience. After the educator has determined these characteristics, scenarios can be constructed to provide the students a consistent set of experiences that require the type of clinical thinking and decision-making that occurs in clinical settings. As the students' knowledge and decision-making capacity grow, the need for more complex and realistic scenarios grows. One way to accomplish this objective is to use a full-sized, highly automated mannequin that exhibits vital signs; has heart, lung, and bowel sounds; has palpable pulses; perspires, vomits, cries, and speaks, among a host of other features. These mannequins can be programmed to display realistic physiologic responses to the actions taken by a student or progress through a series of clinical presentations reflecting a preestablished clinical condition.

Another way to create more realistic scenarios is to use a standardized patient (SP). A standardized patient is a person who might or might not have formal acting experience, but who has been trained to act like a patient with a particular disease or disorder. Standardized patients are taught how to answer questions or are provided a script from which they cannot deviate. They are instructed to interact in a specific way with the provider. Their responses, reactions, and behaviors are maintained in a narrow range in order to provide consistency in the scenario, especially if the scenario is to be offered to several students sequentially. In most educational programs, this type of simulation is ideal. However, it has limitations. First, the realism of the scenario is dependent on the person's ability to act, maintain character, and provide consistency in the scenario. Second, if the scenario requires the patient to exhibit certain physical findings, this might be difficult unless the actor actually has the condition.

Hybrid simulations use a standardized patient for the interactive segments of the scenario, and when physical findings, such as being in labor or having a murmur, cannot be simulated, a partial simulator (for example, birthing simulator or an auscultative model) is used to exhibit the required physical condition or symptoms. Hybrid simulations provide opportunities for the student to assess the patient, including asking questions and receiving responses from a "real" patient. If the student decides that the patient requires a particular skill performed, this skill can be conducted on the manufactured body part attached to the standardized patient.

Standardized patient programs can be costly if the only individuals used are professional actors. A way to reduce cost is to use volunteers such as students, staff members, retired health care providers, and retired persons. It is amazing to discover the number of people who are willing to help teach students in health professions programs for free or for very little money.

Mannequin-based or standardized patient simulations are not the only types of simulations that can be used to deliver content. Screen-based simulations, such as those demonstrating underlying anatomy and physiology and physical assessment techniques evaluating function and structure, are ripe for students to use as learning tools. Numerous online games and tutorials provide information in an engaging and interactive manner, and students can be directed to these sites. An example of this type of simulated game is 6-second ECG, a game that teaches the learner to identify different cardiac rhythms (Skillstat, Inc., 2013). The learner can play the game in which the player must identify the rhythm strips going across the screen in 60 seconds. The ratio of correct to incorrect answers is calculated. Direct feedback ranging between "mastery of content" to "more preparation is needed" is provided.

Other simulation modalities that can be used effectively in the academic setting are computer screen–based simulations (with and without haptic technology devices that provide tactile feedback to the learner) and virtual-reality simulations (computer-simulated environments that simulate the learner's presence in real-world situations). Examples of screen-based simulations that integrate haptic technology to provide content and psychomotor skill training are the Laerdal Virtual I.V. simulator and Virtual Phlebotomy programs. These are comprehensive, interactive, self-directed learning systems that can be used in academic settings to teach both cognitive and psychomotor skills. The learning management systems embedded in this type of simulation product typically allow for use in teaching and testing modes and thus can serve multiple purposes in the academic setting. In the case of a program focused on the knowledge and skills associated with establishing intravenous access, instruction on how to insert a catheter and the issues that should be considered before, during, and after performing the skill are provided via a screen-based computer program. When ready, the learner can move on to practicing actual psychomotor skills of catheter insertion using the haptic device that provides tactile and resistance feedback, with the screen showing the learner's actions. When the learner feels confident, the program provides a scored checklist and a detailed debriefing on performance. A variety of patient situations requiring catheter insertion are provided.

The use of virtual-reality simulations is becoming increasingly popular in academic settings. There are commercially available programs as well as faculty-developed programs. For example, Second Life (an online world that allows interaction between individuals in various settings—www.secondlife.com), Nightingale Isle (a virtual space created to foster collaboration, research, and education for nursing students, educators, and health professionals—www.nightingaleisle.blogspot.com), and Xtranormal (allows anyone to turn words into 3D movies—www.xtranormal.com) provide educators with interactive and highly engaging platforms for developing learning encounters that can accommodate numerous students at one time.

Although a variety of health care settings exist in these virtual worlds, some educators might want to create their own hospitals, clinics, or community centers and to customize their appearance. The same activities that can be conducted in an actual or simulated situation can be created in these virtual worlds. Faculty and students can interact in these settings in a number of ways. They can create avatars (computer-generated representations of themselves) and participate in activities that provide new content or require them to apply newly gained knowledge to patient care scenarios. The level of complexity in virtual-reality settings typically can be manipulated in the same way as face-to-face simulations can be adjusted based on the objectives of the activity. Although there is beginning research on the effect of these programs on actual educational outcomes (Graafland, Schraagen, & Schijven, 2012; Hansen, 2008; Phillips, Shaw, Sullivan, & Johnson, 2010), students—especially those of the millennial generation who have much computer and gaming experience—quickly accept this format and enjoy participating in these simulations. Innovative Nursing Education Technologies (iNET)—a partnership of Duke University, Western Carolina University, and the University of North Carolina Charlotte—provides a website with numerous examples of how this form of simulation can be applied to nursing (http://inet-nurse.org/?p=457).

Serious gaming—the use of a game designed with the specific purpose other than entertainment—is another form of simulation that is being integrated into the academic setting. In health care education, games are being developed to teach specific content, technical skills, and teamwork.

Although games developed for this purpose should be validated before being integrated into the curricula of academic programs, faculty should consider how these simulations might be used to achieve course objectives and acquire competencies. The University of Wisconsin keeps an updated list of online games and simulations for health care (http://healthcaregames.wisc.edu/index.php).

Acquisition and Mastery of Psychomotor Skills

When the ethics of learning skills on real patients began to be questioned, educators knew they had to find a better way, which led to the adoption of simulation. Effective practice includes both technical and cognitive components (Shinnick, Woo, & Mentes, 2011). Simulation presents the unique opportunity for deliberate practice in the quest to obtain mastery of psychomotor skills (Clapper & Kardong-Edgren, 2012).

Educators can use several approaches to assist students in developing their psychomotor skills. The skill can be deconstructed into parts, providing students with smaller tasks that might be more manageable in the beginning. After the student can perform the smaller tasks, the skill is reconstructed into the whole. An alternative can be to have the student watch someone perform the skill and then repeat demonstrate the skill. The educator can walk the student through the skill the first time and then the student tries performing the skill without any guidance. If the student has a question or needs guidance and an educator is not available, the student can use a video that demonstrates the procedure as the guide.

After a student has been shown how to perform the skill, the road to mastery is practice. The student must identify the need to perfect his or her performance. Self-regulated learning is essential in developing competence and maintaining it (Artino et al., 2012). Practicing health care providers have an obligation to self-regulate and seek opportunities to practice in order to maintain a level of proficiency. Promoting this accountability should begin during initial academic preparation for the role of a health care provider. In order for self-regulated learning to be successful, the deliberate practice process must be taught. Critical reflection causes learners to actively seek new learning experiences fueled by the thought that they do not know how to do a skill well enough (Clapper & Kardong-Edgren, 2012).

Deliberate practice is designed for the learner to practice skills. It is good to consider selecting skills for deliberate practice that the learner fears or dislikes practicing because those skills are the ones that often lead to failure or error (Cloud, 2008; Ericsson, 2006). Deliberate practice can result in the learner increasing the speed at which the task is performed, but that is not the goal. The goal is for the learner to master skill performance coupled with the cognitive knowledge and attitudes to anticipate potential problems and the next steps to take if these problems occur (Ericsson, 2006).

It is essential, therefore, that students be provided with adequate opportunities to practice performing skills in a safe environment. Ericsson (2008) proposes that the best training situations in which learners develop mastery most often are those that include immediate feedback, reflection, and correction, followed by opportunities to practice the task again until it can be completed with consistent success. Although a meta-analysis of literature addressing simulation-based medical education (SBME) with deliberate practice compared to results from traditional clinical education found that SBME is superior for acquisition of a range of medical skills (Fraser et al., 2009; McGaghie, Issenberg, Cohen, Barsuk, & Wayne, 2011; Nestel, Groom, Eikeland-Husebo & O'Donnell, 2011), concern about students' ability to transfer knowledge and skills from the learning laboratory to actual patient care areas still exists (Ross, 2012). Learning a skill in isolation without the complexities of real clinical practice is not necessarily sufficient. Educators can create integrated simulated scenarios that provide the contextual learning environment along with clinical scenarios that are either commonly encountered or occur but require application of cognitive knowledge. These simulations should challenge students to think about individual patient characteristics or clinical nuances that might affect the decision to continue on to skill performance or to determine another course of action.

Early Recognition and Rescue of Patients

Failure to identify early signs of deteriorating patient conditions, as well as failure to rescue patients in a timely fashion after a complication has occurred, have been identified by the Agency for Healthcare Research and Quality (AHRQ) as a quality and efficiency issue (AHRQ, 2011). For the last decade, failure-to-rescue has been recognized as a preventable patient complication (Clarke, 2004; Clarke & Aiken, 2003). Level of education, human error, lack of knowledge, and poor performance contribute to the lack of safety. Simulation is a method to address failure-to-rescue events (Schubert, 2012). Exposure to these sorts of situations in a simulated environment enables students to work through potential emergent or infrequent situations that occur in clinical practice so they become proficient in responding. Preparing students to care for patients in these dynamic situations is the goal of all health care educators, and simulation is a powerful tool to achieve this goal. Simulation activities focused on developing cue recognition, clinical judgment, diagnostic reasoning, and managing responses to quickly changing situations can be interspersed throughout the academic program. Situations encountered in clinical practice often are unpredictable and, as such, the behaviors taught to students cannot be so rigid that clinical reasoning is not expected or permitted. In fact, clinical judgments based on the information known and a reasonable understanding of similar situations must be cultivated in students.

In actual clinical settings, patient information is often missing or incomplete, but decisions must still be made. Using unfolding case studies is a popular way to promote clinical reasoning and provide students with opportunities to make decisions about patient needs. In unfolding cases, the fluid nature of clinical reasoning is incorporated in the exercise by using a staged scenario approach. This approach enables students to experience changes in a client's condition based on the planned scenario and the decisions and actions taken by the learner (Baldwin, 2007). A series of scenarios related to the initial case, set in consecutive timeframes, provides the opportunity to react to various situations at each point along a timeline. After the series of cases is complete, the learner is required to reflect on the decisions she made. These exercises provide opportunities to think in ways similar to that required in actual clinical practice.

Regardless of the specific simulation method used, simulation provides effective ways to prepare students for clinical practice. Establishing scenarios in which students encounter commonly occurring abnormal findings prepares students to more quickly recognize subtle variations in physiologic and physical data and prepare them to respond appropriately. Designing scenarios around low-frequency but high-risk situations can prepare students to recognize the signs and symptoms of situations that often result in poor outcomes. When the educators are sure that students' confidence is strong, they can include greater complexity, more complicated patients, greater numbers of patients, and misinformation or misleading information. Deliberately misleading students so they make mistakes might seem to be unethical, but it provides students with opportunities to make mistakes and manage the consequences.

Developing Team-Based and Interprofessional Practice Competencies

Developing the competencies associated with interprofessional practice, including effective communication and teamwork, is recognized as essential to maximizing patient outcomes and improving patient safety (Interprofessional Education Collaborative Expert Panel [IPECEP], 2011). Because communication and teamwork are such important issues, interprofessional collaborative simulations in academic programs typically focus on closed-loop communication, role identity, and leadership. Interprofessional education (IPE) addressing these core concepts, followed by a series of simulations involving commonly encountered clinical situations, can result in greater understanding of team member roles, knowledge base, perspective, and contributions to clinical issues (Robertson et al., 2010). With these improvements, interprofessional collaboration is enhanced resulting in provision of safe and quality care, improved systems, and cost reduction. Participation in simulations with students from other health care disciplines in which effective approaches to interprofessional collaboration are explored is expected to become a core content area for health professional's education (IPECEP, 2011).

Numerous challenges exist when attempting to conduct IPE in academic settings. The most significant challenge is that education in health care programs typically occurs in silos. Course and clinical schedules are often so diverse that it is exceedingly difficult to find a mutually agreeable time to bring students together for IPE (IPECEP, 2011; Robertson et al, 2010). Another challenge can be a lack of administrative leadership support to provide resources for IPE to happen. Many health professions schools are not on academic health science campuses. Thus, the students from one school have no students representing other health care disciplines with whom they can conveniently interact. Regardless of whether the various schools for the different health care professions are located on the same or different campuses, faculty from the schools involved in IPE need to be knowledgeable about the interprofessional competencies as well as the techniques of IPE.

Historically there has been a lack of recognition by accreditors of health professions schools of the vital need to provide substantive opportunities for their students to acquire the competencies for effective interprofessional practice. However, these bodies are increasingly mandating IPE be included in schools preparing health professionals. Simulation is an effective way to meet this requirement. In 2012, the Society for Simulation in Healthcare (SSH) in partnership with the National League for Nursing (NLN) produced a white paper describing the advantage of simulation-enhanced IPE that provides a roadmap to its integration into both academic and clinical settings (SSH & NLN, 2012). Detailed information on the use of simulation in IPE is found in Chapter 8.

An important aspect of learning with simulation is the debriefing that occurs after the scenario is over (see Chapter 5). Debriefing an IPE experience has some unique challenges. During debriefing, discussion and reflection help move the learners to new perspectives, understandings, and skills. In simulation scenarios designed to acquire the competencies associated with interprofessional practice, facilitators in the debriefing need to be sure to focus on the knowledge, behaviors, skills, and attitudes associated with interprofessional practice—not necessarily the clinical situation itself. It is also important for the facilitators to discuss in advance how role-specific questions and reflections will be handled. For example, will there be representatives from the faculty from each school present during the debriefing?

Some simulations associated with team training require little technology in order to be successful. Role-playing activities involving students, educators, or actors do not need to be held in a simulation center. They can be held in the classroom. Simulations used to teach or evaluate communication skills only require another person acting in a particular way for the student to learn how to employ effective communication skills. If the faculty members role-play first, students can observe how they communicate effectively in challenging situations. The students then can be asked to participate in subsequent scenarios. Communication scenarios for students in the health professions typically focus on patient encounters, interprofessional communication challenges, and topics such as breaking bad news. Communication approaches such as active listening skills and the use of nonverbal/ body language can be areas explored in simulations. Debriefing following these simulations can concentrate on challenges encountered and alternative approaches that could be used.

Likewise, scenarios exploring leadership skills can be conducted with little use of technology. Role-playing conducted around a conference table can be used to explore the students' abilities to negotiate, bargain, and build consensus. Scenarios can be conducted using a few students at a time. If the capability exists, additional students in an adjacent room can observe through a one-way window. If video recording is available, simulations can be recorded and viewed in class at a later time or broadcast synchronously to a classroom where students are observing. This provides an opportunity for all students to participate in the scenario by asking student observers to critique approaches and explore various alternatives.

Aligning Technology With Objectives

For the purpose of educating new health care professionals, beyond the ethics, the use of simulators has several significant advantages over the use of actual patients. Simulators allow educators to create the "deliberate practice" training conditions that expedite skills development (Agency for Healthcare Research & Quality [AHRQ], 2013; Ericsson & Lehmann, 1994). Their use makes it possible for educators and learners, rather than patient availability, to set the learning agenda and gives learners "permission to fail" and see the natural consequences of making an error without patients suffering adverse clinical consequences (Gordon, Wilkerson, Shaffer, & Armstrong, 2001). Ultimately, the use of simulators provides greater opportunity for practice (Kneebone, 2003). Using the vast array of available simulators for these purposes requires an educator highly familiar with the capabilities of the simulators in order to achieve the desired educational outcomes.

To create a successful simulation, educators must first have clear learning objectives. With these in mind, it is essential to select a methodology and technology (simulator) with capabilities that are aligned with the objectives. For example, if the objective is to teach students how to record a 12-lead electrocardiogram (ECG), choosing a technology that requires the student to attach leads to a patient's chest is essential. Deciding on whether a full-sized, lifelike mannequin or a static torso should be used depends on the objectives to be achieved. If the objective is to have the student demonstrate appropriate lead placement, either type of mannequin will work. There are a few online programs, which can be accessed free or for a small fee, in which students are expected to place the leads appropriately before the program will allow the student to progress to the next step. However, if the learner is expected to determine if the ECG tracing obtained from the machine is appropriate then a simulator that provides a 12-lead ECG tracing must be used. This can be done with a full-sized mannequin or with actors who have the ECG actually performed on them. This example illustrates why determining the objectives before choosing the simulator is so important.

Another example of aligning technology with objectives is teaching skill acquisition. Task trainers are designed to replicate a part of a system (for example, human body) or process. The learning objectives associated with these simulators are often task specific. Examples include intubation mannequins, IV arms, and surgical device or procedure simulators. The advantages of these devices include standardization, portability, and skill specificity. The disadvantages include a lowered ability to suspend disbelief due to the single task purpose of the trainer. When used in conjunction with integrated simulators or higher technology simulators, this disadvantage can largely be overcome (Beaubien & Baker, 2004).

When learners need to be able to perceive tactile or other stimuli, educators can use haptic systems. This virtual-reality technology offers an opportunity for the learners to practice skills, including surgical techniques, bronchoscopy, and intravenous and central line catheterization. Sensors can be placed within a task trainer to detect pressure and presence during learner activities, such as those associated with learning pelvic exams and surgical procedures (Durham & Alden, 2008). These high-technology simulators lend an added high-fidelity dimension to simulations (Decker, Sportsman, Puetz, & Billings, 2008), but can also increase the overall cost of the simulation experience. Starting with the educational objective in mind helps the educators make cost-effective decisions.

When the ability to contribute a high degree of realism to the simulation scenario is needed, full body simulators of an adult, child, or infant that are capable of responding to certain medications, chest compressions, needle decompression, chest tube placement, and other physiologic interventions and subsequent responses are desirable (Galloway, 2009). Full body simulators help suspend disbelief during a simulation due to the integrated computer technology housed in the mannequin that makes it capable of responding in real time to specific care interventions and treatments.

Role-play can be an effective and efficient simulation method, especially in the realms of team training or changing attitudes (Aldrich, 2005). Role-play, using students, educators, or staff to act out a particular role, can be an effective way to simulate a situation.

Although it is helpful to role-play in a contextually relevant setting (for example, home, hospital, office), it is not essential to do that for the simulation to be effective.

For objectives such as learning how to conduct a physical assessment, take a patient history, communicate bad news, practice a psychiatric intervention, and even perform a pelvic or prostate examination, standardized patients or actors can be the simulation technology of choice. The use of standardized patients has been found to help students gain self-awareness of their communication and clinical strengths and weaknesses, their reactions to stressful situations, and also their biases (Shemanko & Jones, 2008). A well-trained standardized patient with a good script is very effective at suspending disbelief in the scenario and creating a valuable learning experience.

Using Simulation for Instruction or Evaluation

Simulation can be used for instructional or evaluative purposes. Designing an effective and efficient simulation requires clarity of purpose. Is the session being designed as a formative learning experience (to monitor the student's learning and provide feedback) in which learners are allowed to make mistakes and the educator can suspend time, provide needed instruction, and then restart the scenario? Or, is the simulation being used as a summative experience (to evaluate learning by comparing to a benchmark or standard of performance) in which the participant is expected to make clinical decisions and provide safe and competent care with little to no interference from the educator? After clarity about the purpose of the simulation is determined, educators are better able to decide on the most appropriate technology and approach to use in order to achieve the educational objectives and purpose.

The decision to interrupt the flow of the simulation to provide instruction to learners or to enable the learners to work through the entire scenario without direction or interference from the instructor or facilitator dictates how the scenario will be built. This is an important decision that affects the performance and confidence of participants and the perceived success of the simulation. Educators should consider two issues before finalizing this decision. First, consider the level of students participating in the simulation. Will the simulation involve first semester students learning basic tasks or senior students with the knowledge, skills, and abilities to successfully participate without any assistance or direction from the facilitator? If the students are at the beginning level of knowledge development then educators should be prepared to interrupt the flow of the scenario to clarify concepts or to redirect the scenario and should allot time for the interruptions.

The second issue to consider is the educators' ability to respond to all of the possible responses the learners might have to the clinical situation presented. This takes much preplanning with novice learners because the likelihood of them straying from expected approaches is high. However, as the level of learner knowledge and sophistication increases, the alternatives are more easily anticipated and the scenario can be permitted to progress with little to no interruption.

An example of a simulation that can be interrupted so feedback and instruction can be provided is a scenario in which nursing students are learning safe medication administration. In this example, students have had several opportunities to practice the Five Rights of medication administration so they are aware they should perform three medication checks before dispensing the medication. In this simulation, the students are to enter a patient's room in the simulation center; after washing their hands, they are to introduce themselves to the patient; check the patient in the bed is indeed the right patient; and administer the medication. But the students don't do that. They introduce themselves and tell the patient they are going to prepare the medications. They don't check the patient's armband, check the patient's name, or ask the patient for his or her date of birth. Instead, the students move directly to getting the medications from the drawer. Should the simulation be stopped and the students told what has happened or should the simulation be allowed to progress? If the objective of this simulation experience is learning as opposed to evaluation, stopping the simulation and discussing what is happening is appropriate. Before moving forward, the students can be refocused on the correct process and reflect on what they need to know and how they might do things differently. When this is complete, the scenario can be restarted or the group can be moved to a more intensive debriefing session for further exploration.

Although it is easy to see why one would design uninterrupted simulations for evaluation purposes, simulations designed for learning also can be developed to run uninterrupted. These types of simulations are often used in academic environments to allow learners the opportunity to apply the knowledge they have gained, work with others, respond to available data, and experience the natural outcomes of their decisions. When the scenario is completed, a debriefing session is conducted to allow for reflection and to review perceptions of what actually occurred. In the debriefing, facilitators cover the cause and effect of decisions made and actions taken. In addition, facilitators should assure that any problems encountered are explored.

An example of a learning simulation that would be permitted to go to its conclusion is one in which a nurse calls the rapid response team to evaluate a patient who has become progressively more dyspneic, tachycardic, and hypoxic, with a pulse oximetry reading of 86%. To determine if the learners have developed the skills to quickly gather data, assess the patient, and make a decision about whether the patient requires intubation, this scenario is allowed to unfold naturally without interruption. The students recognize the need to increase the patient's oxygen supply and after placing a 100% non-rebreather mask on the patient and not achieving a response, the students decide to call anesthesia to intubate the patient. The students support the patient until intubated. The scenario ends. Afterward, a debriefing session provides participants the opportunity to react to the scenario, reflect on their actions and interactions with the patient and team, and to discuss if alternative approaches to care should have been considered. After all points are reviewed, the facilitator summarizes the important elements and ends the session. Note that the learners in this case were at a point in their education where they should be able to deliver a reasonable amount of quality and safe care. Thus, they are permitted to complete the simulation without interruption.

Simulations can be used for either formative or summative assessment. Either way, the simulations must be designed so they can be implemented in a consistent manner. When students are being tested in high-stakes situations, such as determining their mastery of content or competence, then uniformity is essential.

Objective structured clinical examinations (OSCEs), a form of simulation, have been used in the education of physicians for evaluation of competence since the 1970s (Turner & Dankoski, 2008) and are increasingly being used in other professional disciplines. The overarching philosophy for OSCEs is that all students (candidates) are presented with the same clinical tasks to be completed in the same time frame, and examiners score the students using structured marking schemes, being careful not to introduce bias (Gormley, 2011). During the OSCE, candidates are observed and evaluated as they go through a series of stations in which they interview, examine, and treat standardized patients who present with some type of medical problem. The length of the OSCE station is generally 5 to 20 minutes, and the candidates are expected to participate in the encounter as they would in an actual clinical setting. In some OSCEs, an examiner (usually a licensed professional in the same profession as the student) is present to assess clinical and communication skills using a standardized checklist. Some OSCEs are video recorded and are later assessed by more than one examiner (OSCEhome, 2013).

Conclusion

Many educators assume the only way to use simulation in the academic setting is to have a large facility outfitted with a full array of high-technology simulators. Although nice, this setup is not a requirement to successfully integrate simulation into an academic program. What is necessary is having educators familiar with educational theory who can develop clinical scenarios, select appropriate simulation methods and equipment based on defined educational objectives, and understand how to effectively debrief a simulation-based educational session. Simulation as a teaching and learning strategy has greatly expanded the educator's toolkit. When they're familiar with the full array of simulation methodologies, educators in the academic setting are only limited by their own creativity.

References

Agency for Healthcare Research and Quality (AHRQ). (2011). *National healthcare quality report.* Rockville, MD: Author. Retrieved from http://www.ahrq.gov/research/findings/nhqrdr/nhqr11/

Agency for Healthcare Research and Quality (AHRQ). (2013). *Making health care safer II: An updated critical analysis of the evidence for patient safety practices.* Comparative Effectiveness Review No. 211. (Prepared by the Southern California-RAND Evidence-based Practice Center under Contract No. 290-2007-10062-I.) AHRQ Publication No. 13-E001-EF. Rockville, MD: Author. Retrieved from www.ahrq.gov/research/findings/evidence-based-reports/ptsafetyuptp.html

Aldrich, C. (2005). *Learning by doing: A comprehensive guide to simulations, computer games, and pedagogy in e-learning and other educational experiences.* San Francisco, CA: Pfeiffer.

Artino, A. R., Dong, T., DeZee, K. J., Gilliland, W. R., Waechter, D. M., Cruess, D., & Durning, S. J. (2012). Achievement goal structures and self-regulated learning: Relationships and changes in medical school. *Academic Medicine, 87*(10), 1375-1381.

Baldwin, K. B. (2007). Friday night in the pediatric emergency department. A simulated exercise to promote clinical reasoning in the classroom. *Nurse Educator, 32*(1), 24-29.

Bantz, D., Dancer, M. M., Hodson-Carlton, K., & Van Hove, S. (2007). A daylong clinical laboratory: From gaming to high-fidelity simulators. *Nurse Educator, 32*(6), 274-277.

Beaubien, J., & Baker, D. (2004). The use of simulation for training teamwork skills in health care: How low can you go? *Quality and Safety in Health Care, 13*(Suppl 1), i51-i56.

Bonwell, C. C., & Eison, J. A. (1991). *Active learning: Creating excitement in the classroom.* ERIC Digest. Washington, DC: ASHE-ERIC Higher Education Reports. Retrieved from http://www.eric.ed.gov/PDFS/ED340272.pdf

Clapper, T. C. (2010). Beyond Knowles: What those conducting simulation need to know about adult learning theory. *Clinical Simulation in Nursing, 6*(1), e7-e14.

Clapper, T. C., & Kardong-Edgren, S. (2012). Using deliberate practice and simulation to improve nursing skills. *Clinical Simulation in Nursing, 8*(3), e109-3113. doi:10.1016/j.ecns.2010.12.001

Clarke, S. P. (2004). Failure to rescue: Lessons from missed opportunities in care. *Nursing Inquiry, 11*(2), 67-71.

Clarke, S. P., & Aiken L. H. (2003). Failure to rescue. *American Journal of Nursing, 103*(1), 42-47.

Cloud, J. (2008, February 28). The science of experience. *Time.* Retrieved from http://www.time.com/time/magazine/article/0,9171,1718551-2,00.html

Decker, S., Sportsman, S., Puetz, L., & Billings, L. (2008). The evolution of simulation and its contribution to competency. *The Journal of Continuing Education in Nursing, 39*(2), 74-80.

Durham, C. F., & Alden, K. R. (2008). Enhancing patient safety in nursing education through patient simulation. In R. G. Hughes (Ed.), *Patient Safety and Quality: An Evidence-Based Handbook for Nurses* (Chapter 51). Rockville. MD: Agency for Healthcare Research and Quality (AHRQ). Retrieved from http://www.ahrq.gov/professionals/clinicians-providers/resources/nursing/resources/nurseshdbk/index.html

Ericsson, K. A. (2006). The influence of experience and deliberate practice on the development of superior expert performance. In K. A. Ericsson, N. Charness, P. Feltovich, &. R. R. Hoffman (Eds.), *Cambridge Handbook of Expertise and Expert Performance* (pp. 683-704). Cambridge, UK: Cambridge University Press.

Ericsson, K. A. (2008). Deliberate practice and acquisition of expert performance: A general overview. *Academic Emergency Medicine, 15*(11), 988-994. doi:10.1111/j.1553-2712.2008.00227.x

Ericsson, K. A., & Lehmann, A. C. (1994). Expert performance: Its structure and acquisition. *American Psychology, 49*(8), 725-47.

Fraser, K., Peets, A., Walker, I., Tworek, J., Paget, M., Wright, B., & McLaughlin, K. (2009). The effect of simulator training on clinical skills acquisition, retention and transfer. *Medical Education, 43*(8), 784-789. doi:10.1111/j.1365-2923.2009.03412.x

Galloway, S. J., (2009, May 31). Simulation techniques to bridge the gap between novice and competent healthcare professionals. *OJIN: The Online Journal of Issues in Nursing, 14*(2), Manuscript 3.

Gordon, J. A., Wilkerson, W. M., Shaffer, D. W., & Armstrong, E. G. (2001). "Practicing" medicine without risk: Students' and educators' responses to high-fidelity situations. *Academic Medicine, 76*(5), 469-472.

Gormley, G. (2011). Summative OSCEs in undergraduate medical education. *Ulster Medical Journal, 80*(3), 127-132.

Graafland, M., Schraagen, J. M., & Schijven, M. P. (2012). Systematic review of serious games for medical education and surgical skills training. *British Journal of Surgery, 99*(10), 1322-1330. doi: 10.1002/bjs.8819

Hansen, M. M. (2008). Versatile, immersive, creative and dynamic virtual 3-D healthcare learning environments: A review of the literature. *Journal of Medical Internet Research, 10*(3), e26. doi:10.2196/jmir.1051

Institute of Medicine (IOM). (2011). *The future of nursing: Leading change, advancing health.* Washington, DC: The National Academies Press. Retrieved from www.thefutureofnursing.org/IOM-Report

Interprofessional Education Collaborative Expert Panel (IPECEP). (2011). *Core competencies for interprofessional collaborative practice: Report of an expert panel.* Washington, DC: Interprofessional Education Collaborative.

Kneebone, R. (2003). Simulation in surgical training: Educational issues and practical implications. *Medical Education, 37*(3), 267-277.

Knowles, M. (1996). Adult learning. In R. L. Craig (Ed.), *The ASTD Training and Development Handbook* (pp. 253-264). New York, NY: McGraw-Hill.

Kolb, D. (1984). *Experiential learning: Experience as the source of learning and development.* Englewood Cliffs, NJ: Prentice Hall.

McGaghie, W. C., Issenberg, S. B., Cohen, E. R., Barsuk, J. H. & Wayne, D. B. (2011). Does simulation-based medical education with deliberate practice yield better results from traditional clinical education? A meta-analytic comparative review of the evidence. *Academic Medicine, 86*(6), 706-711. doi:10.1097/ACM.0b013e318217e119

Nestel, D., Groom, J., Eikeland-Husebo, S., & O'Donnell, J. M. (2011). Simulation for learning and teaching procedure skills. *Simulation in Healthcare, 6*(7), s10-s13.

OSCEhome. (2013). *What is objective structures clinical examination, OSCEs?* Retrieved from http://www.oscehome.com/What_is_Objective-Structured-Clinical-Examination_OSCE.html

Phillips, B., Shaw, R. J., Sullivan, D. T., & Johnson, C. (2010). Using virtual environments to enhance nursing distance education. *Creative Nursing, 16*(3), 132-135.

Robertson, B., Kaplan, B., Atallah, H., Higgins, M., Lewitt, M. J., & Ander, D. S. (2010). The use of simulation and a modified TeamSTEPPS curriculum for medical and nursing student team training. *Simulation in Healthcare, 5*(6), 332-337.

Ross, J. G. (2012). Simulation and psychomotor skill acquisition: A review of the literature. *Clinical Simulation in Nursing, 8*(9), e429-e435. doi:10.1016/j.ecns.2011.04.004

Schubert, C. R. (2012). Effect of simulation on nursing knowledge and critical thinking in failure to rescue events. *The Journal of Continuing Education in Nursing, 43*(10), 467-471.

Shemanko, G., & Jones, L. (2008). To simulate or not to simulate: That is the question. In R. Kyle & W. Murray (Eds.), *Clinical Simulation: Operations, Engineering and Management* (pp. 77-84). New York, NY: Elsevier, Inc.

Shinnick, M. A., Woo, M. A. & Mentes, J. C. (2011). Human patient simulation: state of the science in prelicensure nursing education. *Journal of Nursing Education, 50*(2), 65-72.

Skillstat, Inc. (2013). *6-second ECG.* Retrieved from http://www.skillstat.com/tools/ecg-simulator#/-home

Society for Simulation in Healthcare (SSH) & National League for Nursing (NLN). (2012). Interprofessional education and healthcare simulation symposium. Wheaton, IL: SSH. Retrieved from https://ssih.org/uploads/static_pages/ipe-final_compressed.pdf

Su, W. M., & Juestel, M. J. (2010). Direct teaching of thinking skills using clinical simulation. *Nurse Educator, 35*(5), 197-204.

Turner, J. L., & Dankoski, M. E. (2008). Objective structured clinical exams: A critical review. *Family Medicine, 40*(8), 574-578.

Ziv, A., Wolpe, P. R., Small, S. D., & Glick, S. (2006). Simulation-based medical education: An ethical imperative. *Simulation in Healthcare, 1*(4), 252-256.

Using Simulation in Hospitals and Health Care Systems to Improve Outcomes

Jennifer L. Manos, MSN, RN

Thomas E. LeMaster, MSN, MEd, RN, NREMT-P

OBJECTIVES

- Discuss the various opportunities for using simulation in a hospital or health care system.
- Describe how to identify a champion for the simulation program.
- Describe the initial planning for implementation of a simulation program.
- Identify the types of simulators used with different learners and courses.
- Describe the challenges of implementing a simulation program and potential solutions.

Simulation programs situated in clinical settings such as hospitals and health care systems are both similar to and different from those in academic settings. As with simulation programs situated in academic settings, those situated in clinical settings typically have a significant educational component focused on individuals. Some of the uses of simulation in clinical settings include:

- Onboarding of new employees
- Assessing of competency of new or newly employed health care providers
- Assessing and maintaining individual competency
- Building and sustaining high-performing teams
- Testing new equipment for usability prior to implementation
- Testing new clinical services and patient care units
- Assessing processes for latent errors

- Other quality improvement or risk management activities (Agency for Healthcare Research and Quality [AHRQ], 2013; Ulrich, 2013)

A 2013 AHRQ report noted that "the versatility of simulation techniques affords those working to improve patient safety a number of benefits" (p. 441) and the report summarized those benefits:

- Simulation is initiated on command and may be practiced repeatedly.
- Simulation may be particularly valuable in duplicating complex high-stakes scenarios that involve care teams and complex factors that affect performance.
- Errors are allowed in simulation and utilized as a learning experience through reflection and debriefing.
- Simulation may be used to test new technologies, especially ones that involve new learning curves in even the most experienced of clinicians.
- Teams can simulate patient care flow in situ for critical events as well as new facility "usual care" to check for proper equipment (for example, severe hemorrhage drills on various hospital units or in new operating rooms; AHRQ, 2013, pp. 441-442)

The location where simulation activities occur also differentiates clinically based simulation programs from those in academic settings. Simulation programs serving hospitals and health care systems may be based in a freestanding educational building, within the walls of the clinical setting, or even in a mobile van that travels from site to site. Within a hospital or health care system, simulation programs can also exist outside of an actual physical location. They can involve "in situ" simulations occurring in the actual clinical environment (for example, in an operating room, patient care unit, or emergency department).

Simulation programs based in a hospital or health care system are supporting efforts toward improving patient safety, enhancing the educational experiences of staff, and creating a new system to assist in improving overall system performance. Details on using simulation for risk management and quality improvement can be found in Chapter 11.

Leadership

Engaged and active leadership is critical to the success of simulation programs. Hospitals and health care systems need to identify a high-level champion who embraces the value of simulation—for example, a board member or hospital executive—to lead the simulation program. This level of leader can champion the program and help pave the way for the engagement of potential stakeholders, the acquisition of physical space and simulation technology, and the implementation of a new approach to learning within the organization.

The complexity of today's health care environment can make it difficult to implement a change no matter how valuable or appropriate it may be. Changing a system, changing a procedure, or changing a process requires much planning. Not all health care providers in the organization will embrace the idea of using simulation. Therefore, simulation champions need to be kept well informed and involved with their simulation programs. Armed with a thorough understanding of the benefits that simulation can bring to patient safety and the overall quality of patient care services, the champion will be able to facilitate buy-in from the various departments and individuals who can benefit from the simulation program.

Hospitals and health care systems also need to have a simulation planning committee and a steering committee that has decision-making authority. These committees are discussed in detail in Chapter 15.

When considering the organizational reporting structure for the simulation program, consider the message the positioning of the program might send. If the focus of the simulation program is on hospital-wide or system-wide activities, the program should be positioned accordingly within the organization. If the program is based in a specialty department such as emergency medicine or anesthesia, potential users of the program are likely to view it narrowly as offering simulation activities specific to that department or discipline. For example, if the simulation program is based in emergency medicine, potential users, such as nursing services, might be interested in simulation but think the program offers only emergency response scenarios or training.

Simulation programs may be more likely to succeed if they are established to serve all departments and disciplines in the organization rather than just one. If the simulation program is envisioned as serving the hospital or health system, consideration can be given to creating the program as a separate department reporting to a position such as the Chief Quality Officer. Another possibility might be to situate the simulation program within an existing organization-wide department such as education or risk management.

Initial Needs Assessment

Simulation is being incorporated throughout hospitals and health care systems as a learning, high-stakes testing, and quality improvement modality for practicing health care professionals. With the focus on developing a culture of safety within health care, patient safety organizations are calling on hospitals and health care institutions to explore simulation as a means to assist in providing ongoing education and professional development (AHRQ, 2013; Murray, 2010). Simulation provides the opportunity for repeated practice, performance assessment, and potential clinical improvement (Gaba, 2004). Simulation is ideal as an educational modality for a variety of experiences, including high-risk patient conditions. This educational methodology has the potential to improve performance and encourage teamwork with engagement of learners through re-creation of real clinical situations in a safe environment (Senger, Stapleton, & Gorski, 2012).

Performing a needs assessment is a critical step in determining many aspects of the simulation program. Every hospital or health care system has unique learning needs and demands (Beam, 2011). Determining the types of users the simulation program will serve is important for development, growth, and incorporation of simulation into the organization.

A needs assessment is a systematic process for identifying and addressing the needs of the organization, or gaps between current conditions and desired conditions. A needs assessment should be done to focus simulation-based activities and assure alignment with the organization's outcomes, methods, and measures. The needs assessment should consider the type of learners to be served, objectives to be achieved, and the critical elements to be assessed. A needs assessment can be done on an organizational, departmental, unit, course, or population level. It should also be repeated on a regular basis. A systematic assessment of what the simulation program can accomplish will help to guide the overall objectives of the simulation program and curriculum and establish a projected growth plan for simulation within the organization.

Within a hospital or health system simulation program, the types of learners can vary. Examples of specific learner types include registered nurses, physicians, allied health care professionals, unlicensed hospital personnel, students, new graduates, and experienced staff. In addition to identifying learners, based on the assessment, the program should identify how training will occur—interprofessional training, task training, lab-based simulation training, in situ simulation training, use of hybrid simulations, discipline-/specialty-specific training, and so on.

Assuring that the simulation program is developed based on an objective measure of need will allow simulation staff to develop well-designed, effective, and efficient simulation experiences.

Initial Program Development

When the needs assessment is complete, initial program development can begin. The first step in developing a hospital-wide or health care system–based simulation program is to consider the purposes of the program.

- What do you want to accomplish and in what priority?
- Of the needs identified in the assessment, which are the most pressing?
- Do you have to start small due to budget or space limitations, or are you prepared to respond to a broader array of needs initially?
- If you have to start small, can you create a long-term approach to the integration of simulation in a phased-in approach?

The answers to these basic questions will guide your efforts as you begin to develop the program.

Early engagement of stakeholders is important. Develop a list of services to be provided by the simulation program. Consider who might be providing the services currently along with other stakeholders of the simulation program and include them in discussing the development of the program. The key individuals need to understand simulation, the process, and potential benefits. When this is realized, support from the stakeholders will pave the way for program development and eventually facilitating getting learners to use the simulation program.

The next step is to determine the initial objectives of the program. This will drive the development of the program. Who are the learners? Will you be training new staff members in orientation? Developing a simulation program for onboarding new employees such as registered nurses can be an effective method for evaluating competencies and developing person-specific onboarding plans. Will the simulation program be tasked with developing programs to train and maintain high-performing teams such as the trauma team, code team, or the anesthesia department? Simulation is now being used to verify competencies and credential physicians and nurses in specific skill sets prior to beginning clinical rotations or making assignments. Those implementing the simulation program need to determine if it will have a focus on technical or nontechnical skills related to a specific patient safety education program.

When considering in which area to start the simulation program, consider the "low-hanging fruit" concept. Choose a group of learners or a department that understands and desires to participate in simulation education. This might be a small group such as a trauma team or code team. As the learners experience simulation education, their behaviors might change in the clinical environment, and they can share the experience with others. When other departments and learners see the positive changes that are occurring within the teams and hear of positive experiences, interest will be generated. Implementing a program across many groups, especially if they are being forced or mandated to participate in simulation, will lead to additional challenges and potentially failure of the program.

To expose as many learners as possible to the new simulation program, consider implementing simulation experiences where many learners can participate in simulation as a group. Make the experience a part of a course and emphasize a safe learning environment. One possible approach is to implement simulation into nurse orientation. As participants experience simulation and have a positive experience, they are likely to engage their leadership to facilitate a return to the simulation lab.

Developing a Simulation Lab in a Clinical Setting

Obtaining space for a simulation program in a clinical setting can be very challenging. Space for patients and the support services are the priority. That said, providing opportunities to make the environment safer and enhance patient outcomes should also be seen as an important organizational priority. Creating a strong argument for the needs and benefits of the simulation program will be critical to obtaining the necessary space for the program.

The need to replicate patient care environments might be imperative when developing a lab-based clinical simulation program. Consider visiting developed simulation programs to get ideas for your center. You can find a detailed discussion on developing and building simulation centers in Chapter 15.

The Initial Simulation Technology Purchases

Unlike in an academic setting, the initial purchase of simulator technology in a hospital or health care system program might be an unusual purchase. The decision of what equipment to buy should be driven by the goals and purpose of the program. A wide range of simulator technology is available (see Chapter 1 for a full discussion on simulation options) as well as simulation center management software and hardware.

The most expensive simulator might not be the most appropriate, given restrictions of space or available support. A full-body simulator that would be selected for a simulation laboratory setting might need to be different than a simulator that can be used for in situ simulations. The lab environment may be designed to simulate the critical-care environments, operating rooms, or patient care rooms in the hospital. As such, a simulator that exchanges gasses and responds to procedures in real time might be the best choice. Elaborate simulators that are designed for critical-care environments are available. They are, however, expensive. Equipment should be selected based on assessed need, planned use, and space. In situ simulations are often conducted using a tetherless simulator that is self-contained and does not need to be attached to electric or gas sources in order to operate. Most of these mannequins are controlled by a laptop or tablet standing some distance from the simulator, and the mannequins adequately simulate pulses, cardiac rhythms, respiratory movements and breath sounds, and eye opening. In the clinical setting, tetherless simulation devices allow the educator to move the simulator onto patient care units or other locations, which adds realism to the simulation experience and potentially identifies latent (hidden) safety threats to patients, visitors, or staff. There are also haptic simulators for learning ultrasonography and surgical techniques.

> ### Extended Warranties
>
> Organizations will have to make a decision regarding extended warranties for expensive simulators. Some stakeholders might not consider the purchase of an extended warranty important, but the technology used in human patient simulators is unique. When repairs are needed and upgrades are required, having the manufacturer complete the work under a warranty can be more efficient and cost effective than having an organization's simulation staff attempt to complete the work. Questions to consider when reviewing warranties include the turnaround time for service and whether a loaner program for the simulator exists.

Creating Global and Curriculum-Based Objectives

In both academic and clinical settings, developing global and curriculum-specific learning objectives is essential because clearly defined learning objectives help facilitate planning for all aspects of the simulation (Phrampus, 2010). Creating defined objectives focuses the goals of the program as well as course curricula and provides a level of consistency in approach and design. Creating objectives can help determine the priorities for both the health care organization and the simulation program. For example, an objective that aims at increasing the knowledge of general care nurses related to pediatric codes might require a specific pediatric patient simulator whereas development of a difficult airway course for ENT residents might require the purchase of a specific task trainer.

Objectives for a hospital simulation program may differ from objectives related to a simulation program situated in an academic setting. The hospital-based program will be offering experiences primarily to health care professionals with a variety of educational and experiential backgrounds. In addition, the objectives will help determine where the simulation activity will occur—lab-based simulations, in situ simulations, or a combination of both.

Creating "Real" Simulations in a Lab

Creating a simulation center (or lab) in a clinical setting can be challenging, time consuming, and expensive, but it can also provide many benefits to the organization. Organizations can achieve many simulation activities in a lab setting, including simulation-based courses, training for procedural skills, patient safety training, teamwork and communication training, and interprofessional training. For example, due to an initiative to decrease adverse medical events, a hospital-based simulation lab was directed to design specific adverse medical event courses for identified patient care units. The courses were 4 hours in length and included all members of the care team. The simulation experience needed to occur in a safe location that allowed for serious or uncommon scenarios to unfold and for the team to participate in a debriefing designed to identify opportunities for improvement and reflection on practice.

Training in a dedicated simulation lab has both advantages and disadvantages. Several advantages have been identified when hospital staff train in a dedicated simulation lab (Deering, Johnston, & Colacchio, 2011). First, the learning environment is tightly controlled. This can help to standardize the experience for all participants and allows for assessment activities and educational activities to occur. Audiovisual (AV) components are often an essential aspect of the simulation experience and facilitators typically integrate them into the simulation lab. This enables the hospital staff to benefit from video-assisted debriefings that can provide them with the unique experience to assess their own performances and potentially learn from both themselves and colleagues. Additionally, the simulation lab can provide education to a large and potentially diverse group of learners. The group can be predefined and allow for large numbers of care providers to attend specified training at different times to accommodate for scheduling issues. Finally, data obtained during simulations within a designated lab in a controlled environment can be used for research to further the field of simulation in health care.

The most important disadvantage to consider is the potential to frustrate the learners, which can lead to a disengagement and lack of involvement in the simulation (Deering et al., 2011). Unfamiliar equipment, environments that are different than the ones in which they practice, and lack of fellow team members can cause frustration and have the potential to distract the learners from the experience being provided. If the simulation center (or lab) is located at a different site from the hospital, travel time can be a limiting factor. One of the most important disadvantages of providing simulation in a separate lab setting is that the simulation center is unable to identify and fix "systems" issues that are inherent to a particular clinical environment. For example, the simulation lab might not be able to identify latent safety threats that are created by a specific physical space, process, or organizational structure. Such disadvantages can be overcome with planning.

In Situ Simulation: Simulation in the "Real" World

In situ (Latin for "in position") *simulation* is a blended approach to simulation that commonly involves embedding simulators within an actual clinical environment (Rosen, Hunt, Pronovost, Federowicz, & Weaver, 2012). In situ simulations are an important aspect of a hospital-based simulation program because they have the potential to drive deep individual, team, unit, and organizational learning. They allow experienced health care providers to participate in simulation activities within their own clinical environment, which results in more contextually relevant learning and identification of actual process improvement opportunities. In situ simulation provides more realistic experiences than lab-based simulations and thus can provide more accurate evaluation of the patient care units and teams (Patterson, Geis, Falcone, LeMaster, & Wears, 2013).

Hospitals and health care systems that embrace in situ simulation programs provide a means to identify workarounds, knowledge gaps, and latent safety threats that few other methods are capable of matching (Patterson et al., 2013). In situ simulations have the ability to provide learning opportunities to both individuals and teams of health care professionals to reinforce competencies acquired in more traditional learning environments (Rosen et al., 2012). Beyond the educational benefits, in situ simulations provide the opportunity to identify latent safety threats that have the potential to affect patient safety within the organization and stimulate efforts to address them. In a study performed by Geis, Pio, Pendergrass, Moyer, & Patterson (2011), an in situ program developed in a high-risk emergency department identified a total of 73 latent safety threats; a rate of 1 for every 1.2 in situ simulations performed. This use of in situ simulation can close the loop in process improvement by creating an assessment, training, and evaluation system for individual, team, and organizational learning.

Implementing a Hospital-Based In Situ Simulation Program

The first step in implementing a hospital-based in situ simulation program is to determine the outcomes the in situ simulation is designed to target. As discussed earlier, a needs analysis is crucial to uncovering what you want to achieve with an in situ simulation program. Rosen et al. (2012) identified key questions to ask when developing in situ simulation.

- What level of the system is targeted for improvement? Do you want to evaluate individual, team, unit, or organizational improvement?
- Who will participate in the simulation, and who will serve as facilitators or instructors?
- What are the specific objectives for the in situ simulation?
- Where and when will the in situ simulation occur?
- How will the in situ simulation be evaluated?
- How will the information gained from the program be used?

Asking these questions will assist in developing an effective in situ simulation program and in producing the ancillary materials needed (facilitator education, simulators, supplies).

Although in situ simulation is an essential tool in the delivery of education to health care providers, it also has limitations. Considering these issues when developing the program allows the simulation educator to prepare for potential issues before they arise. For example, scheduling and time constraints are a significant issue when developing in situ simulations (Geis et al., 2011; Deering et al., 2012). In addition, as the simulation occurs on the unit, the potential for effecting patient care must be considered. There might also be anxiety generated among the caregivers involved. Finally, when in situ simulation requires the educators and simulators to travel to outlying clinical sites such as clinics, travel time, wear and tear on simulators, and increased workload for the simulation staff must be factored into the effort. Even with the limitations noted, in situ simulation has been shown to provide a valuable experience for the health care provider and the organization (Lighthall, Poon, & Harrison, 2010; Patterson, Blike, & Nadkarni, 2008).

Facilitators need to develop guidelines for running an in situ simulation. This is important because different patient care areas might have specific times when an in situ simulation is not optimal, including but not limited to during patient rounds, shift change, and times of high acuity or high census. For example, in an in situ program developed for a pediatric intensive care unit, the unit and the simulation educator identified a policy that provided specific instructions as to when an in situ simulation should not occur. The parameters include the following:

1. An in situ simulation is *not* to be performed on the unit:

   - If there is a resuscitation in progress or high-risk procedure being performed
   - If there is only one bed open for an admission
   - If there is a low staffing level
   - If it is between 0600 and 0800, 1400 and 1600, 1800 and 2000, and 2200 and 2400 hours

2. In situ simulations are limited to 20 minutes (10 minutes for simulation plus 10 minutes for debriefing).

The policy was communicated to all charge nurses and attending physicians.

Another important point about in situ training is the realization that these simulations have a high probability of cancellation. In providing in situ simulations in emergency departments, Patterson et al. (2013) found a cancellation rate of 28%, although they noted that the cancellation rate decreased as the program matured. As a result, they recommend that overscheduling the number of in situ simulations is necessary in order to achieve the desired total number of simulations. By scheduling more in situ simulations than were potentially needed, the program has a back-up plan in case of unexpected events and cancelations.

Staffing Simulation Programs in the Clinical Setting

As a simulation program grows in the clinical setting, challenges will occur such as inadequate staff to meet demands, insufficient work space and storage space for simulators and supplies, and the need to train new simulation center employees. Simulation educators may need 3 months to 1 year to become comfortable facilitating a simulation scenario. When hiring new staff members, remember the benefit of additional staff will not be appreciated immediately. As the simulation program continues to grow, additional departments will reach out for simulation education. Developing a system early to set priorities will assist in managing the growing demand.

A staffing model to consider initially is one in which all team members are cross-trained in all aspects of simulation. One example is to have the simulation educator trained to set up and run the simulator as well as debrief. Facilitators may also be crossed-trained in the use of the AV equipment. As the program grows and demands increase, team members can remain responsive to learners as new team members are in orientation. Another staffing model is one in which content experts from within the hospital or health care system are trained to be facilitators. This allows the simulation educator time to assist in course development and oversight.

Deciding what staffing model to use will be program specific. Health care providers and staff in the clinical setting will be accepting of simulation if it is relevant and specific to their work. Thus, involving content experts from the disciplines or departments will be important for learner acceptance. You can find detailed information on simulation roles and sample position descriptions in Chapter 13.

Conclusion

The implementation of a simulation program into a hospital or health care system can offer many benefits to the organization, the staff, and patient outcomes. It is a considerable task to undertake, but one that is made easier by committing time and leadership to the planning and development phases.

In growing a simulation program in a clinical setting, hospitals and health care systems must consider the overall outcomes the organization wants to achieve and the needs of the learners. Resources can be found through professional organizations and can assist in the planning and development of a high-quality simulation program. Consider using the peer-reviewed standards for accreditation developed by the Society for Simulation in Healthcare (SSH) (2013). These standards have been specifically created to provide a resource to developing programs as well as those seeking recognition for being in full compliance with the established standards. Although a program may not be ready for accreditation, using standards from accrediting organizations such as SSH will assist in developing the basic infrastructure needed for a successful simulation program.

Having a successful simulation program in a hospital or health care system involves several key steps. Identifying champions at the program and organizational levels should be accomplished early in the development process. Organizations should conduct a needs analysis and use it to identify the global direction of the simulation program. Articulating this direction will facilitate the design of the program and strategic prioritization of activities. After the direction is established, the direction and desired activities will allow those implementing the simulation program to determine the appropriate equipment, simulation modalities, and simulation educational methodologies to employ. In addition, the program will be able to accurately identify budgetary needs as well as a staffing model.

Implementing a successful strategy for the use of simulation in hospitals and health care systems has the potential to be a rewarding experience for simulation educators, the organization, its learners, and ultimately its patients. Simulation has been shown to be effective in assuring safety in other industries that have come to expect ultrasafe performance such as aviation. In health care, simulation programs can result in major improvements in patient care and outcomes.

References

Agency for Healthcare Research and Quality (AHRQ). (2013). *Making health care safer II: An updated critical analysis of the evidence for patient safety practices.* Comparative Effectiveness Review No. 211. (Prepared by the Southern California-RAND Evidence-based Practice Center under Contract No. 290-2007-10062-I.) AHRQ Publication No. 13-E001-EF. Rockville, MD: Author. Retrieved from www.ahrq.gov/research/findings/evidence-based-reports/ptsafetyuptp.html

Beam, B. (2011). Lessons learned from planning, conducting, and evaluating in situ healthcare simulations for Nebraska hospitals. *Nebraska Nurse, 44*(3), 7.

Deering, S., Johnston, L. C., & Colacchio, K. (2011). Multidisciplinary teamwork and communication training. *Seminars in Perinatology, 35*(2), 89-96.

Gaba, D. M. (2004). The future vision of simulation in healthcare. *Quality and Safety in Health Care, 13*(1), i2-i10.

Geis, G. L., Pio, B., Pendergrass, T. L., Moyer, M. R., & Patterson, M. D. (2011). Simulation to assess the safety of new healthcare teams and new facilities. *Simulation in Healthcare, 6*(3), 125-133.

Lighthall, G. K., Poon, T., & Harrison, T. K. (2010). Using in situ simulation to improve in-hospital cardiopulmonary resuscitation. *Joint Commission Journal on Quality and Patient Safety, 36*(5), 209-216.

Murray, J. S. (2010). Walter Reed national military medical center: Simulation on the cutting edge. *Military Medicine, 175*(9), 659-663.

Patterson, M. D., Blike, G. T., & Nadkarni, V. M. (2008). In situ simulation: Challenges and results. In K. Henriksen, J. B. Battles, M. A. Keyes, & M. L. Grady (Eds.), *Advances in patient safety: New directions and alternative approaches* (Vol. 3: Performance and Tools). Rockville, MD: Agency for Healthcare Research and Quality. Retrieved from http://www.ahrq.gov/downloads/pub/advances2/vol3/advances-patterson_48.pdf

Patterson, M. D., Geis, G. L., Falcone, R. A., LeMaster, T., & Wears, R. L. (2013). In situ simulation: Detection of safety threats and teamwork training in a high risk emergency department. *BMJ Quality and Safety in Health Care, 22*(6), 468-477. doi: 10.1136/bmjqs-2012-000942

Phrampus, P. E. (2010). Simulation best practices: Must haves for successful simulation in pre-hospital care. *Journal of Emergency Medical Services, 35*(9), Suppl 4-7.

Rosen, M. A., Hunt, E. A., Pronovost, P. J., Federowicz, M. A., & Weaver, S. J. (2012). In situ simulation in continuing education for the health care professions: A systematic review. *Journal of Continuing Education in the Health Professions, 32*(4), 243-254.

Senger, B., Stapleton, L., & Gorski, M. S. (2012). A hospital and university partnership model for simulation education. *Clinical Simulation in Nursing, 8*(9), 477-482.

Society for Simulation in Healthcare (SSH). (2013). *Informational guide for the accreditation process of healthcare simulation programs.* Wheaton, IL: Author. Retrieved from http://ssih.org/uploads/static_pages/PDFs/Accred/2013_SSH_Accreditation_Informational_Guide_2013.pdf

Ulrich, B. (2013). Leading an organization to improved outcomes through simulation. *Nurse Leader, 11*(1), 42-45.

Using Simulation for Risk Management and Quality Improvement.

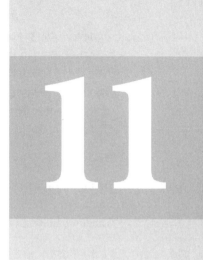

Pamela Andreatta, PhD, MFA, MA
David Marzano, MD
Jody R. Lori, PhD, CNM, FACNM, FAAN

The key tenet for health care providers is "First do no harm" (Smith, 2005). Although modern clinicians might consider the earliest healing methods to be a form of sorcery by today's technology and genome-driven clinical techniques, at their root, all health care practices still depend on human performance and are, therefore, susceptible to human error. Human imperfection will likely remain in perpetuity; however, it is possible to limit errors and associated adverse effects on patients, their families, and practitioners themselves.

The majority of health care professionals have learned through apprenticeships under the tutelage of more experienced clinicians. The apprentice method enables students to learn clinical procedures, techniques, reasoning, and decision-making by observing and subsequently performing these behaviors while providing patient care. Although this method has numerous strengths, its inherent weaknesses include the absence of opportunity for the repetition and deliberate practice so essential

OBJECTIVES

- Discuss how simulation can be used to promote safety in all aspects of health care.

- Examine how simulation can be used to inform quality improvement mechanisms at all levels of the health care system.

- Show how simulation can be used to document evidence of performance skills in health care practices.

- Demonstrate how simulation can be used to reduce risks associated with health care for patients and providers.

for developing psychomotor skills, in favor of subjective preceptors' opinions about performance often in the absence of performance standards, and a lack of preceptor training in teaching and performance assessment. The result is wide variability in the quality of training and subsequently the quality of clinical performance with the potential to adversely affect patient care.

Safety

Simulation affects safety in a number of different health care situations. Most commonly, simulation is seen as an enabler of patient safety. However, there are other domains in which simulation can foster safety, including clinician safety and environmental safety.

Patient Safety

In short, singular reliance on the apprentice-training model of clinical instruction places patients at greater risk for a potential adverse event. Consider the probability that a learner is going to take more time to assess and treat a patient than would a professional provider. Although this delay might not adversely affect many clinical situations, it inconveniences all patients and endangers those with clinical situations that *are* time dependent. For example, a patient presenting with signs and symptoms of a thrombotic stroke requires quick assessment, diagnosis, and administration of potentially lifesaving drugs such as tissue plasminogen activator (tPA).

However, a patient who presents to an emergency department with a stroke faces several obstacles, including timely admission to the emergency department; rapid triage assessment and diagnosis of a potential stroke patient; quick and accurate IV placement; and prompt evaluation by the attending physicians. Experienced clinicians will be able to assess the patient and perform all necessary clinical tasks to restore blood flow to the brain and potentially avert brain damage within 3 hours of onset of symptoms if the patient presents to their care shortly after symptoms become evident. However, numerous potential delays could directly affect patient care in this situation. The nurse triaging the patient could fail to recognize the clinical signs and symptoms of a stroke, which would delay the patient being expedited through the emergency department. The admitting nurse might require multiple tries to place an IV, which would delay the initial evaluation by the physician. A medical student might see the patient and take a detailed but prolonged history and present the findings to a resident, who subsequently performs another examination and presents the information to the attending physician, who then repeats the essential parts of the examination, further adding to the delays. Still more delays can occur as the resident interprets CT scans and lab results and then subsequently reviews and discusses the findings with the attending physician. The resident orders the drugs, but the nurse notes that the order includes an incorrect dosage and must request a new order. Finally, the drug arrives in the correct dose. Unfortunately the time limit for administering the drug has passed due to delayed care; the patient is no longer a candidate and suffers permanent effects from the stroke.

The preceding example illustrates the frustrations that the current training system imparts to all stakeholders—practitioners, trainees, patients, families, and administrators. Fortunately, advances in clinical teaching methods and technologies offer an alternative approach. Simulation-based teaching methods provide an excellent bridge between acquiring clinical skills in a patient-free context and applying clinical skills during patient care. Simulation has been used for clinical training from the earliest days of medical education; early simulations used animals, human cadavers, fruits and vegetables, and manufactured synthetic models designed to replicate an aspect of clinical performance such as suturing or venous access or clinical procedures such as bowel surgery. Advances in computer and imaging technologies have led to training solutions in which hardware and software interfaces merge to provide simulators that function like their clinical correlates. These high-technology simulators include human mannequins, surgical trainers, and virtual-reality constructs, among other hybrid platforms. These simulators enable learners to practice techniques from IV placement, Foley catheter placement, and identification of abnormal physical examination findings to more complex interactions involving team communication, management of disaster drills, and multidisciplinary teamwork. Additionally, many of these high-technology simulators capture performance data that provides feedback to learners about how well they are performing, as well as where they need to further improve to meet expected standards.

The advantages of mastering specific clinical skills in a simulated context prior to working with actual patients are obvious. Not only will the patient benefit from timely and accurate care from those beginning their clinical service, but supervising clinicians will be able to focus on more advanced or critical aspects of clinical care, thus further increasing the overall quality of care for patients. Consider the previous example of the stroke patient. At minimum, simulation-based training would facilitate repeated practice for recognizing the signs and symptoms of a stroke, IV placement, expedited history taking, assessing lab results, and evaluating CT scans. Simulation-based training also facilitates the opportunity for learners and practitioners to rehearse and hone communication skills between the multiple team members involved in patient care, identify and correct any perceived errors, and ultimately decrease the time from admission to administration of correct treatment (Blum, Raemer, Carroll, Dufresne, & Cooper, 2005). The uses of debriefing during these types of team-based simulation activities facilitates the identification and review of actions and behaviors that could potentially lead to error or compromise patient safety (Cantrell, 2008). More importantly, the ability to identify these potential problems prior to their occurrence during actual patient care makes it possible for remedies and retraining to happen before any harm befalls an actual patient, and it ultimately serves to minimize patient risks while at the same time improving clinical efficiencies and quality of care (Barsuk, Cohen, McGaghie, & Wayne, 2010; Hunt, Fiedor-Hamilton, & Eppich, 2008; Hunt, Shilkofski, Stavroudis, & Nelson, 2007; Issenberg, McGaghie, Petrusa, & Scalese, 2005; Van Sickle, Ritter, & Smith, 2006).

Clinician Safety

The apprenticeship model of traditional health care education, in which learning in the context of actual patient care is widely accepted, has clear disadvantages for patient safety. It also has clear disadvantages for clinician safety. The additional stress associated with providing patient care while feeling ill-prepared or incompetent can impose significant negative affective overload that impedes both performance and the learning process (Easterbrook, 1959; Humara, 1999; Mandler, 1979; van Galen & van Huygevoort, 2000; Van Gemmert & Van Galen, 1997). These negative affective elements can affect the performances of both trainees and instructors. Trainees might experience cognitive dissonance as a result of one or more stressors in the environment, including being nervous or fearful of performing tasks or making an incorrect clinical decision (Fletcher et al., 2004; Hassan et al., 2006; Langan-Fox, & Vranic, 2011; Stucky et al., 2009). Instructors might experience stressors associated with divided attention while concomitantly providing patient care and teaching, as well as managing multiple patients and their families (Firth-Cozens, 2003; Lepnurm, Lockhart, & Keegan, 2009; Rutledge et al., 2009; Song, Nakayama, Sato, & Hattori, 2009).

Negative affect has a direct and adverse impact on cognition and psychomotor skills, both of which decline with increased magnitude of the stressors and the number of concurrent stressors (Andreatta et al., 2010; Danboy & Goldstein, 1990; Kirchbaum, Pirke, & Hellhammer, 1993; Schuetz et al., 2008). This increases the risk for clinicians to not only injure the patient but also themselves by performing tasks incorrectly. In addition to increasing the probability for error, these adverse affects put clinicians at risk for incorrect assimilation of the learning context, making it more difficult to build strong knowledge frameworks and consequently extended training periods for discrete cases and in aggregate (Barsuk et al., 2010; Bond et al., 2004; Hunt et al., 2008). Negative affect builds on itself if unmitigated. This is particularly true when stress adversely affects performance in the clinical setting where a trainee is having difficulty, the patient is uncomfortable or annoyed, and the instructor is increasingly concerned about the patient and the amount of time it is taking to perform the clinical tasks. Communication between these constituents, and potentially the patient's family, can further worsen an already stressful context (DiGiacomo & Adamson, 2001).

Health care requires high-quality, reliable, and accurate performance to achieve optimal clinical outcomes. Clinicians are expected to perform to these high standards upon licensure; however they all too often are not afforded adequate opportunity to practice their skills with sufficient frequency to achieve those standards during training. For example, placing an IV catheter requires knowledge of the various instruments and supplies, how each works and connects with the others, manual dexterity to control each instrument and multiple instruments concurrently, all of which must be implemented in a way that does not harm the patient, the clinician, or other clinicians working with the patient.

To achieve mastery in any given area of expertise requires concerted and repeated practice, supported by constructive feedback and assessment (Ericsson, 2004, 2011; McKinley, Boulet, & Hambleton, 2005). This is especially true for psychomotor skills. Clearly, it is unethical to conduct prolonged or multiple attempts at intervention to facilitate learning, or to repeat interventions for the sake of practice in a real clinical setting. Not only would this be uncomfortable for patients, it increases the risk for harm or poor quality care. Simulation provides a contextually accurate environment for practicing techniques without adversely affecting real patients.

Consider the example of an elderly patient, who, after being found feverish and delirious by a family member, is brought to an emergency room in septic shock from an untreated infected toe. The attending physician orders an IV to be placed, and the task is assigned to an intern. The patient is dehydrated, the family is anxious, and the health care team is working intensely to avert the life-threatening situation. This context has multiple levels of embedded stress to which the more experienced providers might be more accustomed; however, for the intern, these stressors, coupled with the unfamiliarity of performing the clinical task, can lead to affective overload that directly—and adversely—leads to cognitive dissonance that impacts task performance. Had the intern been able to practice placing an IV in multiple simulated contexts so that performance became automatic, the impact of the situational stressors could be more easily managed. In that event, any delays in care or prolonging of the task-related clinical engagement that can potentially worsen the clinical situation could be prevented. The likelihood for injury to self and others from incorrectly using instruments or incorrect technique will also be significantly reduced.

In addition, had the team been able to practice performing lifesaving skills together, they might have had sufficient situational awareness to support the intern during the event by using supportive language, providing guidance throughout the task, or even assigning the task to a more seasoned team member because they understood that the difficulty of placing the IV in the critical situation was beyond the intern's abilities. This example is indicative of situations that are not unusual in health care and illustrates how simulation can be used to improve clinician safety.

Environmental Safety

Human performance is instrumental to risk management; however, numerous environmental factors also influence safety in health care. Facilities might be designed to prioritize aesthetics over function; equipment might be integrated into clinical practice without sufficient prior training for personnel; utility hookups might lead to inefficient or unsafe power connections; furnishings and room designs might be inconsistent and confounding; or storage space might be poorly labeled or inadequately maintained. All of these environmental factors require clinicians to divert attention away from patient care in order to assure safety.

Simulation facilitates the optimization of environmental design, as well as orienting clinicians to the environments in which they work (Andreatta, Smith, & Marzano, 2012; Bender, 2011; Dearmon et al., 2012). For example, prior to selecting and integrating new defibrillators, we invited nurses from the entire hospital to test three models using mannequin simulators set up as patients in various room contexts. Each patient simulator experienced cardiopulmonary arrest that required use of the defibrillator. After using the equipment in these simulated contexts, the nurses evaluated each model and noted specific issues that were challenging for them to use. These data informed the purchasing decisions and provided the equipment vendors with suggestions for how to improve some of the design features of their models.

In another example, concerns over patient safety and quality of care led us to design an immersive simulation-based orientation in new hospital facilities prior to transferring the clinical care of actual patients (Andreatta & Marzano, 2013). All clinicians participated in simulated patient care necessitating the use of resources required for patient triage, low- and high-risk antepartum care, normal and urgent intrapartum care, and normal and emergent postpartum care, including surgical interventions. In addition to patient care in the new facilities, participants were paged to consult at each of two institutional emergency departments: pediatric and adult. We asked participants to identify areas of concern, causes for delays, and issues they felt could adversely affect patient care. These data identified several significant quality challenges for which we were able to make specific recommendations for improvement.

Practices and Processes

Hospitals and clinics are busy places, where clinicians, technicians, administrators, and staff who are concerned about time and managing a wide variety of conditions interact with patients and their families. To provide some measure of control and continuity, institutions establish processes, practices, procedures, and protocols—both formal and informal—that serve as a form of governance over actions and activities within and between institutions. These rules and guidelines might be developed proactively or reactively in response to a near miss or adverse event. They are typically created by the risk management administrator in consultation with representatives from the clinical areas impacted by directives; however, institutions rarely have a specific process for reviewing existing processes, practices, procedures, and protocols to determine whether there are conflicting rules, obsolete recommendations, inefficient processes, or directives that are practically impossible to implement. The following section presents examples of how we use simulation to analyze and subsequently inform improvement recommendations for processes in one clinical area of our institution.

Process Analyses

Simulation provides a platform for analyzing both formal and informal institutional practices, and using those analyses for improving associated quality and safety at a system-wide level. Optimally, these types of simulation activities will be supported at the highest levels by institutional management, conducted on a routine basis, and include all clinical specialties and all clinical, administrative, and support staff. Interdisciplinary teams serve this function better than specialty-specific or clinician-focused activities because the idea is to use debriefing to identify those practices with a potential to adversely impact patient care. Capturing and tracking those areas of concern over time will provide a data set from which to analyze trends and reveal the areas requiring review or clarification. Designing interdisciplinary simulated scenarios that require clinicians to implement frequent, infrequent, casual, and critical policies help reveal those areas where improvements can be made. Likewise, simulated scenarios designed to further improve safety and efficiencies in areas where a single discipline manages tasks, decision-making, or other patient activities could benefit discipline-specific behaviors.

Process Improvement

Simulation-based methods are invaluable for identifying areas where excess or deficiencies weaken processes within a health care system. Conducting simulation-based drills designed to require multispecialty, interdisciplinary teams to engage in patient care scenarios is especially useful for identifying weak areas that might otherwise go unnoticed until an adverse or near-miss event occurs. For example, the results of a program involving physicians, nurses, residents, and allied health professionals from emergency medicine, obstetrics, anesthesiology, and neonatology tasked with providing care to pregnant patients presenting to an emergency department (simulated) identified five categories of discrepancies between health system policies and procedures and actual clinical practices by clinicians (Andreatta, Frankel, Boblick Smith, Bullough, & Marzano, 2011). Conflicts and inconsistencies included the use of discipline-specific practices such as jargon, multiple and differing protocols for the same situation, policies that were either unknown or unconsidered, situations in which policy was needed but absent, and policies that were impossible to implement practically. These discrepancies were identified during debriefing sessions that followed the simulated clinical management, and at least one discrepancy was revealed during each session. Importantly, each discrepancy had the potential to lead to errors in patient care or delays in expedited care.

Consider the clinical scenario in which a patient arrives to an emergency department and the resident physician asks the nurse to draw a rainbow. An experienced nurse from that particular emergency department might understand that the order requests that blood be drawn for every color-coded lab vial; however if the nurse is new to the department there might be significant confusion about what the resident is ordering. At best, this could lead to a delay in the order being implemented; at worse assumptions about the order could lead to inaccurate care.

The value of simulation-based activities to facilitate this type of quality improvement is tremendous, if only because it would be practically impossible to discriminate the same information through standard evaluation practices of clinical processes. Current quality monitoring typically involves tracking near-miss and adverse outcomes, such as iatrogenic injury or infection that are reported and analyzed during morbidity and mortality conferences (M & M). Typically, these discussions include participants from one discipline and specialty, thus limiting the ability to analyze system-level weaknesses. Without the information garnered through the types of inclusive simulation described earlier, system-level discrepancies would likely remain hidden until an error brought them to the forefront.

Process Development

In the same way simulation-based activities can help analyze, review, and improve health care practices, they can be used to develop absent, but needed, processes (Andreatta, Perosky, & Johnson, 2012; Schulz, Lee, & Lloyd, 2008). For example, clinical care can rapidly change through the development of a new technology, such as advanced scanning devices or redesigned surgical instruments. In these situations, the processes and procedures that regulate how clinical care is provided might also need to be changed to accommodate the new technology. Rather than guessing how those policies should be changed, clinicians have the opportunity use the technology in simulated contexts to determine how best to approach the creation of clinical and administrative guidelines that impact its uses. They also have the opportunity to test the newly created guidelines with other constituents in the simulated contexts before enacting both the new technology and new process recommendations in the course of real patient care. Referring back to the earlier example of using simulation to select new defibrillators for the health care system, the consensus opinion of those participating in the evaluation was to implement a policy that removed the doors covering the manual controls in order to minimize the likelihood of delays due to unclear operating instructions. Further simulation-based activities confirmed that removing the door removed all confusion about how to access the manual controls without minimizing the clarity of how to operate the equipment in automatic mode.

Professional Development

The uses of simulation to establish performance standards and facilitate performance assessment have the potential to significantly enhance professional development for clinicians at all levels of expertise and in all clinical specialties.

Self-Assessment

When established, performance standards and validated assessment mechanisms provide clinicians with a platform for demonstrating their clinical abilities that is presently difficult to achieve through direct observation of clinical practice, written examination, case logs documenting the numbers and types of clinical activities performed, or examination of the clinical records of treated patients. Simulation levels the playing field by having a common platform (controlled contextual variance), validated assessment instruments (controlled measurement variance), consistent case complexity (controlled clinical variance), and prescheduled performance opportunities (controlled extraneous variance due to fatigue, competing demands, and so on; Andreatta & Gruppen, 2009; Andreatta, Marzano, & Curran, 2011). These levels of control facilitate accurate assessment that informs clinicians whether they need to practice or refresh their skills before they degrade or after they have had a break in continuous practice that might have weakened their skills. These types of assessments do not need to be formal; rather the ability to self-assess privately could lead clinicians to consistently maintain their skills as part of their routine practice and provide evidence of this practice as part of their continuing education toward professional development. The following section discusses this further.

Maintenance of Competency

All licensed health care providers are required to provide evidence that they have maintained their professional competency over time. Currently, specialty boards, state boards, and various other national or international accrediting bodies define the requirements for maintenance of certification (competency; Lewis, Gohagan, & Merenstein, 2007). There might be multiple levels and requirements for the initial granting of licensure, as well as for maintenance of licensure. For example, initial granting of specialty board certification is a multitiered process that includes graduation from an accredited training program, a passing score on a written examination, completion of a specific number of required clinical cases, and finally a passing score on an oral examination administered by examiners from the specialty board. The board certification process primarily assesses cognitive skills, with no measurable performance evidence in either the psychomotor or affective domains. After achieving board certification, practitioners enter into a process referred to as maintenance of certification. Requirements for maintenance of certification vary depending on the discipline and specialty, but typically include successfully reading and answering written questions about a set of predetermined articles and achieving a passing score on a written examination every few years. If successful, the clinician reenters another practice period before repeating the maintenance of certification process. Again, this process assesses cognitive skills only.

The credentialing process examines cognitive skills and assumes that psychomotor and affective performance will positively correlate for multiple reasons, but the primary reason is that it is difficult to measure psychomotor and affective skills in a way that is predictive because few, if any, performance standards are defined for those domains. This is in large part due to two factors: the challenge of assessing performance during real-time clinical care and the variability between clinical cases that confound direct comparison between standards and performance. Simulation provides a platform for resolving this barrier because it facilitates standardized cases, and concomitant establishment of measurable performance standards. As a result, several credentialing bodies have begun to require performance in a simulated clinical context as part of the certification and maintenance of certification processes. For example, the American College of Surgeons (ACS; 2012) now requires that candidates successfully complete the Fundamentals of Laparoscopy that measures psychomotor skills and the American Board of Anesthesiology (ABA; 2012) has mandated simulation-based performance as part of the Maintenance of Certification in Anesthesia (MOCA; Levine, Flynn, Bryson, & Demaria, 2012; Sachdeva et al., 2011).

These examples illustrate the move toward performance-based assessment in the certification and maintenance of certification processes; however, a substantial amount of work remains to be accomplished before these assessment outcomes can be used as competency evidence. Simulation for high-stakes assessment requires rigorous statistical validation to assure that performance measured in a simulated context predicts competent performance in actual clinical practice. However, simulation has the potential to bridge the existing gap between the evidence required by the current certification process and the optimal evidence required to demonstrate competence across all performance domains. The uses of simulation-based assessment have the potential to inform clinical training contexts, certification, maintenance of certification, and reentry and expansion of practice credentialing (Luchtefeld & Kerwel, 2012). One advantage of using simulation-based performance for credentialing processes is that it facilitates assessment in every performance domain. This adds statistical power to the evaluation process because the triangulation of data will provide a greater degree of assurance that the outcomes predict competence.

Privileging, Reentry, and Expansion of Practice

In addition to licensure and board certification, many institutions require additional evidence before granting privileges for clinical practice. These typically include a clinician who has the desired privileges at the institution observing the performance of one desiring privileges or, in more complex areas, the completion of a subspecialty program and its associated credentialing processes. The development of increasingly complex simulations, enhanced contextual fidelity, and precisely validated assessment mechanisms will afford the same level of assurance and standardization to the privileging process as described for the certification process in the previous section.

The perpetual technological and procedural advancements in health care require clinicians to not only maintain their skills, but also to expand them. Simulation provides the opportunity for clinicians to acquire new skills and techniques, acquaint themselves with new technologies and equipment, and practice procedures or clinical tasks that are infrequently performed (Andreatta, Chen, Marsh, & Cho, 2011; Andreatta et al., 2010; Bennett, Cailteux-Zevallos, & Kotora, 2011). Ideally, practitioners should be able to acquire, practice, review, and rehearse their skills prior to performing them in applied clinical care, thus serving as a form of gatekeeping that minimizes risks for clinicians and patients.

Team Development

Individual competence alone is not sufficient. All practitioners work as part of a team, not just as individuals. Team-based factors are known contributors to adverse and sentinel events, and team development efforts have accordingly been recommended as part of quality and safety practices in most hospitals and clinics (Leape & Berwick, 2005). Studies evaluating the extent to which these types of activities will affect actual patient care are ongoing and not yet conclusive, however using simulation to facilitate these types of activities makes logical sense. Team-based performance requires contextually accurate circumstances that cause the types of challenges typical of quality and safety concerns. It would be unethical to enact these types of team exercises in actual clinical practice, so simulation provides the next best alternative. Numerous opportunities are possible, but interdisciplinary cases derived from actual cases from the institution's records have the greatest potential for eliciting relevant team-based factors, as well as minimizing the perception that the case scenario is improbable or contrived (which can reduce the engagement of some clinicians). All aspects associated with individual performance can be considered for team performance as well, and especially the uses of routine performance drills have been shown to have direct effect on clinical performance and patient outcomes (Andreatta, Saxton, Thompson, & Annich, 2011).

Medico-Legal Issues

Simulation can be used effectively in medical and legal issues such as obtaining informed consent and simulating events in preparation for litigation.

Informed Consent

Informed consent is a contract made between a patient and those responsible for the patient's care (Terry, 2007). The contract is made at the time when patients require medical care, which disadvantages patients because they are vulnerable due to a diagnosed medical condition or injury. Patients are asked to sign a form essentially releasing the medical establishment from all responsibility for any and all complications that might occur during the provision of clinical care. Patients are required to choose between signing the contract or not receiving the care required to maintain their health and, in some cases, to avoid death. The process of contracting informed consent involves a physician reviewing the indications for the required treatment or procedure(s) that will be performed, along with any associated risks of the prescribed care plan such as bleeding, infection, and up to and including death. The informed consent process typically takes less than 30 minutes, during which time patients must interpret unfamiliar medical terminology to evaluate the potential risks versus outcomes for their particular medical circumstances. Although patients have become more proactive about asking questions as a result of information available to them through the Internet, chat rooms, and patient information sites, they remain at a disadvantage because of the threat to their health and well-being if they do not agree to the providers' terms, as well as their relative lack of clinical knowledge.

Simulation has the potential to improve this process for patients by providing them with more information presented in a more understandable way, which is also accessible through multiple viewings repeated at will. For example, consider a patient who has been diagnosed with a tumor, which is an indication for surgery. The typical informed consent process includes a surgeon explaining the step-by-step procedure to the patient, but a video-recorded simulation of the key portions of the surgery could be used to actually show the patient the step-by-step process. The surgeon would typically review the potential complication risks using terms such as bleeding, infection, damage to bowel, bladder, ureters, and blood vessels, but a simulator could be used to demonstrate what these complications are, as well as how they would be repaired. Video-recorded simulated procedure could help orient the patient to the preoperative, operative, and postoperative contexts in the same way that hotel websites show guests what to expect on arrival. The patient could be given either a DVD or provided with web access to this information so that the patient could review it multiple times as needed. Additional information could include postoperative information such as how to care for wounds, manage side effects, or perform physical therapy exercises.

Providers could also use simulators to demonstrate their skills while orienting patients to their individual care plans and any associated risks. Mannequin simulators, procedural trainers, virtual-reality models, and standardized patient actors can support the informed consent process by demonstrating to the patients exactly what will take place during their care. Although resource-intensive, these types of simulations could occur through small group activities to review common aspects of care, with private review of individual details. As simulation technologies continue to improve, the ability for clinicians to demonstrate exactly what they will do using a model derived from the patient will likewise further improve the integrity of the informed consent process.

The use of simulation as part of the informed consent process could provide five major improvements to the current system.

- It would likely result in more well-informed patients due to the multiple modalities through which the information is presented: sequential audio, video, text, and illustrations. More informed patients will likely feel more empowered to ask appropriate questions.

- It could allow the patients to review the information at a later date so that if new questions arose they would have the opportunity to ask them prior the scheduled procedure or treatment.

- It could enhance the security of the medico-legal environment for providers by documenting the information provided to patients during the informed consent process.

- It could provide a more standardized informed consent process, eliminating the variability that currently is dependent upon the physician who provides the information.

- Access to these types of simulations—especially if they are in a format that facilitates on-demand access—could decrease the amount of time spent during clinic appointments for these consultations, as well prepare patients to participate in their own care.

Litigation

Litigation is an unfortunate reality of health care practice in many countries. Currently, several factors work against health care providers and institutions when a legal complaint is filed. Documentation is a key factor in a clinical practice defense; however, most lawsuits don't end up in court until several years after the actual event. Medical documentation is rarely sufficient to adequately describe the details around clinical events. Jury members typically do not have medical backgrounds, which disadvantages defendants because lawyers might play on the sympathies of a jury in cases regarding an adverse patient outcome, regardless of whether the outcome was actually a result of a medical error or negligence. This is a situation in which simulation can provide a useful means for reducing costs associated with medical malpractice.

Simulation provides the opportunity for the jury to witness what happened during clinical care, what was typical or atypical about the case, why and how complications could be expected, how they were managed, and why the patient outcome resulted. Rather than listening to verbal interpretations of clinical information that is abstract, the jury would be able to see exactly how things occurred and why decisions were made the way they were (Clifford & Kinloch, 2008). Simulation can allow the jury to see any inherent challenges to a procedure or demonstrate that correct medical practice was delivered, despite the patient outcome. In conjunction to using simulation as part of the informed consent process, the jury could assess whether the patient understood the potential complications of his or her care plan.

Consider the following real-life example. A patient was admitted to the hospital in labor, with expressed desires to have a completely natural labor. Her fetus began to show signs of compromise as demonstrated by a fetal heart rate tracing. The physicians and nurses explained the need for an emergency cesarean delivery to the patient and her partner; however, the patient and her partner refused to consent to the procedure. (Note: In most states, performance of a cesarean delivery without patient consent is considered assault.) The health care team tried to explain the severity of the situation to the patient and her partner for 45 minutes, at which time the patient consented. She was moved to the operating room, the fetal heart tones were no longer present, and the baby was stillborn via cesarean delivery. Despite exhausted resuscitative efforts, the baby could not be revived and was declared dead.

Despite the accurate clinical management of the case, the documentation did not adequately reflect the tone and determination of the patient's refusal to sign the consent. When the first depositions for the legal case were being taken 3 years later, the patient recalled that she and her partner were not adequately informed of the urgency of the situation. Several members of the health care team who were present at the time of the event had moved and were unavailable. During the deposition, the physician reviewed the fetal heart rate tracing under questioning and noted that the patient refused to sign the consent, which led to the delay in performing the cesarean delivery. The jury was left to decide which accounting of events to believe, while facing a grieving couple whose baby died.

Simulation could demonstrate the staging of the actual events that occurred for the jury so that the defendant's lawyer could walk them through the case, step-by-step, demonstrating the actual events and the timeline when information was provided to the patient and when consent was granted. The jury would then be able to deliberate with a realistic depiction of the occurrence, and, along with seeing a grieving patient and her partner, would also see a physician who did everything possible to provide the best care for the patient and her baby within the law. At minimum, the jury would have witnessed the facts and challenges of the case rather than simply heard a description of them in abstraction.

Simulation can also provide a platform for preparing health care workers for the courtroom by helping them learn how the legal system examines the care records and to provide testimony during a malpractice trial. A simulated trial enables participants to learn about all stages of a malpractice suit, including a trial, which prepares them for providing accurate and comprehensive information to the jury (Jenkins & Lemak, 2008). This is an important part of medical education that is lacking, especially given its importance in applied clinical practice.

Conclusion

So how can you begin using simulation to manage and mitigate risk and improve quality and safety at your institution? The best place to start is by working with your quality improvement and risk management groups to identify those areas in which adverse, sentinel, or near-miss events have occurred in the past 5 years and in which any clinical outcomes from your institution are below the national level. Working with these groups will serve multiple purposes. First, you will identify those areas in which improvements will be most visible and therefore easier to capture evidence about any performance effect tied to the simulation activities. Second, you will gain insight into concerns at the institutional level, as well as gain multilateral partnerships in developing objectives and implementing activities. Third, these groups possess the expertise that is critical for analyzing the health care metrics required to evaluate outcomes. Fourth, you will build a collaborative program that can serve the quality and safety needs of the institution itself in all of the ways discussed in this chapter.

Building a culture in which quality and safety are integral components of clinical practice is essential for high-performing health care institutions. Simulation resources and methods provide a framework for introducing and maintaining this type of culture. Lastly, the Society for Simulation in Healthcare (2010) offers guidance for building programs designed to support the acquisition and maintenance of clinician performance factors through processes that have resulted in system-level change at many health care institutions.

References

American Board of Anesthesiology (ABA). (2012). *Maintenance of certification in anesthesiology (MOCA)*. Raleigh, NC: Author. Retrieved from www.theaba.org/Home/anesthesiology_maintenance

American College of Surgeons (ACS). (2012). *Joint statement by the ACS and SAGES on FLS completion for general surgeons who perform laparoscopy*. Chicago, IL: Author. Retrieved from www.facs.org/fellows_info/statements/FLS-certification.html

Andreatta, P., Chen, Y., Marsh, M., & Cho, K. (2011). Simulation-based training improves applied clinical placement of ultrasound-guided PICCs. *Supportive Care in Cancer, 19*(4), 539-543.

Andreatta, P., Frankel, J., Boblick Smith, S., Bullough, A., & Marzano, D. (2011). Interdisciplinary team training identifies discrepancies in institutional policies and practices. *American Journal of Obstetrics and Gynecology, 205*(4), 298-301. doi:10.1016/j.ajog.2011.02.022

Andreatta, P., & Gruppen, L. D. (2009). Conceptualizing and classifying validity evidence for simulation. *Medical Education, 43*(11), 1028-1035.

Andreatta, P., Hillard, M. L., & Krain, L. P. (2010). The impact of stress factors in simulation-based laparoscopic training. *Surgery, 147*(5), 631-639.

Andreatta, P., & Marzano, D. A (2013). *Comprehensive, simulation-based clinical care orientation informed quality and safety mechanisms prior to moving to new hospital facilities.* Abstracts from the International Meeting for Simulation in Healthcare. Orlando, FL. January 2013.

Andreatta, P., Marzano, D. A., & Curran, D. S. (2011). Validity: What does it mean for assessment in obstetrics and gynecology? *American Journal of Obstetrics and Gynecology, 204*(5), 384, e1-6.

Andreatta, P., Maslowski, E., Petty, S., Shim, W., Marsh, M., Hall, T.,...& Frankel, J. (2010). Virtual reality triage training provides a viable solution for disaster preparedness. *Academic Emergency Medicine, 17*(8), 1-7.

Andreatta, P., Perosky, J., & Johnson, T. R. B. (2012). Two-provider technique is superior for bimanual uterine compression to control postpartum hemorrhage. *Journal of Midwifery & Women's Health, 57*(4), 371-375.

Andreatta, P., Saxton, E., Thompson, M., & Annich, G. (2011). Simulation-based mock codes significantly correlate with improved pediatric patient cardiopulmonary arrest survival rates. *Pediatric Critical Care Medicine, 12*(1), 33-38.

Andreatta, P., Smith, R., & Marzano, D. (2012) *Comprehensive clinical care orientation using simulated patients informs quality and safety mechanisms prior to moving to new hospital facilities.* Abstracts from SimHealth 2012, Sydney, AU. September 2012.

Barsuk, J. H., Cohen, E. R., McGaghie, W. C., & Wayne, D. B. (2010). Long-term retention of central venous catheter insertion skills after simulation-based mastery learning. *Academic Medicine, 85*(10), S9-S12.

Bender, G. J. (2011). In situ simulation for systems testing in newly constructed perinatal facilities. *Seminars in Perinatology, 35*(2), 80-83.

Bennett, B. L., Cailteux-Zevallos, B., & Kotora, J. (2011). Cricothyroidotomy bottom-up training review: Battlefield lessons learned. *Military Medicine, 176*(11), 1311-1319.

Blum, R. H., Raemer, D. B., Carroll, J. S., Dufresne, R. L., & Cooper, J. B. (2005). A method for measuring the effectiveness of simulation-based team training for improving communication skills. *Anesthesia and Analgesia, 100*(5), 1375-1380.

Bond, W. F., Deitrick, L. M., Arnold, D. C., Kostenbader, M., Barr, G. C., Kimmel, S. R., & Worrilow, C. C. (2004). Using simulation to instruct emergency medicine residents in cognitive forcing strategies. *Academic Medicine, 79*(5), 438-446.

Cantrell, M. A. (2008). The importance of debriefing in clinical simulations. *Clinical Simulation in Nursing, 4*(2), e19-e23.

Clifford, M., & Kinloch, K. (2008). The use of computer simulation evidence in court. *Computer Law & Security Review, 24*(2), 169-175.

Danboy, A., & Goldstein, A. (1990). The use of cognitive appraisal to reduce stress reactions. *Journal of Social Behavior and Personality, 5*(4), 275-285.

Dearmon, V., Graves, R. J., Hayden, S., Mulekar, M. S., Lawrence, S. M., Jones, L., ...Farmer, J. E. (2012). Effectiveness of simulation-based orientation of baccalaureate nursing students preparing for their first clinical experience. *The Journal of Nursing Education, 52*(1), 29-38.

DiGiacomo, M., & Adamson, B. (2001). Coping with stress in the workplace: Implications for new health professionals. *Journal of Allied Health, 30*(2), 106-111.

Easterbrook, J. A. (1959). The effect of emotion on cue utilization and the organization of behavior. *Psychological Review, 66*(3), 183-201.

Ericsson, K. A. (2004). Deliberate practice and the acquisition and maintenance of expert performance in medicine and related domains. *Academic Medicine, 79*(10 Suppl), S70-S81.

Ericsson, K. A. (2011). The surgeon's expertise. In H. Fry and R. Kneebone (Eds.), *Surgical Education: Theorising an Emerging Domain, Advances in Medical Education 2* (pp. 107-122). New York: Springer Science.

Firth-Cozens, J. (2003). Doctors, their wellbeing, and their stress. *British Medical Journal, 326*(7391), 670-671.

Fletcher, K. E., Davis, S. Q., Underwood, W., Mangrulkar, R. S., McMahon, L. F., Jr., & Saint, S. (2004). Systematic review: Effects of resident work hours on patient safety. *Annals of Internal Medicine, 141*(11), 851-857.

Hassan, I., Weyers, P., Maschuw, K., Dick, B., Gerdes, B., Rothmund, M., & Zielke, A. (2006). Negative stress-coping strategies among novices in surgery correlate with poor virtual laparoscopic performance. *British Journal of Surgery, 93*(12), 1554-1559.

Hillhouse, J. J., & Adler, C. M. (1997). Investigating stress effect patterns in hospital staff nurses: Results of a cluster analysis. *Social Science & Medicine, 45*(12), 1781-1788.

Humara, M. (1999). The relationship between anxiety and performance: A cognitive-behavioral perspective. *Athletic Insight, 1*(2), 1-14.

Hunt, E. A., Fiedor-Hamilton, M., & Eppich, W. J. (2008). Resuscitation education: Narrowing the gap between evidence-based resuscitation guidelines and performance using best educational practices. *The Pediatric Clinics of North America, 55*(4), 1025-1050.

Hunt, E. A., Shilkofski, N. A., Stavroudis, T. A., & Nelson, K. L. (2007). Simulation: Translation to improved team performance. *Anesthesiology Clinics, 25*(2), 301-319.

Issenberg, S. B., McGaghie, W. C., Petrusa, E. R., & Scalese, R. J. (2005). Features and uses of high-fidelity medical simulations that lead to effective learning: A BEME systematic review. *Medical Teacher, 27*(1), 10-28.

Jenkins, R. C., & Lemak, C. H. (2008). A malpractice lawsuit simulation: Critical care providers learn as participants in a mock trial. *Critical Care Nurse, 29*(4), 52-60.

Kirschbaum, C., Pirke, K. M., & Hellhammer, D. H. (1993). The 'Trier Social Stress Test'—a tool for investigating psychobiological stress responses in a laboratory setting. *Neuropsychobiology, 28*(1-2), 76-81.

Langan-Fox, J., & Vranic, V. (2011). Surgeon stress in the operating room: Error-free performance and adverse events. In J. Langan-Fox & C. L. Cooper (Eds.), *Handbook of Stress in the Occupation* (pp. 33-48). Northampton, MA: Edward Elgar.

Leape, L. L., & Berwick, D. M. (2005). Five years after To Err Is Human: What have we learned? *Journal of the American Medical Association, 293*(19), 2384-2390. doi:10.1001/jama.293.19.2384

Lepnurm, R., Lockhart, W. S., & Keegan, D. (2009). A measure of daily distress in practising medicine. *Canadian Journal of Psychiatry, 54*(3), 170-180.

Levine, A. I., Flynn, B. C., Bryson, E. O., & Demaria, S., Jr. (2012). Simulation-based maintenance of certification in anesthesiology (MOCA) course optimization: Use of multi-modal educational activities. *Journal of Clinical Anesthesia, 24*(1), 68-74.

Lewis, M. H., Gohagan, J. K., & Merenstein, D. J. (2007). The locality rule and the physician's dilemma: Local medical practices vs. the national standard of care. *Journal of the American Medical Association, 297*(23), 2633-2637.

Luchtefeld, M., & Kerwel, T. G. (2012). Continuing medical education, maintenance of certification, and physician reentry. *Clinics in Colon and Rectal Surgery, 25*(3), 171-176.

Mandler, G. (1979). Thought processes, consciousness, and stress. In V. Hamilton & D. M. Washington (Eds.), *Human stress and cognition: An information processing approach* (pp. 179-201). New York: John Wiley & Sons.

McKinley, D. W., Boulet, J. R., & Hambleton, R. K. (2005). A work-centered approach for setting passing scores on performance-based assessments. *Evaluation & the Health Professions, 28*(3), 349-369.

Rutledge, T., Stucky, E., Dollarhide, A., Shively, M., Jain, S., Wolfson, T., …Dresselhaus, T. (2009). A real-time assessment of work stress in physicians and nurses. *Health Psychology, 28*(2), 194-200.

Sachdeva, A. K., Buyske, J., Dunnington, G. L., Sanfey, H. A., Mellinger, J. D., Scott, D. J., …Burns, K. J. (2011). A new paradigm for surgical procedural training. *Current Problems in Surgery, 48*(12), 854-968.

Saunders, T., Driskell, J. E., Johnston, J. H., & Salas, E. (1996). The effect of stress inoculation training on anxiety and performance. *Journal of Occupational Health Psychology, 1*(2), 170-186.

Schuetz, M., Gockel, I., Beardi, J., Hakman, P., Dunschede, F., Moenk, S., …Junginger, T. (2008). Three different types of surgeon-specific stress reactions identified by laparoscopic simulation in a virtual scenario. *Surgical Endoscopy, 22*(5), 1263-1267.

Schulz, B. W., Lee, W. E., 3rd., & Lloyd, J. D. (2008). Estimation, simulation, and experimentation of a fall from bed. *Journal of Rehabilitation Research and Development, 45*(8), 1227-1236.

Smith, C. M. (2005). Origin and uses of primum non nocere—above all, do no harm!. *The Journal of Clinical Pharmacology, 45*(4), 371–377. doi:10.1177/0091270004273680

Society for Simulation in Healthcare. (2010). *Accreditation: Frequently asked questions (FAQ)*. Wheaton, IL: Author. Retrieved from http://ssih.org/uploads/committees/Frequently%20Asked%20Questions.pdf

Song, M. H., Tokuda, Y., Nakayama, T., Sato, M., & Hattori, K. (2009). Intraoperative heart rate variability of a cardiac surgeon himself in coronary artery bypass grafting surgery. *Interactive Cardiovascular and Thoracic Surgery, 8*(6), 639-641.

Stucky, E. R., Dresselhaus, T. R., Dollarhide, A., Shively, M., Maynard, G., Jain, S., …Rutledge, T. (2009). Intern to attending: Assessing stress among physicians. *Academic Medicine, 84*(2), 251-257.

Terry, P. B. (2007). Informed consent in clinical medicine. *Chest, 131*(2), 563-568.

van Galen, G. P., & van Huygevoort, M. (2000). Error, stress and the role of neuromotor noise in space oriented behaviour. *Biological Psychology, 51*(2-3), 151-171.

Van Gemmert, A. W., & Van Galen, G. P. (1997). Stress, neuromotor noise, and human performance: a theoretical perspective. *Journal of Experimental Psychology: Human Perception & Performance, 23*(5), 1299-1313.

Van Sickle, K. R., Ritter, E. M., & Smith, C. D. (2006). The pretrained novice: Using simulation-based training to improve learning in the operating room. *Surgical Innovation, 13*(3), 198-204.

Using Simulation for Research

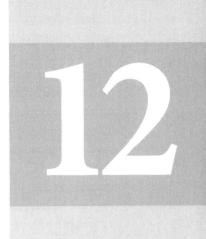

Regina G. Taylor, MA, CCRP

Gary L. Geis, MD

Not all simulation-based interventions produce a straightforward outcome and allow for such an easy assessment as the one noted by Mr. Barry, a Pulitzer Prize-winning American author and columnist. In fact, despite the explosion of publications in the literature centered on simulation-based medical education, you still hear "Show me the proof," or "Where is the evidence?" On the other side, as the use of simulation in health care education has grown, it's not difficult to find those who are confident that simulation-based training improves the treatment of patients. This chapter begins with a review of the current scope of evidence and then discusses how to utilize research in your simulation work.

Definitions

Simulation, in general, is defined as "the imitative representation of the functioning of one system or process by means of the functioning of another" (Merriam-Webster, 2013). Gaba has described simulation as "a technique, not a technology, to replace or amplify real experiences with guided experiences, often immersive in nature, that evoke or replicate substantial aspects of the real world in a fully interactive fashion" (2004, p. i2). Simulation-based training is an instructional technique designed to accelerate expertise by allowing for skill development, practice, and feedback in settings replicating real-world clinical environments (Owen, Mugford, Follows, & Pullmer, 2006).

OBJECTIVES

- Discuss the primary areas of study in which simulation-based training has been the intervention.
- Discuss the design and implementation of simulation-based research.
- Understand the nuances of simulation-based training on participants when research is involved.
- Discuss the impact simulation-based research can have at the bedside.

Simulation technologies in health care include diverse products such as computer-based virtual-reality simulators, high-fidelity and static mannequins, plastic models, live animals, inert animal products, and human cadavers (Cook et al., 2011). Fidelity in simulation has been described as the degree to which the simulator replicates reality (Beaubien & Baker, 2004). The authors of a recent systematic review of high-fidelity simulation-based training (for nontechnical skills within nursing) proposed the following hierarchy of simulation tools in order of increasing fidelity: part task trainers, screen-based computer simulators, virtual-reality simulation, haptic systems, standardized patients, and full-scale simulation, defined as simulation that incorporates a computerized full-body mannequin that can be programmed to provide realistic physiological response to student actions (Lewis, Strachan, & Smith, 2012). They adapted this typology of fidelity within simulation-based education from Cant & Cooper (2010). More specifically, the computer screen–based virtual patient has been defined as "a specific type of computer program that simulates real life clinical scenarios; learners emulate the roles of health care providers to obtain a history, conduct a physical exam, and make diagnostic and therapeutic decisions" (Association of American Medical Colleges, 2007, p. 7). What bearing does this discussion of fidelity have on research within simulation? Most importantly, one does not have to own a high-fidelity simulator or practice in an expensive laboratory to produce valid, important, and sustainable training programs that improve care. In fact, although simulation technology is now a central thread in the fabric of medical education (McGaghie, Issenberg, Petrusa, & Scalese, 2010), this approach was used as far back as the 17th century when simple mannequins were used to simulate the birthing process (Buck, 1991).

Like simulation, research, too, has terms specific to that field. A list of some of the most frequently used terms is found in the nearby sidebar.

Key Terms

Effect size—A statistical calculation that estimates the strength of the association of two or more variables

Meta-analysis—A focused analysis that combines results from different studies with the intent of identifying patterns of agreement and disagreement that might not have emerged in the review of a single study

Reliability—The extent to which a measure is reproducible in other settings

Sample size—The number of participants or observations needed to find a statistically significant difference

Systematic review—A comprehensive review of the current literature on a specific topic

Validity—The extent to which the observed measurement truly measures the outcome or the characteristic it is attempting to measure

Overview of Simulation Research

There is an increasing body of research on the use of simulation and its effectiveness in general and compared to other strategies.

Why Simulation Is an Effective Strategy

Simulation fosters effective learning through active learner engagement, repetitive practice, the ability to vary difficulty and clinical complexity, as well as diagnostic performance measurement and intraexperience feedback (Issenberg, McGaghie, Petrusa, Lee Gordon, & Scalese, 2005; Okuda et al., 2009). The critical factor is that the simulation scenario induces transfer-appropriate processing, that is, those cognitive processes required for performing a task under normal operating conditions (Bolton, 2006; Morris, Bransford, & Franks, 1977). "The most powerful single argument for simulation remains that participation in simulation-based education appears to help to prevent participants from making mistakes in the future, by providing a set of clinical circumstances in which it is permissible to make mistakes and learn from them" (Lewis et al., 2012, p. 88).

In a large, qualitative synthesis of simulation-based medical education, there were 12 features and best practices described: feedback, deliberate practice, curriculum integration, outcome measurement, simulation fidelity, skill acquisition and maintenance, mastery learning, transfer to practice, team training, high-stakes testing, instructor training, and educational and professional context (McGaghie et al., 2010). Using feedback within training is vital; however, determining how to do this and what to include is often variable. The majority of published studies on simulation-based teamwork training utilize face-to-face feedback within a post-training debriefing centered on behaviors observed within the simulations (Weaver et al., 2010). Debriefings that combine process and outcome feedback from multiple sources (such as self, peers, and facilitator) can be useful in presenting the most complete and valid picture of performance (Weaver et al., 2010). An example of the importance of feedback is shown in a study by Edelson et al. (2008). An assessment of in-hospital cardiopulmonary resuscitation (CPR) performance was performed on residents using a novel protocol, including resuscitation with actual performance-integrated debriefing enhanced by objective data from a CPR-sensing and feedback-enabled defibrillator. The simulator-trained group displayed significantly better CPR performance than a historical cohort of residents on a variety of clinical measures, including return of spontaneous circulation, thus demonstrating the effect feedback has on trainee clinical behavior.

Simulation-based training is most effective when used with other educational methods, thus necessitating integration as part of the larger trainee curriculum. Although simulation advances clinical education, it cannot replace or substitute for training grounded in patient care in real clinical settings (Issenberg, 2006; Kyle & Murray, 2008). For instance, as noted by Kneebone, education in "procedural skills should not be divorced from their clinical context and that oversimplification of a complex process can interfere with deep understanding" (2009, p. 954).

Evidence That Supports the Use of Simulation

In a meta-analysis that included more than 600 simulation-based studies, technology-enhanced simulations when compared with no intervention or when added to traditional practice were associated with positive learning outcomes (Cook et al., 2011). This included large effect sizes for health care professional knowledge, skills, and behaviors, as well as moderate effect size for patient-related outcomes. The authors concluded that future work is still needed regarding timing of simulation (when to implement it), selection of simulation technology (that is, task-training or high-fidelity), and cost-effectiveness (Cook et al., 2011).

In a separate meta-analysis published the following year, the same authors compared technology-based simulations to other educational modalities (Cook et al., 2012). Ninety-two studies met inclusion criteria and were analyzed, with most of the comparison being versus lectures, real patients, standardized patients, or small group discussions. Analyses demonstrated that technology-enhanced simulation training was associated with small to moderate effect sizes that were statistically significant for satisfaction, knowledge, process skills, and product skills. However, the effect sizes were larger for skills than knowledge, which led the authors to conclude that hands-on practice—that is, simulation—is more beneficial for higher-order outcomes. No statistical superiority was shown for effects on patient care. Additionally, in the five studies included where cost information was available, technology-enhanced simulation was more costly but also more effective.

In a meta-analysis of the simulation-based training literature surrounding deliberate practice, the authors identified and included 14 studies that compared simulation-based deliberate practice with traditional clinical training (McGaghie, Issenberg, Cohen, Darsuk, & Wayne, 2011). The analysis favored simulation-based deliberate practice for acquisition of medical skills (pooled effect size was 0.71 [CI 0.65, 0.76]), including advanced cardiac life support, laparoscopic surgery, cardiac auscultation, hemodialysis catheter insertion, thoracentesis, and central venous catheter insertion.

In a systematic review of simulation-based procedural training, 81 studies were identified with the majority being at Level IV evidence (n=52) of the National Health and Medical Research Council (NHMRC, 1999) classification, with only 1 Level I (systematic review) study and 5 Level II (randomized control trial) studies (Nestel, Groom, Eikeland-Husebo, & O'Donnell, 2011). However, the most frequent Best Evidence Medical Education ranking was for conclusions probable (n=37). Findings showed that simulation-based procedural training produced a high level of satisfaction among learners and usually led to knowledge and skill improvement, but only in a few studies supported transfer to the clinical environment. Additionally, learning is more likely to occur when there is alignment of the learner, instructor, simulator, setting, and simulation (Nestel et al., 2011). Areas of need identified for future training programs and investigation included principles of instructional design and educational theory, contextualization, transfer of learning, accessibility and scalability, as well as cost-effectiveness.

Evidence That Questions the Use of Simulation

In a large, qualitative review of the simulation-based medical education literature published in 2006, the authors concluded "few published journal articles on the effectiveness of high-fidelity simulations in medical education have been performed with enough quality and rigor to yield useful results. Only 5% of research publications in this field (31/670) meet or exceed the minimum quality standards used for this study" (McGaghie, Issenberg, Petrusa, & Scalese, 2006, p. 795). Furthermore, in a systematic review of the medical literature regarding simulation-based training for surgical skills, 30 randomized controlled trials were identified and included for review. None of the methods of simulation-based training were significantly better than other methods of surgical training (Sutherland, Middleton, Anthony, Hamdorf, & Cregan, 2006). The methodology used within the investigations likely limited the results, including small sample sizes, multiple comparisons, disparate interventions, lack of intensity, limited length of training, lack of allocation concealment and blinding of outcome assessors, and limited validity and reliability of chosen outcome measures. Additionally, assessment of training cost and translation to patient outcomes was noted to be lacking from the literature at the time of this review (Sutherland et al., 2006).

In a systematic review of the simulation-based medical literature regarding nontechnical skill training and patient safety, the authors identified 22 publications. Only 9 included details on the intervention used, and none described the theoretical orientation of the intervention selected (Gordon, Darbyshire, & Baker, 2012). Using a hierarchy to evaluate outcomes developed by Kirkpatrick (1994), outcomes at all levels were investigated, the most common being attitude toward safety. Significant heterogeneity among specific outcome measures was identified. For example, in those 15 studies where attitude was assessed, 11 different outcome measures were utilized. There was uniformity in the content of interventions, which referred to five themes: error, communication, teamwork and leadership, systems, and situational awareness. The authors concluded that this uniformity should allow for development of future investigation, but note that any investigative technique chosen to assess such an intervention should be robustly utilized and well described on publication and that assessing whether such interventions can affect patient outcomes should be considered (Gordon et al., 2012).

In a more recent systematic review of simulation-based training for non-technical skills, Lewis et al. (2012) noted a significant number of studies with equivocal results and multiple design issues. These included lack of information about health care professionals who were not trained, small sample sizes, lack of longitudinal assessment over time, variability in timing of assessments between studies, and limited or variation in the amount of prior simulation experience within or across groups at the time of intervention (Lewis et al., 2012).

Finally, in a systematic review of the medical literature surrounding virtual patient simulation-based intervention, 49 studies were identified: 4 qualitative and 45 quantitative comparison studies; none reported behaviors in practice or effects on patients (Cook, Erwin, & Triola, 2010). When comparing virtual patients to no intervention, pooled estimates significantly favored virtual patients for knowledge, clinical reasoning, and clinical reasoning outcomes. However, when virtual patients were compared to other noncomputer educational interventions, there was no statistical difference in pooled estimates for any of these outcomes.

Outcomes to Strive For

Simulation-based training has often evaluated itself through the use of trainee reaction, such as satisfaction with the training, perceived usefulness, and changes in confidence or comfort. Multiple studies have looked at learning, usually through assessment of knowledge or attitude before and after training, and/or actual behaviors within the simulations and within the clinical environment. For example, improvements in teamwork behaviors and mannequin survival during simulations have been demonstrated after simulation-based teamwork training focusing on trauma resuscitation (DeVita, Schaefer, Lutz, Wang, & Dongilli, 2005; Shapiro et al., 2004). Less well-described have been changes at the bedside or patient-level outcomes, as only 19% of studies in a recent review of the literature assessed patient or organizational outcomes (Weaver et al., 2010). Additionally, in this review, it was reported that the vast majority of studies only collected outcomes immediately after training. The authors felt that "most importantly, our review underscored the need for more thorough and standardized reporting of simulation-based teamwork training programs and efforts to evaluate these programs. Rigorous, detailed reporting is required of clinical effectiveness research—why should we not apply similar standards to research on quality improvement strategies such as simulation-based teamwork training considering their significant role in quality care?" (Weaver et al., 2010, p. 376).

In a recent review, 289 studies were identified and included in a review that compared two or more technology-enhanced simulation training interventions (Cook et al., 2012). Based on the results of their meta-analysis, Cook and colleagues recommend the following features be considered the current best practices for the field, in order of pooled effect size: range of difficulty, repetitive practice, distributed practice, cognitive interactivity, multiple learning strategies, individualized learning, mastery learning, feedback, longer time, and clinical variation. They note that the pooled effect sizes did not always reach significance or approach the effect sizes demonstrated when comparing simulation to no training. Cook and colleagues (2012) recommend that future studies look at comparing simulation to simulation (versus no simulation) and evaluating and comparing costs of different simulation methods, as well as improving interpretation of results through the use of advanced sample size calculation, clear justification of educational significance, and use of confidence intervals.

In January 2011, the Society for Simulation in Healthcare (SSH) held a Simulation Research Consensus Summit (Summit). This Summit selected ten topics of focus regarding research with and about simulation:

- Simulation for learning and teaching procedural skills
- Simulation-based team training in health care
- Engineering/design and integration of simulation systems
- Simulation to research human factors and performance-shaping factors
- Instructional design and pedagogy science in health care simulation
- Evaluating the effect of simulation on translational patient outcomes
- Methods of assessing learning outcomes (formative assessments)
- Research regarding debriefing as part of the learning process
- Assessment and regulation of health care professionals (summative and high-stakes assessments)
- Reporting inquiry in simulation (Dieckmann et al., 2011)

The synthesis of this Summit was described as the major themes for future simulation-based research (Dieckmann et al., 2011). A prominent theme from the Summit was that clarifying any theoretical assumptions about the research topic should probably be the start of any study. More specifically, they encouraged investigators to describe their concept(s) and theory, use explicit definitions/common vocabulary, and elaborate on simulators (including modifications) and scenarios. Following up on this, they concluded that more rigorous data collection and analyses are required, including detailed descriptions of the training of data collectors, application of outcome measures that are valid and reliable, and recognition that simulated and clinical settings differ and that those differences should be accounted for during collection, analyses, and interpretation of the findings.

Designing a Research Project Using Simulation

But how can you be sure that what you are doing with simulation is really improving patient outcomes, increasing knowledge, and changing the way that teams communicate? The best explanation of purpose for simulation-based research that we can find was given by McGaghie et al. (2011, p. 707):

> "The purpose of medical education at all levels is to prepare physicians with the knowledge, skills, and features of professionalism needed to deliver quality patient care. Medical education research seeks to make the enterprise more effective, efficient, and economical. Short- and long-run goals of research in medical education are to show that educational programs contribute to physician competence measured in the classroom, simulation laboratory, and patient care settings."

Integrating research into simulation curriculum can help demonstrate the impact of the training on these key concepts as well as a variety of other valuable questions. "Improved patient outcomes linked directly to educational events are the ultimate goal of medical education research and qualify this scholarship as translational science" (McGaghie, 2010, p. 19cm8). The idea of conducting research can be an intimidating and daunting task, but with a clear and well-developed study, the process becomes much simpler.

Where to Start

When you are beginning a research project, the first step is to identify the question to be answered. In our daily work, questions arise all the time and can range from wondering if the simulation training changes how we perform procedures to whether learners retain the knowledge gained in a course. These are often very broad questions that could be studied in a variety of ways, so the question will need to be clarified into a focused and specific question that is relevant, feasible and answerable (Bragge, 2010).

Before training, perform a needs analysis to determine who to train, what to train, and how best to train, including analyzing the organization, the tasks, and the individual (Weaver et al., 2010). This includes obtaining a baseline determination of proposed outcomes and deciding whether simulation-based training is the correct strategy. In a recent qualitative analysis of the published simulation literature, very few studies report information regarding how training needs were determined (Eppich, Howard, Vozenilek, & Curran, 2011). Eppich and colleagues note that "the tripartite contribution of the individual, the team, and the organization must fundamentally inform any educational strategy aimed at producing effective, functional teams" (Eppich et al., 2011, p. S15). In their review of the medical simulation literature regarding simulation-based teamwork training, these authors stress multiple concepts, the initial one being performance of a needs assessment prior to training development.

In the process of refining a research idea into a well-defined research question, the population, intervention, comparison, outcome (PICO) framework is often utilized (Schardt, Adams, Owens, Keitz, & Fontelo, 2007). The PICO framework is a simple approach that clearly identifies the Population problem, the Intervention, the Comparison, and the Outcome (see Table 12.1). Defining each of these key pieces drives the development of the research from a broad idea into a smaller, more specific research question that will influence the development of the research design and methods (Bragge, 2010).

Table 12.1 PICO Framework

Population problem	What is the problem that you are trying to improve?
Intervention	What are you going to do to change or improve the problem?
Comparison	What are the alternatives to your intervention?
Outcome	What change do you expect to see as a result of your intervention?

The UTOST model, which is similar to the PICO framework, describes five research variables used in quantitative research designs (Shadish, Cook, & Campbell, 2002). Investigators decide on the unit (U) of analysis (that is, individual, team); treatment (T) or intervention (that is, simulation-based training); observations (O) (that is, outcome measurements); setting (S) where the research is conducted (for example, laboratory, in situ); and time (T) (that is, duration of training, timing of assessments).

After the question has been clearly identified and a PICO or equivalent framework completed, it is important to conduct a comprehensive literature search to determine what work has been done in this area and what questions still remain unanswered. Using the PICO framework when reviewing the existing literature will make the search more targeted and efficient. A literature search will help guide the refinement of the question and will enable you to build on the research that has already been done. As you continue to plan the research study, the literature that has been published can serve to identify effective approaches to designing a successful study as well as appropriate measures that can be utilized, and you can use this information to revise the PICO question as you gain more knowledge.

Aims, Objectives, and Hypotheses

After you have identified the question using the PICO or equivalent approach and learned what work has been done in the area of interest through a comprehensive literature search, the next step is to begin thinking about the objectives, aims, and hypotheses of the research to be done. The aims of the study are the goals of the research formulated into succinct and focused points. Simply put, the purpose of the study is clearly outlined in the aims of the study. Although this might sound simple, the specific aims of the study will drive the creation of the study protocol; determine the type of study design used; the study outcomes; and how you will measure change in those outcomes (Hanson, 2006). Throughout the research project, keep the specific aims at the forefront so that the study remains focused and the goals of the project remain clear. The specific aims along with the study objectives, which detail how the aims will be carried out, shape the study protocol and set the stage for what the research will involve (Stone, 2002). For each specific aim there should also be a hypothesis, which is a statement of what you believe the study results will show based on your intuition, knowledge, and experience (Boissel, 2004). The hypothesis should be written prior to any research activities taking place in order to preserve the validity of the project and the outcomes.

Identifying Measures

Although the aims clearly state the purpose of the study and the objectives detail how you will carry out those aims, the outcomes are the things that you expect to change as a result of the study. This can be difficult to determine in simulation-based research because the differences you expect to see are not as easily defined as they are in other areas of research. For example, if you are studying the effect of an investigational drug on a specific type of cancer, there are many things that you could study, but the most obvious outcome would be the rates of death for those patients who received the drug versus those who did not receive the drug. When it comes to basic investigational drug studies, the outcomes are often clear and easily categorized (Boissel, 2004). In simulation-based research, outcomes are frequently centered on concepts that are more difficult to assess and require additional tools and measures.

In general, research outcomes for simulation-based research fall into four main categories: technical, nontechnical, safety, and satisfaction. Technical outcomes assess the participant's ability to perform a skill, such as demonstrating proficiency in central venous catheterization. These outcomes are typically seen in a task training curriculum but they can also be included in other types of simulation-based research. This is often measured with a competency validation checklist or a competency validation using in-person observation or retrospective video review. Nontechnical skills are cognitive and interpersonal skills utilized in treating patients such as communication, teamwork, and knowledge (Gordon et al., 2012). Outcomes related to safety focus on improving the safety of the care delivered and the prevention of medical errors. These outcomes are often closely entwined with nontechnical skills and are frequently included together. Finally, outcomes related to satisfaction focus on the participant's satisfaction with the course and might include things such as confidence in skills following the simulation-based training, perceived importance of the training, and quality of the training.

Another way to classify and assess outcomes of educational training is by the set of four descriptors developed by Donald Kirkpatrick (1994). These are now widely used to evaluate the impact of interventions in education and are described as participation (level 1), attitudes (level 2a), knowledge and/or skills (level 2b), behavior (level 3), organizational practice (level 4a), and benefit to patients (level 4b).

Kirkpatrick actually initially described them as steps, not levels, and listed the four steps of evaluation as reaction, learning, behavior, and results. As simulation-based training moves forward, translation of educational concepts from the laboratory setting will need to be assessed at the bedside, within the institution, and within the health care community. Kirkpatrick's four-level evaluation model provides a framework for this assessment.

Outcome Measures

When identifying the outcomes to be included, the researcher needs to ensure that the outcomes accurately reflect the aims and objectives of the study and that they are measurable (Kendall, 2003). Measuring outcomes can present many challenges, but devoting time to identifying appropriate measures improves the overall quality and feasibility of the research project. There are numerous measures available for use, including published checklists, questionnaires, and surveys that have been used in previous research endeavors. Outcome measurement of simulation-based health care education is vital, but it needs to be valid and reliable. This data is used by facilitators and educators during and after simulations to instruct the learner, but they are also to measure the effectiveness of the education. Three primary sources of simulation-based training evaluation and research data exist: observational ratings of learner performance, learner responses, and haptic sensors captured and recorded by the simulators (McGaghie et al., 2010). Assessment based on direct observation should be an essential component of outcomes-based education and certification (Crossley, Humphris, & Jolly, 2002; Shumway & Harden, 2003). Prior to including a measure in a research project, the researcher needs to carefully scrutinize the measure in several key areas, including validity, reliability, and feasibility. The first step in doing this is to review the original article in which the measure was developed in order to clearly understand how the measure was created. Important questions to consider include how the measure was derived, the population used in the original study, and the validity and reliability of the tool.

To enhance the quality of evidence in health care education, published research should include the assessment or intervention; methods of implementation; and evidence for reliability, validity, and educational outcomes (Reed et al., 2005). Validity relates to the extent to which the observed measurement truly measures the outcome or the characteristic it is attempting to measure (Lachin, 2004). In other words, does the tool really measure what it is supposed to measure? For example, if you develop a tool to assess the communication of a team, do the items actually measure communication? The reliability of a measure refers to the extent to which a measure is reproducible in other settings (Lachin, 2004). If you were to use a measure developed in a different setting to measure the same outcome, a reliable measure would have the same results in this new setting with a new set of circumstances. When selecting a measure to use, select a measure that has been demonstrated to have strong validity and reliability.

Although many published measures can be easily accessed, sometimes you might need to develop your own measure to accurately assess the outcomes in your study. Developing a measure is a science firmly grounded in the psychometric principles of validity and reliability. Before embarking on developing a measure, consult with an expert in the area that you are studying, discuss the development of the measure with experts in psychometrics, and develop a clear plan for creating and deriving the measure. Without thoughtful planning and preparation, the research question that you aim to answer might not be appropriately assessed, which could jeopardize the validity of your findings.

Identifying a measure that demonstrates both validity and reliability is only the first step. Applying a measure in a controlled laboratory environment is quite different than integrating the measure into the simulation environment. You can't control all of the potential factors that might occur in the simulation training that could negatively affect the use of the tool. The best method for determining if the measure you have selected can be feasibly used in the project you have designed is to conduct a small pilot test. This helps to identify any issues that might arise when you use the measure in the actual research setting.

For example, one of your outcomes focused on nontechnical skills is to assess how team members communicate needs. To measure this, you have decided to count the number of requests made during a simulation-based training using video review. Before deciding on this measure, you view videos from previous trainings and realize that due to the limitations of the videos, you are unable to hear all of the requests that were made. After testing this measure, it is clear that it is not feasible to use the tool in the way that you have planned. If a small pilot test of a measure shows that it is not feasible, it might be easy to adapt the plan and use the measure in a different manner. In this example, perhaps you could have a member of the study team present at all of the trainings with the responsibility of counting all of the requests made by team members. Failing to pilot a measure could result in data that is not valid or prevent data from being collected and could compromise the results of the research.

Lessons Learned

As you begin the research process, identifying potential pitfalls can save you a lot of time and a lot of headaches. This sidebar describes a few of the lessons that our team has learned from our projects.

Leadership

When identifying the staff who will work on the project, assigning clear roles and identifying responsibilities is essential to the success of the project. The principle investigator (PI) is responsible for overseeing the project and maintaining the integrity of the work. As the study progresses, the PI should hold the team accountable for completing the work as well as keeping the team motivated and engaged in the project.

Scope of the Project

When beginning a project, it's easy to want to answer all of the questions you have or collect a large amount of data because it might be helpful in the future. As you plan your project and refine your research question, remember that research is a process and each study builds upon the previous work that's been done. It's important to keep the scope of the project focused so that it is feasible and it addresses the specific question(s) that you have. More questions will arise throughout the project; keep a list of these questions that could be included in the secondary analyses or could be the focus of future projects.

Feasibility

Before you officially begin your project, a small pilot test can be invaluable in identifying issues before they arise. The data collected in the pilot test should not be included in the final data for analysis, but it can provide helpful insight into the feasibility of your project. It will allow you to test the measures that you have chosen as well as the simulation-based education. This pilot can simply involve running through one training with volunteers or asking staff to complete a survey that you have developed. Following the pilot test, the study team should meet to review any issues that were identified and develop a plan for addressing these issues.

Timeline

Research always seems to take longer than anticipated with regulatory reviews, challenges in identifying and recruiting participants, and identifying the resources and staff needed for the project. During the planning process, create a detailed timeline with realistic goals and continue to monitor the progress and update the timeline throughout the study.

Special Concerns for Research With Students and Employees

Many laws and regulations governing health care research are there in order to protect the rights and welfare of human subjects. The Code of Federal Regulations: Protection of Human Subjects (U.S. Department of Health and Human Services [DHHS], 2009) and the Belmont Report (U.S. DHHS, 1979) both detail the requirements for human subjects research conducted in the United States, including the ethics review process and the informed consent process. As the vast majority of simulation-based training, and thus investigation, involves health care professionals, requirements of human subjects research are applicable. All research involving human subjects must be reviewed, approved, and monitored by an institutional review board (IRB) or ethics board in order to protect the rights and welfare of the research participants. The IRB is a great resource for investigators and study staff.

Conducting research in the educational setting can introduce new questions in human subjects protection. The Code of Federal Regulations is targeted toward investigational drug and device studies, which are often very different from simulation-based research. Simulation-based research typically includes two groups of vulnerable populations: employees and students. The regulations require additional protections for these two groups because they might be at increased risk of coercion or undue influence. These additional protections might include assurance that individual performance will not be reported to leadership, a more rigorous informed consent process, or a recruitment plan detailing how individuals will be approached for participation.

For projects that are solely being conducted for research purposes, the line between research and education is clear; however, when research is being conducted in conjunction with ongoing education, it becomes more difficult to determine how to best protect the rights of the research participants. In projects being done for research purposes only, participants are involved in the project on a completely voluntarily basis and typically a full informed consent is required. In contrast, research can be integrated into simulation-based training that is part of the participant's ongoing continuing education. Often, the research is investigating the impact of the course rather than the performance of the participants, or put more simply; the course is the subject of the research, not the participants in the course. Examples would include effectiveness of the intervention for team-level outcomes, such as teamwork behaviors or workload, or department-level outcomes, such as the identification of latent threats to patient safety. For these types of research, differentiate the tasks that are being completed for research purposes from those that are part of the education. The requirements of the federal regulations still apply, but the approach might need to be altered.

When you are using this hybrid approach that combines research and education, the simulation training might be a required part of ongoing continuing education; however, participation in research cannot be made mandatory. Participants should be informed that research is being conducted and fully informed of their rights as participants. Completing procedures that are solely part of the research is voluntary and the participants may decide not to complete these procedures. An example of this would be a training course for new staff that is part of their orientation. The research is examining the change in knowledge, a provider-level outcome, in key areas, as well as the retention of that knowledge over time. To measure this, the participants complete a knowledge test before the course to determine the baseline level of knowledge and then complete a similar test immediately following the training and again 3 months later. Because the knowledge tests are being completed only for research purposes, completion of these tests would be voluntary whereas all other activities are a mandatory requirement of the orientation. In this instance, the participants would need to be informed of the research project and consent would need to be obtained before any of the knowledge tests are completed.

In studies where the results are significant, findings often lead to changes within clinical teams and spaces, as well as influence the type and timing of future training. If the institution wants to reassess team-level or department-level outcomes, this would likely not require consent. However, if the institution wanted to reassess individual-level or patient-level outcomes, then application to the IRB and informed consent most likely would be required. This might be institution dependent, as some of this work may fall into quality assurance or performance improvement.

Team Measures Versus Individual Measures

Depending upon the measures you have chosen, you might be collecting data related to an individual or data related to a team or a unit. Research examining competency typically examines individual performance and the measures are generally individual measures. On the other hand, if you are studying team communication, you would likely utilize a measure that examines the entire team. When considering which type of measure to use, revisit the aims, objectives, and outcomes of the study and make sure the approach appropriately addresses those outcomes. Both approaches have benefits in regard to statistical analysis, feasibility of data collection, and protection of the participant's rights. Individual measures offer the ability to match the participant's data throughout the study, which might provide more statistical power when assessing for changes following the training. But collecting individual data might not be feasible if the outcome is related to how the team performs as a whole.

Team-based measures introduce more complexity when you are analyzing the data. Due to logistical issues, the composition of a team cannot be easily controlled, which might introduce variation in the teams that you are comparing. One team might have several very experienced nurses who function at a high level, and the next team might have more novice nurses, which could affect the performance of the team. It is also difficult to match the teams over time in studies examining the retention of skills. From a regulatory perspective, team-based measures can introduce new concerns. If you are assessing the team as a whole, what happens if one member of the team does not want to participate in the research? Do you exclude the data for the entire team or are there alternative ways that you can assess the team without including one person? For measures completed by the participant, such as a knowledge test or satisfaction survey, it might be feasible to exclude a team member, but it becomes more complex if you are observing the behaviors of the team as a whole, such as communication skills. When analyzing the data, you may collect information on an individual level but then analyze it as a team or a unit so that individual performance is not assessed in an effort to protect the anonymity of the individual participants.

Informed Consent

The expectation for all research involving human subjects is that a full informed consent will be obtained from every participant; however, in some cases this process can be altered given some requirements are met and a justification for altering the consent process is provided. The primary methods of altering the informed-consent process in educational research are a waiver of documentation of informed consent and/or a waiver of informed consent. Both of these alterations require that the study present no more than minimal risk to the participants and that the waiver would not increase this risk. A waiver of documentation of consent is typically seen when the consent document is the only document linking the participant to the research study. The participant would still be provided with the information contained in the consent form but the document would not be signed. In other cases, the participant might be provided the information about the study and his or her rights as a participant, and the completion of research-related activities is considered consent. This often occurs when a survey is sent to participants. You present information about the research project and the rights of the participants at the beginning of the survey, and by responding to the survey, the participant is agreeing to participate in the study.

A waiver of informed consent is granted when it would not be feasible to obtain consent from participants due to the nature of the research. This is often seen when records are retrospectively being reviewed, including the review of medical records for patients. An investigator might want to examine the effect of the simulation-based training on the care of patients in the clinical setting. In order to accomplish this goal, the investigator plans to review the medical records of patients that were treated during the course of the training program. A waiver of informed consent may be approved in this case because it would not be feasible to retrospectively consent patients that were treated months after discharge from the hospital, and the waiver would not increase the risk to the patients.

Anonymity, Confidentiality, and Privacy

Simulation-based training is an attractive educational approach because it provides a safe but realistic environment to practice skills and receive timely feedback. When you are collecting data on the performance of these skills, it is vital that participants feel confident that the data collected will not be used in ways they did not approve. Students and employees might fear that information collected might be used in evaluating their performance in their training programs or be reported to their employers. Taking steps to protect the privacy and confidentiality of the data can reassure participants that the data will only be used to evaluate the outcomes of the research. This can be done by limiting the amount of identifiable data collected as well as limiting the number of people that have access to this data. Utilizing more team-based measures can also increase confidentiality, although this approach can have some drawbacks as previously discussed. Another option might be to collect data in an anonymous manner, which can often be done when using a survey or questionnaire that is completed by the participants. This enables the participants to feel confident that their responses cannot be linked to them.

Coming Full Circle: Translating Simulation-Based Research to the Bedside

As noted earlier in the chapter, in Kirkpatrick's model the highest levels of evidence show results at the patient-level, not the health care professional level. Translational science is usually defined as biomedical or biomedical engineering research designed to accelerate movement of results from the laboratory to the patient bedside (McGaghie et al., 2011). Simulation-based research qualifies when its outcomes are measured and demonstrated at the bedside, within the institution, and within the health care community. Investigators should reference the guidelines for designing and reporting quality improvement (QI) initiatives published by Davidoff, Batalden, Stevens, Ogrinc, & Mooney (2009) as they offer explicit guidance for detailed, comprehensive QI reporting and publication.

There is increasing proof that simulation-based health care education can translate from the laboratory setting to the clinical environment by improving health care professional behaviors and patient outcomes. This has been demonstrated through response by inpatient code teams, surgical operating room performance, and neonatal outcomes complicated by shoulder dystocia (Draycott et al., 2008; Seymour, 2008; Wayne et al., 2008).

An example of translational research within simulation-based training is the work of Jeffrey Barsuk and his fellow investigators over the course of four studies surrounding central venous catheter insertion. Initially, this group showed improvements in procedural skill in a cohort of simulation-trained residents compared with historical controls (Barsuk, McGaghie, Cohen, Balachandran, & Wayne, 2009). The subsequent studies showed that simulation-trained residents had higher success rates and fewer complications at the bedside compared with historical controls (Barsuk, McGaghie, Cohen, O'Leary, & Wayne, 2009), as well as decreased catheter-related bloodstream infections compared with the same unit prior to the intervention and another unit during the intervention (Barsuk, Cohen, Feinglass, McGaghie, & Wayne, 2009). Finally, these same authors demonstrated cost-effectiveness of simulation-based training via cost savings from reduced catheter-related bloodstream infections (Cohen et al., 2010). This work exemplifies translational science by combining simulation-based training within an institution with rigorous research methodology from a group of investigators to create feasible, valid, reliable and sustainable training resulting in benefit at the bedside.

Conclusion

Simulation-based health care education and training is a relatively new field; however, over the past decade the number of publications has increased exponentially. The topics discussed in this chapter can help you place your ideas, interests, and potential studies into context with what has been shown, while at the same time can provide you with a framework for developing future research studies about simulation and with simulation.

How do you know what you are doing is important, effective, and sustainable? We suggest application of the principles discussed in this chapter toward your next class as a way not only to assess the training, but to spur improvements within the training and excitement about research in your facility. Keep the scope of the assessment small and the outcomes measures simple. Start by performing a quick needs assessment of your learners, and then search the medical education literature for an outcome measure that fits what your learners feel they need from the class. Apply this outcome measure during or after the simulation as a part of your debriefing session. Have your educators reflect on the feasibility and validity of the instrument and then discuss reliability between the assessors. This will enable you to practice creating simulation-based research projects by answering a simple research question in a feasible but valid manner. Then take what you learned and apply it to your current curriculum or to develop a new course.

References

Association of American Medical Colleges. (2007). *Effective use of educational technology in medical education: Summary report of the 2006 AAMC Colloquium on Educational Technology.* Washington, DC: Author.

Barsuk, J. H., Cohen, E. R., Feinglass, J., McGaghie, W. C., & Wayne, D. B. (2009). Use of simulation-based education to reduce catheter-related bloodstream infections. *Archives of Internal Medicine, 169*(15), 1420-1423.

Barsuk, J. H., McGaghie, W. C., Cohen, E. R., Balachandran, J. S., & Wayne, D. B. (2009). Use of simulation-based mastery learning to improve the quality of central venous catheter placement in a medical intensive care unit. *Journal of Hospital Medicine, 4*(7), 397-403.

Barsuk, J. H., McGaghie, W. C., Cohen, E. R., O'Leary, K. J., & Wayne, D. B. (2009). Simulation-based mastery learning reduces complications during central venous catheter insertion in a medical intensive care unit. *Critical Care Medicine, 37*(10), 2697-2701.

Beaubien, J., & Baker, D. (2004). The use of simulation for training teamwork skills in health care: How low can you go? *Quality and Safety in Health Care, 13*(Suppl), i51-i56.

Boissel, J. P. (2004). Planning of clinical trials. *Journal of Internal Medicine, 255*(4), 427-438.

Bolton, A. E. (2006). *Immediate versus delayed feedback in simulation-based training: Matching feedback delivery timing to the cognitive demands of the training exercise.* (Doctoral dissertation). Orlando, FL: University of Central Florida.

Bragge, P. (2010). Asking good clinical research questions and choosing the right study design. *Injury, 41*(Suppl1), S3-S6.

Buck, G. H. (1991). Development of simulators in medical education. *Gesnerus, 48*(Part 1), 7-28.

Cant, R. P., & Cooper, S. J. (2010). Simulation-based learning in nurse education: A systematic review. *Journal of Advanced Nursing, 66*(1), 3-15.

Cohen, E. R., Feinglass, J., Barsuk, J. H., Barnard, C., O'Donnell, A., McGaghie, W. C., Wayne, D. B. (2010). Cost savings from reduced catheter-related bloodstream infection after simulation-based education for residents in a medical intensive care unit. *Simulation in Healthcare, 5*(2), 98-102.

Cook, D. A., Brydges, R., Hamstra, S. J., Zendejas, B., Szostek, J. H., Wang, A. T.,…Hatala, R. J. (2012). Comparative effectiveness of technology-enhanced simulation versus other instructional methods: A systematic review and meta-analysis. *Simulation in Healthcare, 7*(5), 308-320.

Cook, D. A., Erwin, P. J., & Triola, M. M. (2010). Computerized virtual patients in health professions education: A systematic review and meta-analysis. *Academic Medicine, 85*(10), 1589-1602.

Cook, D. A., Hatala, R., Brydges, R., Zendejas, B., Szostek, J. H., Wang, A. T.,…Hamstra, S. J. (2011). Technology-enhanced simulation for health professions education: A systematic review and meta-analysis. *Journal of the American Medical Association, 306*(9), 978-988.

Crossley, J., Humphris, G., & Jolly, B. (2002). Assessing health professionals. *Medical Education, 36*(9), 800-804.

Davidoff, F., Batalden, P., Stevens, D., Ogrinc, G., & Mooney, S. E. for the SQUIRE development group. (2009). Publication guidelines for quality improvement studies in health care: Evolution of the SQUIRE project. *British Medical Journal, 338*, 402-408.

DeVita, M. A., Schaefer, J., Lutz, J., Wang, H., & Dongilli, T. (2005). Improving medical emergency team (MET) performance using a novel curriculum and a computerized human patient simulator. *Quality & Safety in Health Care, 14*(5), 326-331.

Dieckmann, P., Phero, J. C., Issenberg, S. B., Kardong-Edgren, S., Ostergaard, D., & Ringsted, C. (2011). The first research consensus summit of the Society for Simulation in Healthcare: Conduction and synthesis of the results. *Simulation in Healthcare, 6*(Suppl), S1-S9.

Draycott, T. J., Crofts, J. F., Ash, J. P., Wilson, L. V., Yard, E., Sibanda, T., Whitelaw, A. (2008). Improving neonatal outcome through practical shoulder dystocia training. *Obstetrics & Gynecology, 112*(1), 14-20.

Edelson, D. P., Litzinger, B., Arora, V., Walsh, D., Kim, S., Lauderdale, D. S.,…Abella, B. S. (2008). Improving in-hospital cardiac arrest process and outcomes with performance debriefing. *Archives of Internal Medicine, 168*(10), 1063-1069.

Eppich, W., Howard, V., Vozenilek, J., & Curran, I. (2011). Simulation-based team training in healthcare. *Simulation in Healthcare, 6*(Suppl), S14-S19.

Gaba, D. M. (2004). The future vision of simulation in health care. *Quality & Safety in Health Care, 13*(Suppl 1), i2–i10.

Gordon, M., Darbyshire, D., & Baker, P. (2012). Non-technical skills training to enhance patient safety: A systematic review. *Medical Education, 46*(11), 1042-1054.

Hanson, B. P. (2006). Designing, conducting and reporting clinical research: A step by step approach. *Injury, 37*(7), 583-594.

Issenberg, S. B. (2006). The scope of simulation-based healthcare education. *Simulation in Healthcare, 1*(4), 203-208.

Issenberg, S. B., McGaghie, W. C., Petrusa, E. R., Lee Gordon, D., & Scalese, R. J. (2005). Features and uses of high-fidelity medical simulations that lead to effective learning: A BEME systematic review. *Medical Teacher, 27*(1), 10-28.

Kendall, J. M. (2003). Designing a research project: Randomized controlled trials and their principles. *Emergency Medicine Journal, 20*(2), 164-168.

Kirkpatrick, D. L. (1994). *Evaluating training programs: The four levels.* San Francisco: Berrett-Koehler.

Kneebone, R. (2009). Simulation and transformational change: The paradox of expertise. *Academic Medicine, 84*(7), 954-957.

Kyle, R. R., & Murray, W. B. (Eds.). (2008). *Clinical simulation: Operations, engineering, and management.* Burlington, MA: Academic Press.

Lachin, J. M. (2004). The role of measurement reliability in clinical trials. *Clinical Trials, 1*(6), 553-566.

Lewis, R., Strachan, A., & Smith, M. M. (2012). Is high fidelity simulation the most effective method for the development of non-technical skills in nursing? A review of the current evidence. *The Open Nursing Journal, 6,* 82-89.

McGaghie, W. C. (2010). Medical education research as translational science. *Science Translational Medicine, 2*(19), 19cm8. DOI:10.1126/scitranslmed.3000679.

McGaghie, W. C., Draycott, T. J., Dunn, W. F., Lopez, C. M., & Stefanidis, D. (2011). Evaluating the impact of simulation on translational patient outcomes. *Simulation in Healthcare, 6*(Suppl), S42-S47.

McGaghie, W. C., Issenberg, S. B., Cohen, E. R., Barsuk, J. H., & Wayne, D. B. (2011). Does simulation-based medical education with deliberate practice yield better results than traditional clinical education? a meta-analytic comparative review of the evidence. *Academic Medicine, 86*(6), 706-711.

McGaghie, W. C., Issenberg, S. B., Petrusa, E. R., & Scalese, R. J. (2006). Effect of practice on standardised learning outcomes in simulation-based medical education. *Medical Education, 40*(8), 792-797.

McGaghie, W. C., Issenberg, S. B., Petrusa, E. R., & Scalese, R. J. (2010). A critical review of simulation-based medical education research: 2003-2009. *Medical Education, 44*(1), 50-63.

Morris, C. D., Bransford, J. D., & Franks, J. J. (1977). Levels of processing versus transfer appropriate processing. *Journal of Verbal Learning and Verbal Behavior, 16*(5), 519-533.

National Health and Medical Research Council (NHMRC). (1999). *A guide to the development, implementation, and evaluation of clinical practice guidelines.* Canberra, ACT: Author.

Nestel, D., Groom, J., Eikeland-Husebo, S., & O'Donnell, J. M. (2011). Simulation for learning and teaching procedural skills: The state of the science. *Simulation in Healthcare, 6*(Suppl), S10-S13.

Okuda, Y., Bryson, E. O., DeMaria, S., Jr., Jacobson, L., Quinones, J., Shen, B., & Levine, A. L. (2009). The utility of simulation in medical education: What is the evidence? *Mount Sinai Journal of Medicine, 76*(4), 330-343.

Owen, H., Mugford, B., Follows, V., & Pullmer, J. (2006). Comparison of three simulation-based training methods for management of medical emergencies. *Resuscitation, 71*(2), 204-211.

Reed, D., Price, E., Windish, D., Wright, S. M., Gozu, A., Hsu, E. B.,...Bass, E. B. (2005). Challenges in systematic reviews of educational intervention studies. *Annals of Internal Medicine, 142(12 pt 2),* 1080-1089.

Schardt, C., Adams, M. B., Owens, T., Keitz, S., & Fontelo, P. (2007). Utilization of the PICO framework to improve searching PubMed for clinical questions. *BMC Medical Informatics and Decision Making, 7,* 16-21.

Seymour, N. E. (2008). VR to OR: A review of the evidence that virtual reality simulation improves operating room performance. *World Journal of Surgery, 32*(2), 182-188.

Shadish, W. R., Cook, T. D., & Campbell, D. T. (2002). *Experimental and quasi-experimental designs for generalized causal inference.* Boston, MA: Houghton Mifflin Co.

Shapiro, M. J., Morey, J. C., Small, S. D., Langford, V., Kaylor, C. J., Jaminas, L.,...Jay, G. D. (2004). Simulation based teamwork training for emergency department staff: Does it improve clinical team performance when added to an existing didactic teamwork curriculum? *Quality & Safety in Health Care, 13*(6), 417-421.

Shumway, J. M., & Harden, R. (2003). Association for Medical Education in Europe. AMEE Guide No. 25: The assessment of learning outcomes for the competent and reflective physician. *Medical Teacher, 25*(6), 569-584.

Simulation. (n.d.). In *Merriam-Webster's online dictionary.* Retrieved from http://www.merriam-webster.com/dictionary/simulation

Stone, P. (2002). Deciding upon and refining a research question. *Palliative Medicine, 16*(3), 265-267.

Sutherland, L. M., Middleton, P. F., Anthony, A., Hamdorf, J., & Cregan, P. (2006). Surgical simulation: A systematic review. *Annals of Surgery, 243*(3), 291-300.

U.S. Department of Health and Human Services (DHHS). (1979). *The Belmont Report: Ethical principles and guidelines for the protection of human subjects of research.* Washington, DC: Author. Retrieved from www.hhs.gov/ohrp/humansubjects/guidance/belmont.html

U.S. Department of Health and Human Services (DHHS). (2009). *Code of Federal Regulations Title 45, Part 46.* Washington, DC: Author. Retrieved from http://www.hhs.gov/ohrp/humansubjects/guidance/45cfr46.html

Wayne, D. B., Didwania, A., Feinglass, J., Fudala, M. J., Barsuk, J. H., & McGaghie, W. C. (2008). Simulation-based education improves the quality of care during cardiac arrest team responses at an academic teaching hospital: a case control study. *Chest, 133*(1), 56–61.

Weaver, S. J., Salas, E., Lyons, R., Lazzara, E. H., Rosen, M. A., Diazgranados, D.,...King, H. (2010). Simulation-based team training at the sharp end: A qualitative study of simulation-based team training design, implementation, and evaluation in healthcare. *Journal of Emergencies, Trauma, and Shock, 3*(4), 369-377.

> *"All the world is a stage,*
> *And all the men and women merely players.*
> *They have their exits and entrances;*
> *Each man in his time plays many parts."*
>
> *—William Shakespeare*

Defining Roles and Building a Career in Simulation

Carol Cheney, MS, CCC-SLP, CHSE

Karen Josey, MEd, BSN, RN, CHSE

OBJECTIVES

- Describe the basic roles essential to simulation.
- Know the basic skills needed in simulation.
- Identify different position titles and sample position descriptions utilized in simulation centers.
- Understand certifications and resources that might assist in advancing a career in simulation.
- Define the four Society for Simulation in Healthcare simulation educator competencies.

The roles and job descriptions of individuals involved in simulation are evolving rapidly. In many cases, a single person will serve many roles within the simulation spectrum. This chapter provides an overview of the roles needed to design and deliver a successful simulation program. Whether you are on a limited budget with a small center or have a huge multihub center and an unlimited budget—where you can amass a "dream-team list" of employees—you still need to cover all the basic roles.

All individuals working in simulation must understand and be well versed in simulation as well as being competent in their clinical or technical roles. In other words, being an expert on the da Vinci surgical robot or advanced cardiac life support might have little bearing on a simulation educator's ability to successfully design, operate, and run a simulation scenario or simulation center. In many cases, the initial designers of the simulation center or simulation proposal are the administrator, the facilitator, debriefer, educator, simulation curricula designer, and delivery expert, as well as supportive roles such as the scheduler. One person may do it all—or in many cases is required to do it all. Either way, after someone embarks upon the simulation journey, that person is then considered the resident simulation expert at the facility, department, or location served.

Simulation in health care is a specialty with knowledge and competencies most people do not inherently possess. Many individuals working in simulation have to learn on the job, with assistance from conferences and workshops such as the International Medical Simulation in Healthcare Conference, the International Nursing Association for Clinical Simulation and Learning (INACSL), and the Society for Simulation in Healthcare (SSH). Additional educational sources might come from fellow pioneers, from publications, or through programs offered by large university-based simulation centers.

Simulation Program Roles

For the purpose of this discussion, the functions needed for operations of simulation programs and centers will be discussed as roles typically found in the simulation community. Position titles and position descriptions vary depending on a variety of reasons, including the budget, staff, and resources allocated (see the accompanying Job Title Examples sidebar). Although larger programs might have multiple individuals in each of the roles, smaller simulation programs might consolidate the roles into individual positions. Because simulation is a relatively new specialty, it is especially important for organizations to clearly define the roles and responsibilities of each simulation position and for individuals considering positions in simulation programs to understand what is expected by the organization. Two sample position descriptions are provided at the end of this chapter in Tables 13.1 and 13.2.

The following questions are often asked of the simulation teams. Thus, team members need to have a strong knowledge base as to how these things are accomplished in relation to the programs they serve:

- What is simulation and how does it apply to adult learning?
- How can simulation be utilized with existing education or in building new learning opportunities?
- What equipment is best for the learning objectives?
- How are simulation scenarios built?
- How are effective and measurable goals written?
- How do you conduct an effective debriefing?
- How do you facilitate group and individual learning?

- How do you gain buy-in for a simulation program?
- What makes simulation any more effective than anything else?
- Why should I even consider simulation?

Job Title Examples

Simulation Specialist
Simulation Educator
Human Factors Engineer
IT Support
Clinical Educator
Simulation Program Manager
Data Analyst
Simulation Coordinator
Technical Simulation Specialist
Simulation Operations Manager
Simulation Technician
Clinical Skills Simulation Educator

Administrator/Leader/Coordinator Role

Any operational department that has more than one employee typically has to have a leader. If there are no employees outside of the simulation educator/specialist, then that person may serve as the program leader. Whether the simulation specialist is the program leader or if you have a separate leader/administrator, the typical responsibilities of leadership include budgeting, performance reviews, staffing and scheduling, and service contracting. If simulation is a newer resource to the organization, the leader often markets and communicates capabilities and benefits of simulation utilization. Simulation specialists in our organization (Banner Health) work closely with others in the clinical education environment and often with other teams. They often have opportunities to advance into leadership roles in the organization or in other departments. Many simulation accreditation centers require administrative or operational leadership as well as medical leadership. A dedicated medical or clinical director for simulation might be necessary depending on the size of the simulation program. There are undergraduate and graduate degree programs, conferences, national organizations (such as American College of Healthcare Executives), and extensive sources and opportunities to develop leadership skills.

Simulation Scenario/Curricula Development Role

The individuals in this role build the curricula into a simulation scenario. This also is a crucial role in simulation, as most educators do not know how to incorporate their curricula or desired objectives into a simulation. "The development of appropriate scenarios is critical in high-fidelity simulation training" (Alinier, 2011, p. 9). The curricula may be developed by a subject matter expert (SME) or someone in simulation who has that subject matter expertise. The simulation educator might be the educator, the SME, and the simulation programmer all in one. Alternatively, the simulation educator might build scenarios based on information provided by the SME. At the Banner Health Simulation System, both of these situations commonly occur. Although simulation educators might have subject matter expertise in some clinical areas, no one can be an expert in all clinical practices. The excitement for some simulation educators is the exposure and opportunity to work with many different experts.

The simulation educator must have a comprehensive knowledge of what needs to be considered, evaluated, and demonstrated in the learning environment to ensure positive learning outcomes. Knowing the resources available and the likely educational needs might influence whether a simulation educator is hired with specific clinical knowledge in any one given area. Knowledge of current technology available to use in simulation is also valuable in assisting curriculum incorporation into simulation.

There are many tools and sources for scenario building; many are available via the Internet. By searching the Web for "simulation scenario templates," you will find a multitude of links to scenario template examples from universities such as Duke University, simulation alliance and interest groups such as California Simulation Alliance (CSA) and Oregon Simulation Alliance (OSA), and many other sites. It is beneficial to look at as many tools as you can find from various centers and vendors and then either customize them to fit specific needs of the organization or ask for permission to use a template if you find one that is perfect as it is. How the simulation scenario and curricula are built varies on the length and complexity of the clinical scenario and desired outcomes.

Scenarios should have specific learning objectives (Fanning & Gaba, 2007). Skills for building a scenario or simulation curricula include goal/objective writing, sequencing, and many of the skills that are foundational in an education degree.

The most skilled bedside clinician does not necessarily have the foundational knowledge of adult learning theory, hierarchy of learning and goal and objective writing, measures, evaluation, and assessment. The simulation educator has to understand all of these concepts to successfully design and develop simulations. An instructional designer can be instrumental in helping design not only the objectives within the simulation but also any other aspects of the curricula that might be needed to promote learner achievement (Brown & Green, 2005) If you have the resources to build a "dream team" then you might consider an instructional designer. The National League for Nursing (NLN) states nurse educators need to "be up to date" on simulation and technology (NLN, 2011). Nurse educators can design curricula or can be the SMEs, facilitators, evaluators, and debriefers. *Simulation in Nursing Education* (Jefferies, 2007) is a resource for nursing faculty to incorporate simulation into nursing education.

Subject Matter Expert Role

Having access to an SME is essential in building a simulation scenario. The SME may not be knowledgeable about simulation at all. For example, a physician who does not have any educator or simulation experience can be an SME. The simulation educator can assist in developing the curricula into an effective simulation to include evaluation and assessment. When it comes to using simulation, one of the team needs to be an expert or have comprehensive and applied knowledge of simulation in order to put the subject matter into an effective simulation scenario. Examples of clinical SMEs include direct care nurses, nurse educators, clinical nurse specialists, paramedics, physicians, and other individuals, depending on the training needs. It would be improbable to employ every type of clinical SME for the comprehensive learning that is required in a practice environment; however, it is wise to set aside some budget dollars in case a contract or payment for expert individuals is needed to assist with the simulation.

Programming/Simulation Operator/Driver Role

The real work begins when the simulation educator learns to program and run (or "drive") the simulation equipment. The equipment or "trainers" used for simulation can vary from simple to complex and from low technology to high technology. The training tool might be as simple as a latex or plastic body part that neither acts nor reacts (task trainer), or as complex as a high-technology, full-body mannequin that has heart, lung, and bowel sounds and can breathe, sweat, and blink. Either way, the simulation educator has to know how to use these simulators or trainers, when to use them, and which simulator or trainer will work best for the job at hand.

> Remember that the highest technology tool does not always equate to the best scenario for the specific learning objective.

Many of the high technology mannequins today are becoming much more "plug and play" than the mannequins of yesterday. If the simulation educator has any general computer knowledge, the magic begins as soon as the mannequin is powered up. Most individuals learn to run the mannequin on the fly. Typically, running the mannequin does not involve comprehensive programming; instead it involves adjusting blood pressure, heart rate, or respiratory functions at the moment the change is needed as the scenario or learning opportunity occurs.

More comprehensive programming enables the simulation educator to build a scenario in the software that causes the mannequin's physiological state to progress, react, and respond depending on time or the actions of the learner. Programming can become very complex if there is a need to have multiple patient scenarios running over long periods of time. For example, Banner Health has an onboarding process in which multiple patient scenarios run simultaneously for 4 to 6 hours. Determining the trending of each simulated patient's responses has to be timed, and in some cases complex storyboards have to be written to manage the complexity of coordinating multiple simulated patients. This is important so the learner who cares for these simulated patients is not tasked with handling too many patient situations at one time, and events transpire more realistically as happens in the real environment. Therefore, having comfort with computers and many Microsoft Windows-based applications and technology, in general, is essential for programming and driving the simulators.

The vendor of the simulator/mannequin can be a great resource, and it's often where simulation newcomers learn the tools of their trade. Many of the vendors provide courses in basic and advanced programming for their simulators. Also, some universities and educational conferences partner with various vendors to offer programming classes and training. Programming and driving the simulators are foundational for any simulation program and are at the heart of the definition of the key player—the simulation educator.

Facilitator Role

The role of facilitator is important for almost any non-web-based simulation learning opportunity. It is crucial that the facilitator provide a supportive climate and create trust (Fanning & Gaba, 2007). The facilitator is typically the person who sets the stage for the scenario. The facilitator guides and directs, asks open-ended questions, rephrases, uses silence, or ad libs during the training session. Facilitators typically provide the pre-briefing of the scenarios and might review general scenario objectives. The facilitator may need to jump in and guide the scenario or a learner if the wrong path is taken or the scenario has derailed completely. Facilitation is a skill set that educators need to possess to create meaningful learning environments. Facilitators ask open-ended questions to guide the group to self-reflect and assimilate learning. Facilitative skills include clarification, allowing time for answering questions and solving problems, paraphrasing, and staying on track using the objectives as a guide (Fanning & Gaba, 2007).

Debriefer Role

The debriefer role requires training and practice to be effective. Debriefing is a facilitative method that guides the learner(s) to sustain or improve performance through self-reflection and to obtain deeper understanding through self-guided discovery and feedback. Debriefing can also be more directive, when needed, in order to obtain the goals of the objectives in the simulation (Archer, 2010). Debriefing might include viewing a previously recorded event and then discussing it as a group; alternatively, it might simply follow the event whether recorded or not. The debriefer should understand the overall goals of the scenario as well as techniques such as using open-ended questions, using guided reflection, and drawing out quiet individuals in a group setting. Debriefing is a vital part of simulation, influencing learning and self-discovery, and is at the heart of many adult learning theories as being the most effective part of learning.

Sometimes the debriefing occurs at the same time as the facilitation. The facilitator might stop the scenario and then provide some debriefing to help correct the course of action if learners are going down the wrong path or the learning objective is getting lost. The debriefing role may be assumed by any number of individuals. This is certainly a role with which the simulation specialist must be familiar and knowledgeable. Typically, the person who "owns" the scenario is the one who does the debriefing; the simulation educators/specialists debrief on the curricula they develop, such as onboarding education that is provided in the simulation center by the simulation staff.

Training for debriefing has become more readily available in the world of simulation. A "how-to" guide is a great help to share with an individual performing the debriefing if it is not the simulation educator doing so. There are resources such as conferences, articles, and so on that can assist educators in the art of debriefing. Detailed information on debriefing can be found in Chapter 5.

Evaluator Role

Evaluation is an essential part of any educational program whether it uses simulation or not. Evaluation occurs on many levels and is interwoven throughout any learning process. Perceptual evaluation of the learner is important, but if you consider Kirkpatrick's (1998) hierarchy (reaction, learning, behavior, and results), this is only the beginning. *Feeling* comfortable or even confident performing is different than *being* competent in performance. Generally, the role of the evaluator in a simulation program greatly benefits from individuals who understand how to evaluate without influencing responses and outcomes, and who are familiar with metrics to evaluate if learning has occurred. An even higher level of evaluation is to determine if that learning has generalized to other environments.

Evaluation can be formative or summative and the person in the evaluator role must understand the difference and rationale for both. Many simulation programs are asked to perform high-stakes evaluation, which is an entirely different skill set than what many practice-based educators are familiar with. Checklists are a common method of evaluation. Some great reading on the art and science of creating and utilizing checklists includes Atul Gawande's *Checklist Manifesto* (2010). Gawande speaks to good and bad checklists and describes what a good checklist entails. A good checklist addresses "the most critical and important steps—the ones that even the highest skilled professionals using them could miss" (p. 120). Gawande suggests using a one-page checklist format with five to nine items and that "wording should be simple and exact" (p. 123). He notes that using checklists consistently can be a valuable resource in education and in patient safety. Simulation educators also benefit from some knowledge of psychometrics. A human factors engineer or instructional designer would be ideal to evaluate on a cognitive, psychomotor, and affective domain, but individuals with evaluation knowledge and ability can also perform this function.

Researcher Role

Organizations, associations, and societies that lead and promote excellence in simulation speak to professional growth, patient safety, standards of practice, and research. "Research will be a key factor in advancing the field of simulation to the benefit of patients and healthcare professionals" (Issenberg, Ringsted, Ostergaard, & Dieckmann, 2011, p. 155). This role can be a vital one in some simulation environments, especially in academic settings where research is expected. In other settings, it can be a luxury due to the time and effort it takes to be dedicated to research. It is a specialty role that requires specialized skill sets and high-level education and experience. Research is a standard in and of itself in these organizations that are leading simulation. SSH and INACSL both promote research in their mission statements.

Data Analyst Role

The data analyst is an important position to assist in aggregating data and the aforementioned evaluation metrics to demonstrate utilization and outcomes. Most clinical educators and trainers do not succinctly capture data on low-level measures like attendance or perceptual feedback, let alone measures of learning or skill generalization. Attendance data as to how many nurses or physicians or students utilize the center, why they use it, how they perform, and so on can be valuable information in addressing use and operations in the evaluation of center usage. The purpose of the data analyst role is to assist in the creation of databases and automation of different types of psychometric tools, such as checklists, evaluations, assessments, and test scores. An individual with a comprehensive understanding of Excel, Access, database software, and tools is an incredible asset. This person does not have to be clinical. In fact, a nonclinical person can add a fresh perspective to the team.

Technical Support Role

The first thing almost anyone new to simulation learns is how to set up the equipment or mannequins. Set up includes connections of lines, tubing, and compressors as well as start up and shut down of computers. Many simulation centers use a technician to fill this role—someone who might not have formal education as a health care provider. The individual in the technician support role might program and run the simulator, but a clinical resource might be needed to assist the technical support person to understand how to adjust the clinical parameters. Other responsibilities might consist of preparing and applying moulage, cleaning up, performing routine maintenance, assuring that all equipment is working properly, and running system diagnostics from the mannequin to the computer systems. Moulage is a specialized area of simulation that is very time consuming. It takes training and practice to learn the many formulas, compounds, and "items" to produce realistic moulage that helps to immerse the learner into the simulation. You also need to understand which compounds and materials could affect the integrity of the mannequins or equipment so as not to permanently damage or stain their resources.

Troubleshooting equipment is another aspect of technical support. This can include installing software upgrades, problem solving a compressor issue, or intervening when equipment does not function as intended, such as when a lung won't inflate.

Often, the greater understanding of the technology and equipment one has, the greater the opportunities to modify the equipment and creatively develop or re-create clinical issues without purchasing separate mannequins or trainers. Individuals with an advanced understanding of the equipment and technology can often perform quick repairs if there is an equipment malfunction without waiting for separate technical support to arrive or having to abort the scenario altogether. This knowledge can be a critical element in operations.

Learning the ins and outs of the mannequins and other simulation technology can be very rewarding. Although there are simulation workshops that focus on basic and advanced aspects of technical support, novices often learn these skills on the job as well as learning more advanced problem solving with the help from vendor technical support. In many cases, the simulation educator also fills the technical support role. Depending on the size and complexity of the simulation program, simulation educators might also have an information technology (IT) support person or other support staff to assist them in maximizing the use of the available simulation equipment.

Audiovisual Role

The audiovisual (AV) role is another vital role that's important to smooth operations. A person who can assist with videorecording and teleconferencing capabilities will increase efficiencies in the program. Many high-technology simulators include an audiovisual recorder that allows for recording and immediate playback opportunities. The IT support role might assist with this if the simulation center has that availability. Some programs have separate AV teams to help with this equipment.

Scheduler/Administrative Assistant Role

The scheduler and administrative assistant roles are extremely time-consuming functions. Some type of scheduling or management system is needed to document the needed space and resources for simulations. In addition, someone is needed to operate it. Inventory, purchasing, data collection and entry, monitoring supply levels, and receptionist duties can take time away from the simulation team's main function of simulation education. Scheduling is not limited to coordinating designated simulation space. The varied people resources, equipment, and numbers of participants to juggle can become a job of its own. Sometimes the mannequins have their own "social" calendar and are loaned out of the simulation space. Receptionist responsibilities and coordination of scheduling simulations are huge functions that can be combined and will lead to a smoother-functioning center when someone is designated to this role. It is often more cost effective to employ a nonclinical person to perform these functions, which allows the clinical or simulation experts to focus on their areas of expertise.

Other Roles and Skill Sets in Simulation

Other roles in simulation include human factors engineers, clinical educators, simulation program managers, administrators, medical simulation technical specialists, simulation coordinators, simulation specialists, standardized patient educators, and simulation technicians.

Job postings typically include the skill set needed for the position. A standardized patient educator job posting may be specific to the skills needed to run this aspect of simulation, including orientation, training, and supervision of teaching and assessment of training using standardized patients. Many different roles and responsibilities have been discussed that lend to the general competency of a simulation educator. An additional item that is useful to understand as a simulation educator is the various ways to increase fidelity of a simulation. Some ways include but are not limited to the use of confederates and standardized patients. Using confederates, actors, or standardized patients are other means to design effective simulations. A *confederate* is a person who is scripted to bring realism to the simulation by providing extra challenges, such as a family member or an ambulance worker. A *standardized patient* is a trained actor who portrays a patient in a consistent scripted manner. The use of these individuals can greatly add to the realism and complexity of a health care scenario; however, it takes time and highly specialized knowledge in order to train the actors to deliver behaviors for the learner to experience the desired learning outcomes (Barrows, 1993). There are many articles that speak to the value and the process of using confederates in simulation. Standardized patient programs require a completely different understanding of operations, flow, personnel, and training of these individuals. A simulation educator might not be involved in a standardized patient program, but it is important to understand the relationship and general concepts.

Other job postings in simulation include skill sets that encompass market research to include current practice and trends in simulation training, public relations, budgeting, grant writing, and finding funding sources for both operations and research applications. Responsibilities in job postings might include:

- Giving tours
- Promoting the program to external organizations
- Developing the website
- Developing simulation employee education
- Coordinating and developing the simulation program
- Providing summaries of operational expenses
- Collecting class attendance data
- Tracking equipment usage
- Evaluating, maintaining, and repairing simulation training technology and equipment
- Ensuring compliance with the Occupational Safety and Health Administration (OSHA) and hospital regulations
- Developing policy
- Understanding electronics, digital IT/AV systems, production and software, support and media application

Health Care Simulation Educator

The health care simulation educator's position might encompass many of the roles described previously in this chapter, or it might involve only one role. The requirements are often based on the size of the program in which the health care simulation educator is employed.

SSH defines a health care simulation educator as an individual who is involved in delivering health care–related simulation education interventions or an individual who directly oversees or administers health care–related simulation educational interventions (SSH, 2012). Health care simulation educators seeking certification from SSH are evaluated in the following areas:

- Professional values and capabilities
- Knowledge of educational principles, practice, and methodology in simulation
- Implementing, assessing, and managing simulation-based educational activities
- Scholarship
- Spirit of inquiry and teaching

SSH certification for health care simulation educators is described more fully in Chapter 14.

Resources to Get Started and Advance

Many associations and organizations dedicated to health care simulation give resource assistance to those new in the field and support those who have experience to keep up to date on trends and publications as well as research. These organizations are easily accessed online and offer memberships and opportunities for collaboration. NLN has an online simulation e-learning site called the Simulation Innovation Resource Center (SIRC), which offers courses such as designing and developing simulations, debriefing, simulation research, and curriculum integration (http://sirc.nln.org/). Universities and annual conferences also cover many of these same items and include operational topics, research, debriefing, and evaluation methods, to name only a small number of opportunities available. Interservice/Industry Training Simulation and Education Conference (I/ITSEC) has social media support and puts on a modeling, simulation, and training

annual conference and promotes cooperation among users of simulation (http://www.
iitsec.org).

The American College of Surgeons is a resource for medical surgical simulation. SSH,
a multidisciplinary organization, and INACSL are two organizations that have standards
for simulation practice and performance that can be extremely helpful in guiding one
who is looking for a job in the simulation field. These organizations provide links on their
websites to other simulation societies, including international resources. Their journals,
Simulation in Healthcare and *Clinical Simulation in Nursing Journal*, are available to members and can be accessed online.

Other support for simulation educators includes career centers that have job postings specific to simulation as well as links to many simulation centers, such as the Winter
Institute for Simulation Education and Research (WISER). Many of these groups have social networks that include Listservs and use Facebook forums that are specific for health
care professionals who are interested in simulation. News, blogs, and newsletters are also
available. Some state and local organizations to help support those locally are also available in some areas. There are modeling and simulation programs present in many different industries for education and training; however, these programs are typically tracks for
various types of engineers and programmers.

Going to workshops, conferences, and webinars; engaging in vendor education; and
visiting simulation centers are other ways to get started in this field. SSH has a comprehensive literature review for the Certified Healthcare Simulation Educator (CHSE) that
can be accessed by anyone interested in simulation. Certifications demonstrate expertise in best practice and standards that are a foundation of performance that encompass
"knowledge, skills, and abilities."

Conclusion

Educators of any sort wear many different hats depending on the needs and the populations they serve. The basic roles identified in this chapter can be of assistance to you when
compiling a job description for a simulation center or applying for a simulation job position. Roles discussed include technical setup and support, AV, SME, facilitator, debriefer,
programmer/driver, scenario/curricula developer, and evaluator. Other support roles are
data analyst, researcher, scheduler and administrative assistant, as well as someone to

moulage, play the confederate, and train standardized patients to use in simulations. Job titles and positions can be a combination of the roles discussed in this chapter depending on the need and budgets of a simulation center. Being certified as a simulation educator can assist you in demonstration of qualification and expertise in simulation. Many resources exist that may assist in learning what the current needs and trends are in the simulation world. There is no shortage of opportunities in the roles and positions available in the specialty of simulation.

> People always have many different roles to play. The crucial thing is to be determined to make a wholehearted effort in everything and be fully engaged in what we are doing at any given moment. The secret to successfully fulfilling a variety of roles is to concentrate fully on the task at hand and give it our best effort with enthusiasm, maintaining a positive, forward-looking attitude and not worrying. –Daisaku Ikeda

Table 13.1   Sample Position Description—Simulation Director

Banner Health Position Description

Position Title: Simulation Director

POSITION SUMMARY

This position has system responsibility for the standardization of simulation education and training to achieve system organizational strategies and initiatives; ensures professional practice through design, development, and implementation of simulated and innovative business solutions; seeks opportunities to trial creative ideas and processes in a safe and professional environment; partners and collaborates with leadership and physicians throughout the organization to design and implement simulated learning and development opportunities, and oversees and has responsibility for all simulation training centers and simulation programs. Instrumental in the creation and implementation of local and system policies related to simulation environments and practices. Recruits and manages staff, interprets policies, oversees regional and system simulation and innovation strategy development and overall system management of simulation and innovation programs and technologies; ensures for effective participation to achieve full integration of system-wide simulation structure and practice.

Table 13.1 Sample Position Description—Simulation Director *(cont.)*

ESSENTIAL FUNCTIONS

1. Engages system, regional, and facility stakeholders in establishing a vision for simulation and innovation and in following the path to achieve that vision. Develops and implements simulation and innovation strategies to establish and assure that our facility work environments and cultures support leaders, physicians, and employees to excel in the performance of their roles, provides quality patient care, and ensures patient safety throughout the organization.

2. Demonstrates an understanding of key organization strategies and initiatives and ensures the simulation resources and programs are aligned accordingly. Assures the integration of system simulation and innovation activities to achieve system strategies and objectives. Maintains key stakeholder involvement in development and sustainability of simulation services.

3. Directs the preparation of annual simulation and innovation operating and capital expenses, manages financial budget and procurements, and assures responsible use of allocated budget. Responsible for the preparation, writing, and management of simulation- and innovation-generated grants, research and commercial projects. Assumes marketing and communication efforts to support simulation and innovation service growth and effectiveness.

4. Provides direction and support to the simulation and innovation team. Selects, onboards, and develops a high-performance, customer service–oriented team. Establishes effective staff, physician, and leadership partnerships throughout the organization. Performs as a change agent. Establishes visibility and credibility. Leads and participates on assigned committees and teams. Supports an environment and infrastructure that promotes professional growth and development. Functions as a member of the regional clinical services leadership team; partners with counterparts in guiding and directing simulation activities.

5. Develops and implements strategic simulation and innovation services and opportunities to support the achievement of workforce goals, quality initiatives, and clinical practice. Oversees the clinical and operational aspects of simulation and innovation. Incorporates resources and establishes standards supporting the continuum of clinical practice, patient safety, and evidence-based practice.

6. Evaluates simulation learning effectiveness using standardized outcome measurements. Identifies and acts on research opportunities. Utilizes performance measures and organizational needs to drive simulation and innovation plans and strategies. Provides leadership and oversight in the collection, review, and analysis of data.

7. Incorporates technology to provide remote/distance simulation experiences. Integrates simulation and innovation services with learning technologies including the organization

learning management system and e-learning technology opportunities. Establishes a sentry function in order to identify opportunities for early adoption of enabling technologies and in support of the evolution of clinical practice.

Performs all functions according to established policies, procedures, regulatory and accreditation requirements, as well as applicable professional standards. Provides all customers of Banner Health with an excellent service experience by consistently demonstrating our core and leader behaviors each and every day.

NOTE: The essential functions are intended to describe the general content of and requirements of this position and are not intended to be an exhaustive statement of duties. Specific tasks or responsibilities will be documented as outlined by the incumbent's immediate manager.

SUPERVISORY RESPONSIBILITIES

DIRECTLY REPORTING

May include simulation managers, simulation coordinators, and educators at all simulation training centers.

MATRIX OR INDIRECT REPORTING

None

TYPE OF SUPERVISORY RESPONSIBILITIES

Assigned full authority for employment actions including selection, training, coaching, and performance reviews.

Banner Health Leadership will strive to uphold the mission, vision, and values of the organization. They will serve as role models for staff and act in a people-centered, service excellence–focused, and results-oriented manner.

SCOPE AND COMPLEXITY

Maintains accountabilities toward achieving system strategies and initiatives. Balances vision with detail. Position must be effective in strategic thinking and maintain a high level of accountability while demonstrating the ability to engage others in the work. Must demonstrate the ability to influence others to achieve objectives. Must possess critical-thinking skills with ability to prioritize needs rapidly. Requires an understanding of regulatory guidelines, policies, procedures, and standards of practice.

Table 13.1   Sample Position Description—Simulation Director *(cont.)*

PHYSICAL DEMANDS/ENVIRONMENT FACTORS

OE—Typical Office Environment: (Accountant, Administrative Assistant, Consultant, Program Manager)

Requires extensive sitting with periodic standing and walking.

May be required to lift up to 20 pounds.

Requires significant use of personal computer, phone, and general office equipment.

Needs adequate visual acuity, ability to grasp and handle objects.

Needs ability to communicate effectively through reading, writing, and speaking in person or on telephone.

May require off-site travel.

MINIMUM QUALIFICATIONS

Must possess a strong knowledge of health care as normally obtained through the completion of a master's degree in a health care–related field.

Must possess at least 10 years of acute clinical experience and at least 5 years of managerial experience.

Requires current knowledge and experience with strategic development, program development, operations and learning solutions. Demonstrates understanding of adult learning principles. Excellent presentation, facilitation, and computer technology skills required. Strong organization and communication skills required. Ability to take initiative, problem solve, and improve processes required. Extensive reading, verbal communication, writing, presentation, financial/statistical analysis, and experience in integrating information technology.

PREFERRED QUALIFICATIONS

Minimum 2 years in a position with primary responsibility for design and delivery of learning content preferred.

Additional related education and/or experience preferred.

Used with permission of Banner Health.

Table 13.2 Sample Position Description—RN Simulation Specialist

Banner Health Position Description

Position Title: RN Simulation Specialist

POSITION SUMMARY

This position implements education programs for several service line workforce needs to achieve successful simulation education and training. Plans, designs, implements, and evaluates simulation-based learning and development outcomes to support the achievement of workforce goals, facility and regional strategies, and initiatives. Provides expert consultation and critique to simulation development.

ESSENTIAL FUNCTIONS

1. Serves as an internal consultant for simulation design. Designs workforce learning and development outcomes that support facility strategies and initiatives. Conducts assessment of current and projected workforce development needs and provides efficient, effective, high-quality programs and services in response. Provides guidance on clinical issues for various service line areas. Serves as a resource for policy and procedures, standards of care, and external agency requirements.

2. Coordinates and assists in all development of scenarios and training in conjunction with faculty and staff to integrate simulation usage into clinical curriculum. Researches, plans, implements and evaluates curriculum content and sequence. Incorporates proficient clinical practice, safety, and patient-centered care in all educational scenarios. Programs, tests, and runs scenarios with faculty, assuring that faculty and equipment are prepared for teaching scenarios.

3. Directly responsible for the development and delivery of employee development programs and designated learning programs that attract new recruits, retain current staff, and improve quality of care. Ensures timely delivery and integration between plan objectives and design in order to obtain intended program impact and stakeholder/participant satisfaction while managing required resources effectively.

4. Uses advanced knowledge to execute setup, programming, maintenance, use, disassembly, and troubleshooting of simulation equipment. Demonstrates and teaches technical and philosophical aspects of operating and programming simulators to staff. Develops a schedule of simulator activities to include periodic review and maintenance of equipment.

5. Implements, interprets, and evaluates learning goals and objectives. Implements assessment tools to be integrated as competency measures in all aspects of simulation-based education. Evaluates learning effectiveness using standardized outcome measurements. Uses performance measures and workforce needs to drive education plans and learning strategies.

Table 13.2   Sample Position Description—RN Simulation Specialist
(cont.)

6. Manages and leads program development of new systems, applications, software conversions and upgrades, and media integration maintaining partnerships and troubleshooting. Identifies opportunities for technology improvement and integration into health care education.

7. Conducts regular evaluations and critiques of programs, soliciting recommendations from both internal and external customers.

8. Provides consultation for research projects; guides and/or directs process. Effectively translates research outcomes into actions, working with others to improve overall quality and cost effectiveness of patient care.

Performs all functions according to established policies, procedures, regulatory and accreditation requirements, as well as applicable professional standards. Provides all customers of Banner Health with an excellent service experience by consistently demonstrating our core and leader behaviors each and every day.

NOTE: The essential functions are intended to describe the general content of and requirements of this position and are not intended to be an exhaustive statement of duties. Specific tasks or responsibilities will be documented as outlined by the incumbent's immediate manager.

SUPERVISORY RESPONSIBILITIES
DIRECTLY REPORTING
None

MATRIX OR INDIRECT REPORTING
None

TYPE OF SUPERVISORY RESPONSIBILITIES
N/A

Banner Health Leadership will strive to uphold the mission, vision, and values of the organization. They will serve as role models for staff and act in a people-centered, service excellence–focused, and results-oriented manner.

SCOPE AND COMPLEXITY

This position designs simulation-based clinical training programs for all levels of clinical staff and providers for both internal and external facilities. This position is also responsible for research and applicable grant funding.

PHYSICAL DEMANDS/ENVIRONMENT FACTORS

DP—Typical Direct Patient Care environment: (Nutrition Rep, Chaplain, RN)

Able to stand, walk, bend, squat, reach, and stretch frequently.

Possess physical agility and adequate reaction time to respond quickly and appropriately to unexpected patient care needs.

Needs adequate hearing and visual acuity, including adequate color vision.

Requires fine motor skills, adequate eye-hand coordination, and ability to grasp and handle objects.

Able to use proper body mechanics to assist patients in ambulating, transferring in and out of bed, chair, or wheelchair.

May be required to lift up to 75 pounds.

Must use standard precautions due to threat of exposure to blood and bodily fluids.

Needs ability to communicate effectively through reading, writing, and speaking in person or on telephone.

May require periodic use of personal computer.

NOTE: All patient and exposure encounters are simulated, but require exercise of caution as required in actual patient care settings.

MINIMUM QUALIFICATIONS

Must possess a strong knowledge of clinical care, education, and/or technology as normally demonstrated through the completion of a bachelor's degree in nursing, health care, education, technology, or related field.

Requires a current RN license.

Must possess a strong knowledge and understanding of clinical care as normally demonstrated through 5 years of recent experience in an acute care setting. Requires 2 years experience using adult learning principles. Requires the ability to facilitate shared understanding and creative team processes. Develops collaborative relationships that foster synergy, creative solutions and successful results. Must have excellent written and oral communication skills.

Table 13.2	Sample Position Description—RN Simulation Specialist *(cont.)*

Must also have familiarity with programming and troubleshooting software.

PREFERRED QUALIFICATIONS

Master's degree in nursing, health care, or adult learning preferred.

Additional related education and/or experience preferred.

Used with permission of Banner Health.

References

Alinier, G. (2011). Developing high-fidelity health care simulation scenarios: A guide for educators and professionals. *Simulation and Gaming, 42*(1), 9-26.

Archer, J. C. (2010). State of the science in health professional education: Effective feedback. *Medical Education, 44*(1), 101-108.

Barrows, H. S. (1993). An overview of the uses of standardized patients for teaching and evaluating clinical skills. *Academic Medicine, 68*(6), 443-451

Brown, A., & Green, T. D. (2005). *The essentials of instructional design. Connecting fundamental principles with process and practice* (1st ed.). Upper Saddle River, NJ: Prentice Hall.

Fanning, R. M., & Gaba, D. M. (2007). The role of debriefing in simulation-based learning. *Simulation in Healthcare, 2*(2), 115-125.

Gawande, A. (2010). *The checklist manifesto: How to get things right.* New York: Picador Henry Holt and Company.

Issenberg, S. G., Ringsted, C., Ostergaard, D., and Dieckmann, P. (2011). Setting a research agenda for simulation-based healthcare education: A synthesis of the outcome from an Utstein Style Meeting. *Simulation in Healthcare, 6*(3), 155-167. doi: 10.1097/SIH.0b013e3182207c24

Jeffries, P. (2007). *Simulation in nursing education: From conceptualization to evaluation.* New York: National League for Nursing.

Kirkpatrick, D. L. (1998). *Evaluating training programs: The four levels* (2nd ed.). San Francisco, CA: Berrett-Koehler.

National League for Nursing (NLN). (2011). *Simulation and technology.* Retrieved from www.nln.org/facultyprograms/simulation_tech.htm

Society for Simulation in Healthcare (SSH). (2012). *SSH certified healthcare simulation educator handbook.* Wheaton, IL: Author. Retrieved from http://ssih.org/uploads/static_pages/PDFs/Certification/CHSE_Handbook.pdf

"My meaning simply is, that whatever I have tried to do in life, I have tried with all my heart to do well; that whatever I have devoted myself to, I have devoted myself to completely; that in great aims and in small, I have always been thoroughly in earnest."

–Charles Dickens

Credentialing and Certification in Simulation

Andrew Spain, MA, NCEE, CCP-C
Joseph O. Lopreiato, MD, MPH

OBJECTIVES

- Summarize how simulation is being used in the credentialing of health care personnel.

- Identify the importance and value of certification in simulation.

- Describe various requirements for using simulation to create a certification process that meets accreditation criteria.

- Discuss the development and value of the Certified Healthcare Simulation Educator (CHSE) certification program.

Credentialing is an accepted part of life in academic and health care settings. The process of credentialing typically involves a systematic approach to verifying qualifications, including assessment of whether an individual has the knowledge, skills, and abilities required for a specific position. According to the Institute for Credentialing Excellence (ICE) (formerly the National Organization for Competency Assurance), the term "credentialing" should be used as an "umbrella term to include professional certification, certificate programs, accreditation, licensure, and regulation" (ICE, 2013a, p. 1). A number of different credentialing methods have been established to meet the needs of various service sectors and professional disciplines. These forms include licensure, accreditation, certificate programs, and certification (ICE, 2013a). In health care, simulation often plays an important role in each of these forms of credentialing. In addition, simulation is increasingly being used as a mechanism for assessment of personnel for the purpose of granting or retaining clinical privileges.

Licensure

Many health care professions have multiple steps to obtain licensure, some of which involve the use of simulation to verify competencies or skills. For instance, a paramedic candidate is required to demonstrate competence by successfully completing a number of skill stations as part of the National Registry of Emergency Medical Technicians practical examination (www.nremt.org). Upon successful completion of the skills assessment and a written examination, the candidate becomes a nationally registered paramedic and can submit the registry certificate to the home state as part of the process to become licensed.

The United States Medical Licensing Examination (USMLE) (www.usmle.org) is another example of simulation being used as part of the process to obtain a license as a health care provider. This multiple-part examination assesses "the ability to apply knowledge, concepts, and principles, and to demonstrate fundamental patient-centered skills" (USMLE, 2012, p. 1). A portion of this examination requires candidates to demonstrate their professional, interpersonal, and technical skills through the use of simulated patient encounters.

Accreditation

Accreditation is mentioned briefly here, as it is a recognized form of credentialing. According to the Society for Simulation in Healthcare (SSH), accreditation is "a process whereby a professional organization grants recognition to a simulation program for demonstrated ability to meet pre-determined criteria for established standards" (SSH, 2013a, p. 27). The role of accreditation in health care simulation is to ensure quality through the assessment of simulation programs and centers. This form of credentialing is focused on programmatic level competency and performance rather than the individual performance that is the focus of licensure, certificate programs, and certification.

SSH has developed standards for simulation programs in health care and an accreditation process for simulation programs (SSH, 2013b). There are standards in the following areas:

- Core standards and criteria
- Assessment standards and measurement
- Research standards and measurement

- Teaching/education standards and measurement
- Systems integration: Facilitating patient-safety outcomes

The SSH Accreditation Standards, Accreditation Instructional Guide, Accreditation Self-Study, Accreditation Application, and a current list of accredited simulation programs are available on the SSH website (www.ssih.org/accreditation).

The American College of Surgeons (ACS) also has an accreditation program for education institutes, including simulation-based education/training centers (ACS, 2012).

Certificate Programs

In health care, the terms *certificate* and *certification* are often used interchangeably, but certificate programs and certification programs are distinctly different. There are also different types of certificate programs:

- Certificates of attendance or participation
- Assessment-based certificates

"Certificates of attendance or participation are provided to individuals (participants) who have attended or participated in classes, courses, or other education/training programs or events. The certificate awarded at the completion of the program or event signifies that the participant was present and in some cases that the participant actively participated in the program or event. Demonstration of accomplishment of the intended learning outcomes by participants is NOT a requirement for receiving the certificate; thus, possession of a certificate of attendance or participation does not indicate that the intended learning outcomes have been accomplished by the participant" (ICE, 2010, p. 2).

An assessment-based certification program, on the other hand, "is a non-degree granting program that (a) provides instruction and training to aid participants in acquiring specific knowledge, skills, and/or competencies associated with intended learning outcomes; (b) evaluates participants' achievement of the intended learning outcomes; and (c) awards a certificate only to those participants who meet the performance, proficiency or passing standard for the assessment(s)" (ICE, 2010, p. 2).

Certificates are awarded after successful completion of a specified course or training session, whereas professional or personnel certification is usually a voluntary process involving an external review that assesses an individual's knowledge, skills, or abilities in a specific area. The primary focus of assessment-based certificate programs is to facilitate the accomplishment of intended learning outcomes, whereas the primary focus of certification is to provide an independent assessment of the knowledge, skills, and/ or competencies required for competent performance of an occupational role or specific work-related tasks and responsibilities (ICE, 2010). In addition, oversight for certification programs is provided by an autonomous governing body composed of representatives from relevant stakeholders, while this is not required from assessment-based certificate programs (ICE, 2010).

The use of simulation in certificate-granting programs has become much more prevalent in health care. In these programs, simulation can be used to teach, assess, remediate, and evaluate. Certificate programs can be nationally recognized or locally developed. An example of a nationally recognized simulation-based program that provides a certificate is TeamSTEPPS by the Agency for Healthcare Research and Quality (AHRQ) (http:// teamstepps.ahrq.gov/). An example of a locally developed program that uses simulation for teaching and evaluation of a specific competency would be a chemotherapy program developed by a hospital for its registered nurse staff.

Many disciplines, many specialties, and many aspects of health care have certificate programs. Some certificate programs exist to teach educators how to use simulation for the purpose of health care education or to improve their skills as simulation educators. Having a certificate from a course may demonstrate exposure to content and/or actual demonstration of competency at completion of the program. However, when presented with any certificate, especially one related to simulation, you need to determine the credibility of the issuing organization, the conditions of the course, and the actual requirements to receive the certificate. For example, a certificate might be given to document that the learner attended a course (certificate of attendance) or it might only be given when the learner has demonstrated achievement of the course objectives.

Evaluation

Whether embedded in a certificate-granting program or being used to determine a health care professional's fitness to be granted specific privileges to practice in a clinical setting, using simulation for evaluation requires special attention. When simulation is used for the purpose of high-stakes assessment or evaluation of competency, educators and facilitators need to ensure appropriate, consistent, and fair processes are in place. They need to carefully consider elements such as providing an environment conducive to testing, providing a consistent evaluation experience, and using a reliable and valid tool with proven inter-rater reliability when developing and implementing these types of evaluation programs. Simulation-based credentialing and privileging programs require special attention to ensure the developers and evaluators are well versed in the appropriate simulation techniques to achieve these purposes. See Chapter 6 for further information on using simulation for evaluation.

Professional Certification

The concept of certification in the education and health care sectors is not something new, at least in the United States. In this context, certification is a process of verifying and recognizing individuals who meet an established set of standards. In many medical, nursing, and allied health fields, specialty certification is now an expected part of professional development. Often individuals must have a minimum set of certifications in order to be eligible for certain roles or positions. For instance, physicians, nurses, and other health care providers working in a trauma center or emergency room are often expected to obtain and retain specific emergency or trauma certifications. Simulation has now been integrated into almost every specialty certification program in health care.

Although a number of certificate programs exist that have applicability to health care simulation educators (HSEs), more comprehensive and globally recognized certifications in this specialty have only recently been developed. The rapid rate of growth in simulation-based education for health care students and professionals has created challenges to establishing core knowledge, skills, and competency standards that are fundamental to the creation of a well-constructed certification program.

Principles of Professional Certification

Some knowledge of the principles of certification is valuable in understanding the role of certification for HSEs. Competence has been defined as "an expected level of performance that integrates the knowledge, skills, abilities, and judgment" (American Nurses Association [ANA], 2010, p. 12).

- "Knowledge encompasses thinking, understanding of science and humanities, professional standards of practice, and insights gained from context, practical experiences, personal capabilities, and leadership performance.
- Skills include psychomotor, communication, interpersonal, and diagnostic skills.
- Ability is the capacity to act effectively. It requires listening, integrity, knowledge of one's strengths and weaknesses, positive self-regard, emotional intelligence, and openness to feedback.
- Judgment includes critical thinking, problem solving, ethical reasoning, and decision-making" (ANA, 2010, pp. 12-13).

Of the many evaluation methods used for certification, the most common by far is the multiple-choice question examination designed with a rigorous process and using psychometric principles to establish the required level of competency to be demonstrated. This is not to say there are not alternative approaches to evaluation for certification. Individuals can be certified based on their work and professional history, for instance through a review of a curriculum vitae. However, these forms of evaluation might have subjective problems, such as poor inter-rater reliability or bias based on personal preference. As a result, multiple-choice questions are the most easily supported knowledge assessment method in certification programs.

Standard procedures and processes for certification have been established and published by accrediting organizations such as the National Commission for Certifying Agencies (NCCA), the International Organization for Standardization (ISO) (www.iso.org), and others, such as the American Board of Nursing Specialties (ABNS) (www.nursingcertification.org), that focus on discipline-specific certifications or address specialty areas of practice. Organizations that accredit certification programs establish requirements to ensure fair treatment of candidates. Standards typically include effective governance, identification of resources, inclusion of stakeholders in the certification process, use of valid and psychometrically sound assessment instruments, and establishing rules for recertification (ICE, 2013b). Organizations such as ABNS also provide lists of available certifications as well as resource materials for individuals considering certification (ABNS, 2013).

One final principle of certification is the real-world impact of the process. Initially, when certification programs are introduced to a field, the early adopters view it as a verification of their knowledge and work experience and as a means to seek recognition within their community. As certification programs mature, employers and institutions begin to demand certification as a prerequisite to employment or as an early goal for new employees. Higher salaries might be provided as a reward for a certification, or the loss of a certification might result in suspension from, or even total loss of, a job for which the certification is required. This reinforces the importance of taking an evidence-based approach when integrating the use of simulation into certification-preparation programs. The potential impact of preparation programs increases when certifications are required for employment.

Value of Professional Certification

A question often asked is, "What's the value of certification?" If simulation educators are seeking to become certified, they need to be able to articulate possible benefits of certification. These benefits include the following (Henderson, Biel, Harman, Wickett, & Young, 2012):

- Protection of the public
- Greater confidence in professional competence
- Increased autonomy in the workplace
- Enhanced marketability, employability, and opportunity for advancement
- Improved monetary rewards
- Better compliance with regulations and conditions of third-party payers
- Raised public opinion
- Lowered risk

A Professional Certification Program for Health Care Simulation Educators

Recognizing the value of certification, SSH began work on the creation of an international certification program in 2009. The initial period of work was focused on identifying the knowledge, skills, abilities, and attitudes for which all modalities of simulation had common ground and practice. This was not an easy task given the variety of simulation modalities available. These include task trainers, standardized patients, mannequins, virtual-reality devices, computer simulations, and combinations of these elements. The end result was the development of SSH's *Certification Standards and Elements* (hereafter the Standards) (SSH, 2012). The Standards were developed using a consensus approach involving several meetings of health care simulation subject matter experts (SMEs) from North and South America, Europe, and the Asia-Pacific region. These SMEs represented a wide variety of professional societies and stakeholders including SSH, the Society in Europe for Simulation as Applied to Medicine (SESAM), the NLN, the Association of Standardized Patient Educators (ASPE), the International Nursing Association for Clinical Simulation and Learning (INACSL), the Australian Society for Simulation in Healthcare (ASSH), the Brazilian Association for Simulation in Healthcare (ABRASSIM), the Canadian Network for Simulation in Healthcare (CNSH), and the Dutch Society for Simulation in Healthcare (DSSH). This multidisciplinary group of international SMEs met and agreed to create clear expectations in a field where little had existed previously. They shared information, such as INACSL's standards for simulation, created foundational documents, and established a unique collaborative approach to be used in the development of the certification program. The group agreed that the Standards would embrace simulation principles and theories essential for practitioners in the field, regardless of the method of simulation employed. The initial Standards were summarized into four core categories:

- Professional Values and Capabilities
- Knowledge of Education Principles, Practice, and Methodology in Simulation
- Scholarship—Spirit of Inquiry and Teaching Implementing, Assessing
- Managing Simulation-Based Educational Interventions

Practice Analysis

To meet recognized standards for creating a certification examination, it was necessary to conduct an analysis of the typical work experiences in the field. A practice analysis (also called a job analysis) constructs:

> "a detailed description of current practice in a job or profession. Information from the practice analysis is used at all stages of examination development, including the creation of test specifications, item writing, and examination construction. The practice analysis provides the link between test content and real-world practice; it ensures that the examination is job related, and in this way provides the foundation for examination validity" (Professional Exam Services, 2003, p. 4).

To complete the practice analysis, an outside vendor with expertise in the activity was engaged to work with the SMEs to compile a list of knowledge, skills, and abilities (KSAs) expected of a Healthcare Simulation Educator (HSE). The sources for this list included job descriptions as well as articles and research that reflected upon the function of an educator in the health care simulation community. The work resulted in the addition of a fifth core category of standards related to managing overall simulation resources and environments and the development of a multiple-choice question examination blueprint (SSH, 2011).

When the practice analysis was complete, a survey was sent out to almost 11,000 individuals believed to be active in simulation (members of simulation, education, and professional organizations). The survey shared the results of the practice analysis and asked the respondents to comment on the following questions in regard to the compiled list of KSAs:

- Is it important?
- Is it written clearly?
- Is it performed by practitioners regularly?
- Is it redundant with other tasks?
- Does it belong where it is in the outline?
- Is it testable?

A total of 1,100 useable responses were received. Of the respondents, 94% had a bachelor's degree or higher, and 98% had more than one year of experience in simulation education. From the responses, the following important information was obtained:

- Feedback on the practice analysis: 99% of the respondents indicated that the survey either completely or adequately described the critical tasks required of the competent HSE
- Feedback on missing or unclear items
- Weighting of the importance of each category (domain weight)

With this information in hand, the group of SMEs finalized the list of KSAs, clarifying and improving where needed based on the feedback of the survey, and they determined the final weighting of each of the domains in preparation for the development of the examination. Weighting was given as follows:

- Display Professional Values and Capabilities (4%)
- Demonstrate Knowledge of Simulation Principles, Practice, and Methodology (34%)
- Educate and Assess Learners Using Simulation (52%)
- Manage Overall Simulation Resources and Environments (6%)
- Engage in Scholarly Activities (4%)
  (SSH, 2011)

Examination Development

The final step in the development of the certification program was to develop the examination. This task required the dedicated work of a number of interdisciplinary SMEs to generate questions, review answers, and develop a reference list. The general process for writing the questions was as follows:

1. Generation of question and answers

   - Questions had to be tied to each item on the test blueprint
   - Questions needed to be supported by a direct reference (for example, a journal article)

2. Review of questions

- Improvement of question stems and selections (for example, no negatives, no humorous distractors)

3. Compilation of items into two examination forms

- For security purposes, two forms of the examination were developed

4. Initial review of the forms by a group of SMEs

- To ensure each form met the requirements of the test blueprint (weighting)

5. Final review of the forms by a separate group of SMEs

- Further review of items and approval of items

Certification Launch

After years of study, discussion, and debate, and with the necessary groundwork completed, the Certified Healthcare Simulation Educator (CHSE) program was launched in June 2012. Initially, a pilot phase of 200 applicants allowed psychometric assessment of the test and establishment of the passing point, or cut score. The process used to determine the cut score was a modified Angoff method, a certification industry–accepted process. This method captures the input of the SMEs who review the data from the reviewed item performance, and it also reviews the overall performance of each examination. Each SME must review the data and establish a passing rate for each item. Through a combination of the input from this group of SMEs and the statistical data available for the items and forms, a final cut score was set for each form. Additionally, further work was completed to ensure that no matter which form candidates have when taking the examination, they have an equally successful chance to pass. There is empirical evidence to support this method, ensuring exam validity and reliability (Tiratira, 2009).

The pilot phase was completed and the examination opened to all who met the eligibility criteria. You can find information on becoming a CHSE at the SSH website (www. ssih.org/certification). Upon completion of the certification process, including achieving a passing score on the examination, the HSE is certified as a CHSE and is awarded the CHSE credential. The certification is good for 3 years. Renewal of the certification re-

quires maintaining practice requirements and fulfilling professional development requirements or taking the CHSE examination (SSH, 2012).

Future of Certification in Health Care Simulation

Although it is difficult to predict what the future holds for HSE certification, many things
are known. The practice analysis data revealed a number of educators who have been
doing education and, more specifically, education in simulation, for many years. These
individuals clearly exceed the basic competency level of performance recognized with the
CHSE process, and a need exists to recognize their enhanced KSAs through a higher level
of certification. An advanced level of certification for individuals such as these is being
developed. There is also initial work on the development of a certification program for operators, technicians, and technologists in health care simulation. Certifications for others
involved in simulation in health care are likely as well. For example, administrators and
those who support the technical and infrastructure needs of HSE are integral elements of
simulation programs. If these groups will desire or require certification in the future and if
so how they might become certified are open questions.

No matter the level of certification, it is very clear that professional certification programs for the simulation specialty will need to remain flexible and adaptive as the field
of health care simulation grows. The rapid growth that is being experienced is wonderful
news in almost all ways, but it results in a mandate to continually reevaluate the practice
of HSEs. The typical time period before a repeat practice analysis is needed ranges from
5 to 7 years for established certifications in stable industries. It is possible that, with the
amount of research and growth that exists in HSE, the next practice analysis will occur
earlier than this time frame.

The development of certification programs for educators in health care simulation has
helped to create opportunities for those seeking professional development in the field.
With the publishing of the Standards and the examination blueprint, existing certificate
programs will likely adapt their educational objectives to ensure that individuals who
complete those programs will have success when seeking certification as a health care
simulation educator.

Conclusion

With increasing emphasis on improving patient safety and enhancing patient outcomes by assuring competence of providers, credentialing and certification are certain to continue to be important areas of interest for all health care organizations. Educators who engage in health care simulation will be challenged to integrate simulation into various activities associated with credentialing—either by developing educational programs that leverage the use of simulation to address maintenance of competency or by using simulation techniques to assess the competency of providers for purposes of privileging.

In this setting, the demand for certification of health care professionals is likely to increase. Educators in health care simulation will now have the opportunity to demonstrate their competence and expertise by seeking certification themselves. By becoming certified, the HSE professional can become a better practitioner of the science and art of simulation and demonstrate that expertise for others to see.

References

American Board of Nursing Specialties (ABNS). (2013). *ABNS   About us.* Aurora, OH: Author. Retrieved from http://www.nursingcertification.org

American College of Surgeons (ACS). (2012). *Accreditation, verification, and quality improvement programs. Simulation-based education/training centers.* Chicago, IL: Author. Retrieved from http://www.facs.org/acsqualityprograms/index.html

American Nurses Association (ANA). (2010). *Nursing: Scope and standards of practice* (2nd ed.). Silver Spring, MD: Author.

Henderson, J. H., Biel, M., Harman, L., Wickett, J., & Young, P. (2012). *A look at the value of professional certification.* Washington, DC: Institute for Credentialing Excellence.

Institute for Credentialing Excellence (ICE). (2010). *Defining features of quality certification and assessment-based certificate programs.* Washington, DC: Author. Retrieved from http://www.credentialingexcellence.org/p/cm/ld/fid=4

Institute for Credentialing Excellence (ICE). (2013a). *What is credentialing?* Washington, DC: Author. Retrieved from www.credentialingexcellence.org/p/cm/ld/fid=32

Institute for Credentialing Excellence (ICE). (2013b). *National Commission for Certifying Agencies (NCCA) Accreditation.* Washington, DC: Author.

Professional Exam Services. (2003). Practice analysis: The foundation of examination validity. *PES News, 2*(1), 4-6.

Society for Simulation in Healthcare (SSH). (2011). *SSH Certification examination blueprint.* Wheaton, IL: Author. Retrieved from https://ssih.org/certification

Society for Simulation in Healthcare (SSH). (2012). *SSH Certification standards and elements.* Wheaton, IL: Author. Retrieved from https://ssih.org/certification

Society for Simulation in Healthcare (SSH). (2013a). *SSH accreditation process.* Wheaton, IL: Author. Retrieved from https://ssih.org/accreditation/how-to-apply

Society for Simulation in Healthcare (SSH). (2013b). *SSH certified healthcare simulation educator handbook.* Wheaton, IL: Author. Retrieved from https://ssih.org/certification

Tiratira, N. (2009). The basic Angoff method and the item response theory method. *The International Journal of Educational and Psychological Assessment, 1*(1), 39-47.

United States Medical Licensing Examination (USMLE). (2012). *2013 USMLE Bulletin of information.* Philadelphia, PA: Federation of State Medical Boards (FSMB) and National Board of Medical Examiners (NBME). Retrieved from http://www.usmle.org/pdfs/bulletin/2013bulletin.pdf

"We shape buildings; thereafter, they shape us."

–Winston Churchill

Developing and Building a Simulation Center

Beverly Dorney, MS, RN, NE-BC, EDAC
Cynthia Walston, FAIA, LEED AP
Sharon Decker, PhD, RN, ANEF, FAAN

OBJECTIVES

- Describe a planning and assessment process that supports the purpose and objectives of the simulation center.

- Establish planning parameters to generate the simulation center facility requirements and operational pro-forma.

- Develop a simulation center project based on current health care planning practice and the most recent facility planning parameters for a clinical simulation laboratory.

The preceding chapters have covered the fundamentals and key concepts in simulation. There is little doubt the role of simulation is becoming commonplace at colleges and universities, but its use is growing at teaching hospitals as well as in community settings. Now that you understand the concepts and benefits of simulation, how do you go about designing and building a center? This chapter covers the needs assessment—physical plant, personnel, and resource considerations—to develop a simulation center.

Although the use of simulation in health care can be traced back over 100 years, the facility planning and technologies used to optimize educational and practice outcomes from simulation have changed a great deal with recent advances in technology. Simulation centers have become standard in health care academic and practice settings. As an indicator of the growth in simulation, membership of the Society for Simulation in Healthcare has experienced a 16-fold increase since 2004 (Huang et al., 2012). Although educators have focused on development of course curricula and improved the techniques of simulation, there has been little development of facility planning guidelines on merging people systems, technology systems, and physical space to create an environment best suited to support the objectives of simulation. The opportunity to create a new simulation environment comes rarely and raises the expectation to "do it right" and optimize the use of resources for the project and for the ongoing program. This chapter focuses on the planning needed to create a new simulation center or renovate an existing simulation center.

Planning a simulation center for health care is a combination of planning a health care environment along with planning for pedagogy and research. No widely accepted simulation facility planning parameters exist. The best way to obtain information on simulation facility planning is often to tour and benchmark existing programs.

In contrast, in the field of health care architecture, architects have well-established space program and planning parameters based on actual performance of the buildings and clinical programs. These planning parameters are based on the expected workload volumes, clinical programs, and technologies. Workload volumes include the number of patients, types of patients and their families, and throughput expectations. Throughput might include length of stay for an inpatient or number of visits per exam per year in an emergency department. Outpatient care requires a different environment than inpatient care, and an oncology program needs different resources from a rehabilitation program. The architect uses evidence-based planning to develop the space program and eventual design for the desired clinical outcome and patient experience.

A clinical simulation laboratory is a costly venture to build and operate, so decisions need to be based on justified need. Typical construction costs for new build-out in existing structures range from $200 to $250 per square foot. Equipment costs, fees, permits, and inspections can be double or triple this cost, depending on the complexity. There is also the continuing cost of operating the facility with staffing, supplies, maintenance of facility and equipment, and upgrades of technology. It is imperative to make decisions wisely to justify resources.

First Things First

Developing and building a simulation center requires a structured planning approach such as the one depicted in Figure 15.1.

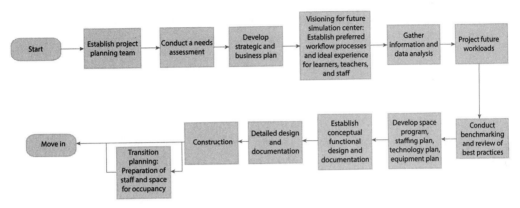

Figure 15.1   Simulation center planning approach.

Planning Team: Steering Committee and Design Team

The first step is to create a diverse planning team, including center leadership, educators, facility engineers, audiovisual/Information Technology (AV/IT) specialists, and simulation technologists. This in-house team will become the steering committee for the project. The steering committee represents the institution as the owner or client. This group should be kept fairly small as it is a decision-making entity.

After the steering committee defines the project parameters in the needs assessment, a design team—consisting of the architect, engineers, AV/IT consultants, center leadership, and key users—should be engaged. The role of the design team is to translate the needs assessment and project objectives into a program of spaces and then bring this forward through the design and construction phases described later in this chapter. One lesson learned by the authors was a project in which AV/IT was not in the initial meetings, and their expert input later reversed some of the planning that had taken place.

Design excellence is built around a collaborative team in search of the best ideas. The architect, working with the steering committee, users, and other consultants on the site, offers leadership to the process that establishes a cooperative effort. This leadership should be particularly adept at working with multiple and sometimes conflicting interests and incorporating their individual goals and ideas into the design. This is achieved through a series of interactive user work sessions. The project will benefit by involving teachers and students in the planning process during conceptual and design phases. The owner should anticipate and commit the time required to be involved in the process.

Needs Assessment

This section, and the next section about strategy, will help guide the planning team in making the first decision, which is, "Is a simulation center needed to meet strategic and service goals?" The initial outlay of capital and the ongoing operational costs are no small investment, thus a purposeful and thoughtful process is needed to answer this first question.

When conducting the needs assessment, begin with a strengths, weaknesses, opportunities, and threats (SWOT) analysis. Determine the attributes of the organization—both the strengths (S) and weaknesses (W). What are your current and perceived strengths that would assist in achieving your objective? This could include personnel currently employed, your reputation, location, partnerships, and research projects. Identify any weaknesses that might hinder your success. Be realistic. Identified weaknesses could include lack of financial support, scheduling issues, personnel, and space. Next, think about external factors that present opportunities (O) or threats (T) for the endeavor. Opportunities could include national recognition of the pedagogy of simulation, available research or technology funding, and recognition of simulation by accreditation agencies. Threats if the endeavor was not implemented might include issues related to patient safety, recruiting, and the mission of the organization.

A needs assessment should reflect input from key stakeholders and potential users, both internal and external, of the facility. A survey should be developed to obtain information related to:

- All potential simulation center users (determines if the center should be discipline-specific or have an interprofessional focus)
- Proposed number and type of users (for example, undergraduate nursing students, graduate nursing students, licensed practitioners, technologists)
- Proposed simulation typology (for example, advanced patient simulators, standardized patients, haptic devices, partial trainers, 3D immersive)
- Potential hours of use (inquire if users expect to access the facility during the evenings and/or weekends)

Data obtained from the needs assessment will assist in designing space appropriately, determining the appropriate personnel for the facility, and estimating the type and amount of equipment, mannequins, simulators, and AV infrastructure needed to support the center's purpose.

Vision and Strategy

A building design is based on the expected functionality. Architects refer to this as "form follows function." There should be clear strategic and programmatic objectives driving the plan for the new or renovated center. The strategic goals for a technical school are different from the experiential objectives of a graduate nursing program or hospital-based center. The curriculum objectives drive the use of the required technology, size of simulation class, length of simulation episodes, number of simulation episodes, preparation for the episodes, and follow-up evaluation and review of the episodes. In our experience, which is supported by survey findings (Dorney, Mancini, & Walston, 2012), early center planners initiated their simulation centers by adapting to space available rather than having the opportunity to take a more strategic facilities planning approach. Early centers might have had more or less space than needed because they "made do" with the space provided for the new center. In the real world, new programs and services are often given a start by taking over some available space. Even if using a predetermined space is the first opportunity to open a center, follow through on a planning process as outlined. The end plan clarifies any variances and future requirements to align the program strategy and goals with the facility space and design. The planning team should be prepared to answer a number of questions to inform the planning and design of the new center. Design of the environment will be impacted by the number of people in the space, the technologies and equipment to be used, the level of flexibility and adaptability in use of space, and the desired experience for the learners and teachers. The simulation center emulates a health center with enhanced infrastructure to support the IT and AV systems used.

To understand the functional attributes that will impact the facility design, the planning team needs to answer the following questions:

- What is the strategic plan for the simulation center?
- What are the goals for the simulation center?
- What are the measures of success for the simulation center?
- What functions will occur within the center? Who are the learners? What are they learning?

Describe and define the typical simulation episode:

- What type of simulation episodes will be provided in the center?
- How many episodes by type per session?
- What is a session?
- How many learners in each episode?
- What is the duration of the episodes by type?

The simulation episode will have features similar to a patient care episode. The diagnostic and procedure codes used to describe a patient care episode relate to the resources the care episode is likely to use, the level of care intensity required, and the length of stay. The health care architect can accurately project the type of spaces, the number of spaces, the support spaces, and so on that will be needed to care for the projected patient workload. For example, the health care planner can project the size of an emergency department and number of exam rooms that will be needed to support a projected number of patient visits because of the growing body of evidence-based information available to guide the planning for the new emergency department. As episodes of simulation are better defined and categorized into types, planning for the simulation center will become more evidence-based.

- What type of equipment will be needed to support the learning objectives of the simulation episode?
- What type of human simulators or task trainers/devices will be used?
- What infrastructure (power, data, wireless, AV, medical gas) is needed to run the simulation?
- Will the simulation center use standardized patients? What is the desired experience expected by the patient actors?
- Describe the staffing and the support the staff will need to run the center. What technologists will be needed to support and run the simulation? Where and what role will the educators have during the simulation episode? What level of privacy is needed for the simulation episode?
- What level of realism is needed to accomplish the learning objectives? Will spaces be finished out in the detail of real hospital spaces? Will the space be a sound stage, fully flexible, using virtual environments? Will real medical gases

be used? Will the space have alternative uses, such as to support a flex capacity plan in an emergency?

- What technology will be used in the next 5 years? How is the program expected to grow? What new teaching and research programs are anticipated?

- Will there be external users from partnerships and contracts who use the center? Who are potential outside users?

- What is the desired experience for the learners? Will student support spaces such as lounge, locker, or study spaces be provided in the center?

- How will the technologies and equipment be maintained and managed?

- How will materials and people flow in and out of the center? How will supplies be managed?

- Where will the center be located to optimize adjacency and functional relationships and provide easy access for learners? Will it be centralized? Is mobile capability important?

As the planning team answers the questions, the center's guiding principles and ideal workflow processes will emerge. The guiding principles and ideal workflow will impact planning and design of the new center.

Gathering Information and Benchmarking

A facility-focused survey of nine simulation centers was conducted in preparation for a presentation at the Southern Region meeting for Society of College and University Planners in the fall of 2012 (Dorney et al., 2012). The purpose of the survey was to investigate the facility features and performance of the facilities in support of the current programs using the centers. Centers across the nation differ in size, shape, affiliations, partnerships, and operational/organizational structure. The survey included centers at a technical college, colleges of nursing and medicine, allied health professions schools, and a hospital. Regardless of the size, shape, and type of programs served, the surveyed centers all reported successful programs and have experienced program growth.

The SSH accreditation program stipulates that "simulation is conducted in an environment that is conducive to accomplish the Program's teaching, assessment, research, and/or systems integration activities" (SSH, 2013, p. 10). When seeking accreditation, centers submit a "narrative description of the facility detailing the environment for education, functionality and intended use of the rooms" (p. 11) and floor plans. The accreditation survey also requests information to support that the program provides an adequate number and variety of simulation offerings to develop and maintain expertise, including a list of courses and targeted learners and educators, number of participants, learner contact hours, and anticipated trends in use of simulation with anticipation of expansion or changes in use. The Association of American Medical Colleges (AAMC) 2011 survey notes common types of spaces in medical school and teaching hospital centers, including debriefing, training/scenario, exam/standardized patient rooms, partial task trainer/procedure, office, observation, control room, conference room/classroom, storage/equipment room, and mixed use area (AAMC, 2011). Examples of center floor plans are shown in Figure 15.2.

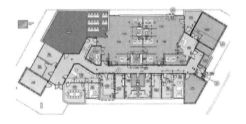

Common to all:
Simulation areas,
Conference/debrief/classroom,
Equipment and storage,
Control,
Limited administrative space

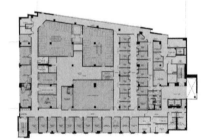

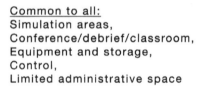

SPACE DESIGNATION

SIMULATION
OFFICE
CONTROL
SUPPORT
DEBRIEFING
CIRCULATION/PUBLIC

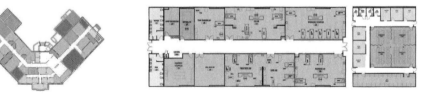

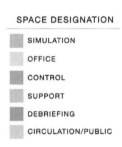

Figure 15.2   Examples of center floor plans.

Space Requirements

The space where actual simulation occurs varies a great deal, depending on the purpose of the simulation and level of realism and attention to detail.

Large Learning Lab

Large "lab-like" spaces accommodate several positions. A "position" is defined as an area where the "patient" receives care—for example, an inpatient bed, an exam room table, and an emergency room stretcher space including space for the care providers. These large rooms accommodate several care positions and are used most often to emulate acute care, emergency care, critical care, and pediatric care areas with head walls and appropriate bedside equipment (see Figures 15.3 and 15.4). These spaces are very flexible in use for high-tech or low-tech simulation encounters. Most have AV systems to record encounters. There might be direct observation from a control room. There is room to accommodate three to six people around each simulation encounter position. Surveyed centers reported encounter space within the large learning labs ranged from 110 square feet to 225 square feet per position and evaluated this size to be about the right size. Some centers are using large screens with photos to create a mock-up and details of a "real" room or outdoor environment. Hospital centers desire their simulation areas to be very similar to the actual patient care environment, using hospital standard medical equipment and carts. The key to these large simulation areas is flexibility to use in various ways.

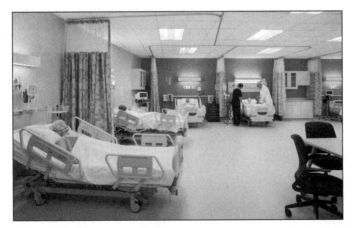

Figure 15.3   Large lab with multiple stations. Courtesy of Texas A&M Health Science Center.

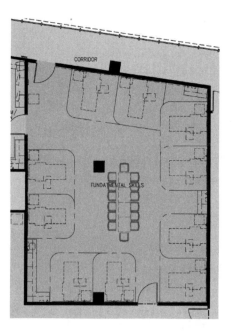

Figure 15.4 Example floor plan of a large lab. Courtesy of FKP Architects.

Medium Learning Lab

Medium-sized rooms accommodate teams for resuscitation encounters or surgery and procedural encounters (see Figure 15.5). These rooms may be 350 square feet to 600 square feet and provide AV systems for recording and playback of the session. Encounters within this space often focus on teamwork and collaboration as well as the technical skills of the learner. This size room may also accommodate several simulation encounters if the room is designed for flexible use.

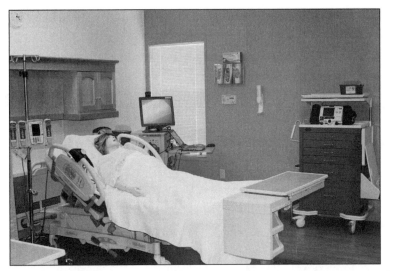

Figure 15.5   Medium-sized lab. Courtesy of UT Arlington Smart Hospital.

Small Rooms

Small rooms accommodate a single simulation position, such as an inpatient room or procedure room, and range in size from 150 square feet to 300 square feet. This size room would accommodate team training and be supported by the AV system.

Exam Rooms

Exam rooms accommodate a single encounter, such as standardized patient exam. These rooms are typically 110 square feet to 150 square feet and accommodate a "patient" plus two or three people. These rooms are supported by AV systems and are typically detailed and finished out with real medical equipment.

Conference Rooms/Classrooms/Debriefing Rooms

Conference rooms or classrooms vary in size to accommodate various sizes of groups. Typically conference rooms need to accommodate 2 to 10 people. Schools might need these rooms to accommodate large groups of 60 people or more, often using moveable walls to add flexibility in use. Debriefing sessions as well as preparation and learner staging for upcoming simulation encounters may occur in small or large rooms. These spaces provide AV systems linked to the simulation AV/learning system. There may be an opportunity on a college campus to recruit collaboration from the media arts department in the design of the AV system.

Debriefing rooms come in a variety of sizes as shown in Figures 15.6 and 15.7.

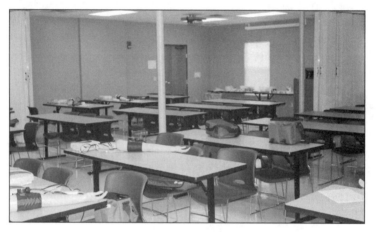

Figure 15.6   Large training space with movable partitions. Courtesy of UT Arlington Smart Hospital.

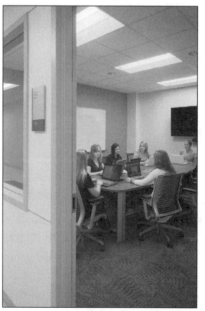

Figure 15.7   Debriefing room. Courtesy of Texas A&M Health Science Center.

Storage Areas

Storage areas are needed for equipment and supplies. From 35% to 50% of the simulation center space should be dedicated to storage. Older centers provided less space for storage, but post-occupancy evaluations informed planners to increase the amount of space dedicated to storage and maintenance of equipment. Most centers use a portion of storage space for the repair and maintenance of the mannequins. Bed and stretcher storage is required. Storage spaces must support various sizes of equipment from small pieces and parts to large adult-sized mannequins with computer systems in storage cases (see Figures 15.8 and 15.9). Existing centers frequently report that the need for storage is underestimated, especially as programs grow and add services. Center directors recommend that storage be flexible for the wide range of supplies and equipment used in the center and to accommodate the flexibility of rooms to be multipurpose. The storage area should be able to support storage of carts that can move to simulation areas for stocking, staging, and preparation for the encounters. This process is similar to preparations made for surgical cases and use of "case carts" to prepare the operating room (OR), including use of preference sheets.

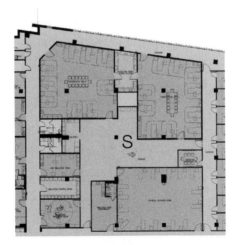

Figure 15.8   Storage accessible from multiple rooms. Courtesy of Texas A&M Health Science Center.

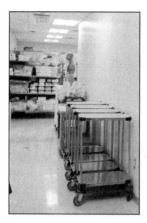

Figure 15.9   Storage for room case carts and supplies. Courtesy of Texas A&M Health Science Center.

Control Areas

Control areas might be centralized rooms handling multiple simulation areas or decentralized rooms controlling only one or two simulation spaces. These rooms are computer control rooms requiring appropriate air conditioning and workstation spaces for the simulation technologists and instructors. An example of a control area is shown in Figure 15.10.

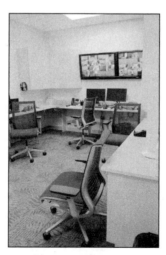

Figure 15.10   Centralized control room. Courtesy of Texas A&M Health Science Center.

Administrative Support Spaces

Offices for the directors, educators, and technologists vary depending on the programs the center supports. Administrative staff and technical personnel tend to use "touch down" or hotel office spaces, conference rooms, and shared offices.

Space Program

The space program or program of requirements describes the purpose of the center, projected utilization, operational relationships, space requirements, and other basic information relating to the fulfillment of the organization's objectives, The program includes a description of each function; the operational space required for each function; the numbers, types, and areas of all spaces; the special design features; and the services required. This program is developed to support the program goals and curriculum demands. The size of each space is defined by net square feet or net square meters, which is the area within the walls of the room. Room size is primarily driven by the purpose of the space and the number of people, the medical equipment, and AV equipment within the space. During space programming, the planning team begins to establish functionality within the space and relationships to adjacent spaces, as well as required equipment and technology that will be used within the spaces. Ideally, the space program is based on the needs and demands of the simulation center programs, not the wishes and desires of individual persons. A diverse planning team reduces risks in planning and increases engagement of those who will use and support the center. A budget can be drafted after the space program is established by using a cost-per-square-foot of types of spaces. Ranges of areas for the primary rooms in a clinical simulation laboratory are shown in Table 15.1.

Table 15.1   Space Program

Space Description	Net Square Footage Range per Space	Notes
Multi-position Simulation Lab	110–225 ft^2 per position	For example, six positions in the lab would need 660–1,350 ft^2 net. Add more space if there will be collaboration space within this lab.
Single-position Simulation Lab	150–300 ft^2	Partial task trainer, procedure room.

Table 15.1 Space Program *(cont.)*		
Space Description	*Net Square Footage Range per Space*	*Notes*
Operating Room Simulation Lab	400–800 ft²	Depending on detail, this might also serve as trauma room or a labor/delivery/recovery room.
Exam/Standardized Patient Room	110–150 ft²	Typically these rooms are detailed to replicate an exam room.
Debrief/Conference/ Classroom	20–30 ft² per person	Consider flexible rooms with moveable partitions.
Observation	400–500 ft²	Many centers do not provide direct observation rooms.
Control Room	200–400 ft²	Centralized or decentralized, size depends on number of technicians/educators accommodated.
Storage/Equipment	400 ft² and larger	35% to 50% of the simulation space.
Office	100–150 ft² each	

This is not a comprehensive list of rooms and spaces. The actual space program will reflect the functional requirements and people to be accommodated by the space—for example, a lobby and reception space might be required or might not be required if adjacent space is available and shared. For example, one hospital center repurposed available space for the simulation center and was able to reduce center space by using nearby conference rooms, lobby, and restrooms.

Conceptual Design

The goal of this phase of design is to translate the space program into a three-dimensional physical solution. The conceptual design should establish the design aesthetic/image, flow and plan, adjacencies, materials, systems, and overall functional layout/flow for all areas of the project. This set of documents might then be priced to set the probable construction and project cost. It is essential that the owner be aware of the responsibilities of the owner role during this phase. Because all major design decisions are being made, the planning team must be aware of the product, process, and required time commitment to carry out the design processes. At the end of conceptual design, the design phase is generally complete. Any significant adjustments to the design beyond this phase require leadership approval and additional costs. In general, it is more expensive to make changes after the project is begun.

Detailed Design

In the detailed design or the construction document phase, the design concepts and functional requirements established for the project are expanded and documented in a form suitable for pricing. They are subsequently utilized as the road map for constructing the project. All significant design decisions that impact the interior and exterior of the building must be made by this time. The design focus now moves from planning, information gathering, and setting the major design concepts to development of the details that convey the established design. The architect will include the consulting engineers, IT specialists, and the planning team to create the detailed floor plan and documents for the construction of the center. There is limited involvement of the users in this phase of the project.

Construction and Transition Planning

Although the center is under construction, you need to begin transition planning and get ready to occupy the new center. Although many new ideas and processes are created during the design and planning for the new center, you need to create a detailed plan to actualize the new processes and prepare the people who will run and use the center. The planning team provides the continuity and leadership required for success.

Staffing and Resources

The staffing plan includes roles and responsibilities based on the program demands. Preparation of staff begins with the design of the center. Survey findings show a wide variance in staffing patterns (Passiment, Sacks, & Huang, 2011). Centers associated with university programs (that is, medical schools and nursing schools) tend to have more dedicated full-time equivalents (FTEs) than hospital-based centers (Huang, et al., 2012).

Personnel needs for the center are determined by multiple factors, including the mission of the center, the budget, the size of the center, hours of operation, and the types of simulation pedagogy available in the center. All centers need a director and/or coordinator (title is dependent on the institution). Some centers will have one position that combines the responsibilities listed in Table 15.2. For schools this might be designated as a faculty appointment that allows participation in curricular and instructional decisions. In a survey of centers, Dorney, Mancini, and Walston (2012) found that full-time staff of the surveyed centers ranged from two technologists at the technical college to 6 to 8 staff at the larger university centers; the hospital-based center had two FTEs with added part-time support from various other departments. All programs had directors of their programs with full-time technical personnel. Some programs also employed full-time faculty instructors. Centers recommend that their staff support the development of simulation encounters that are easy to use by the course instructors and use little direct technologist time during the actual simulation encounter. Examples of personnel and responsibilities are shown in Table 15.2. You can find additional detailed information on roles in Chapter 13.

Table 15.2	Personnel and Responsibilities
Position/Title	**Potential Responsibilities**
Director	Organizational and fiscal management
	Research development
	Faculty development
	Performs evaluation and ensures program quality and determines areas of improvement
Coordinator	Management of day-to-day activities
	Scheduling of space, equipment, simulators, and so on
	Inventory control
	Curriculum integration
	Assists with evaluation and quality improvement
Information Technologies	Supports all hardware and software, including audio/visual system, user and simulation workstations, and peripheral devices
	Compiles data from all assessment encounters (standardized patients, advanced patient simulators, hybrid experiences)
	Supports appropriate integration into institution's network

Position/Title	Potential Responsibilities
Standardized Patient Coordinator	Recruits, trains, schedules, supervises, and monitors the standardized patients
	Coordinates case development, design, and monitoring of simulations that integrate standardized patients
	Performs evaluation and ensures program quality and determines areas of improvement
Simulation Technician	Provides technical support for simulation setup and delivery
	Maintenance and repair of equipment, mannequins, and simulators
	Maintains agreements with vendors
	Operates simulators for educators according to center's policies
	Programs simulators
	Maintains inventory of equipment, mannequins, and simulators
Unit Coordinator	Orders supplies, equipment, mannequins, simulators as requested by director and/or coordinator
	Maintains inventory of assets and supplies
	Assists with setups and cleaning
Business Assistant/ Receptionist	Maintains files and records
	Schedules meetings
	Takes minutes
	Answers the telephone
	Maintains utilization statistics

Funding and Planning Resources

Whether funding for the center is proposed to be through internal funds, partnerships, or from donors, a pro-forma financial statement must be developed. If the initial funding for a center is obtained through a donor, the process is usually initiated and managed by the institution's department for development or foundation. Be extremely careful to adhere to all policies related to approaching donors. The pro-forma financial statement should provide a fiscal overview of the project and include current funding, required funding, proposed use of these funds, and potential business opportunities (forecasting) for the center. An example of items that need to be addressed in the pro-forma are shown in Table 15.3.

Table 15.3 Financial Pro-forma	Year 1	Year 2	Year 3	Year 4	Year 5
INCOME					
Consultation					
Utilization fees					
Partnerships					
Grants					
Donors					
GROSS					
OPERATING EXPENSES					
Administrative Expenses					
Salaries					
Benefits					
Maintenance and Operations					
Utilities and Telephone					
Equipment					
Simulators/Mannequins					
Supplies					
Agreements					
Travel					
TOTAL OPERATING EXPENSES					
NET PROFIT					

Funding sources for medical and nursing schools and teaching hospitals (Passiment, Sacks, & Huang, 2011) commonly include the following:

- Medical school
- Nursing school
- Teaching hospital
- University
- State government and federal government
- Grants/foundations
- Philanthropists
- Revenue generated by courses and service to groups

There are various partnerships across the country in which service providers and educators have come together to operate a shared center. The government has special interest in studying ways to reduce costs while increasing productivity and quality in service settings and schools for health care providers. Government funding for simulation research has increased recently; there is also a role for simulation centers in researching new methods for education and training.

A patient simulator and the hardware and software system to capture the session cost around $100,000 per simulation position (not including the medical equipment or furnishings) in 2013 dollars. Operational costs vary widely. In the 2011 survey "Medical Simulation in Medical Education: Results of an AAMC Survey," ongoing operational costs for 57% of simulation centers in teaching hospitals was less than $250,000 at the low range (Passiment, Sacks, & Huang, 2011). At the high range, 11% reported annual operating costs of $1,000,000 to $2,000,000. Only 22% of medical schools reported operating budgets of less than $250,000, and 15% reported operating budgets between $1,000,000 and $2,000,000.

Resources

Although this chapter gives an overview of the planning process, key questions to answer, and space planning to guide design for a clinical simulation center, a growing source of potential resources for the planning team exists. The National League for Nursing (NLN) Simulation Innovation Resource Center (SIRC) provides an online course: Designing

Simulation Centers (NLN-SIRC, 2013). A simple Google search uncovers a number of sites for the planner to review. Although much has been published regarding the large academic-associated centers, demand is growing in smaller organizations where simulation will benefit learners in pharmacy programs, physical rehab, health care technical training programs, and community hospitals.

Lessons Learned

The survey of simulation centers by Dorney, Mancini, and Walston (2012) found many lessons learned. The things the surveyed centers liked most about their centers were:

- Functionality
- Easy access
- Ease of use
- Flexibility
- High instructor satisfaction
- Integration of simulation programs, such as standardized patient program with the technical simulation program
- Team collaboration and partnerships

Surveyed centers suggested that future planning include:

- More storage space, especially to accommodate program growth
- Improved layout to better support efficient work flow
- Student support space
- A growth strategy to support program expansion
- Inclusion of many in the planning process, such as experts, users, faculty, facility engineers, environmental services and security, and students who have experienced simulation in learning

A number of centers were challenged to meet the complex scheduling demands and preferred preparations of the many courses supported in their centers. Centers also have increasing choices available when choosing a simulation management system, one to capture and manage the simulation events as well as the operational tasks such as resource management and scheduling.

Conclusion

It is clear that demand will increase to educate and train health care providers. It is also clear that the education and training must produce competent providers using new techniques and processes for lower cost yet more effective outcomes while extending the valuable resources of our educators. Health care is delivered by teams of providers who need highly developed team skills. Simulation centers in the future will reflect the latest technologies and the latest research on learning; many will be interprofessional centers of learning.

Hospital-based and academic simulation centers are being used to develop high-performance teams, enhance professionalism, and provide scenarios for providers to improve communication and coordination skills necessary to improve patient safety. Hospitals are creating or renovating multiuse rooms near the point of service—such as on inpatient units where mobile simulation is supported—as well as typical classroom use. Large and small programs are requesting space to support simulation.

For example, a hospital might repurpose old space to support simulation. The older building floor-to-floor heights might not support high-tech patient care, but the older space might be an ideal location for a simulation center. The renovated space might take advantage of existing hospital services such as cafeteria, restrooms, office spaces, and meeting rooms. However, challenges might include methods to accommodate public traffic flows near inpatient care services and simple internal circulation and signage to facilitate finding one's way to the center.

Future centers will extend the benefits of simulation by being more mobile and adaptive to various environments so that more providers can conveniently participate in learning through simulation. At the same time, the technology used within the simulation center will continue to evolve rapidly.

The future holds opportunities for virtual simulation where the health care environment is simulated within a virtual environment and the learner is surrounded by avatars who respond using artificial intelligence. Not all success in simulation will be related to highly technical systems but will include the right mix of high-fidelity and high-touch experiences. Considering these trends will help you plan efficient and effective simulation centers for the future.

The planners for the next generation of simulation centers will have improved access to evidence-based planning. Planning teams will take advantage of the experience of health care planners and leaders in education working together to design and implement simulation centers that will successfully support the vision and experience of the users. As several leaders suggested when responding to the survey by Dorney, Mancini, and Walston (2012), be purposeful in planning and don't let your facilities or your technology dictate your program.

References

Association of American Medical Colleges (AAMC). (2011). *Medical simulation in medical education: Results of an AAMC survey.* Washington, DC: Author. Retrieved from https://www.aamc.org/download/259760/data/medicalsimulationinmedicaleducationanaamcsurvey.pdf

Dorney, B., Mancini, M. E., & Walston, C. (2012). *Maximize resources in your simulation center to transform medical education.* Society for College and University Planning Southern Conference. Raleigh, NC.

Huang, G. C., Sacks, H., Devita, M., Reynolds, R., Gammon, W., Saleh, M.,…Passiment, M. (2012). Characteristics of simulation activities at North American medical schools and teaching hospitals: An AAMC-SSH-ASPE-AACN collaboration. *Simulation in Healthcare, 7*(6), 329-333.

National League for Nursing (NLN) Simulation Innovation Resource Center (SIRC). (2013). *Designing simulation centers.* New York, NY: National League for Nursing. Retrieved from http://sirc.nln.org

Passiment, M., Sacks, H., & Huang, G. (2011). Medical simulation in medical education: Results of an AAMC survey. Washington, DC: Association of American Medical Colleges. Retrieved from https://www.aamc.org/data/

Society for Simulation in Healthcare (SSH). (2013). *SSH accreditation self-study guide: Accreditation standards and measurement criteria.* Wheaton, IL: Author. Retrieved from https://ssih.org/accreditation/

The Future of Simulation in Health Care

Pamela R. Jeffries, PhD, RN, FAAN, ANEF

Eric B. Bauman, PhD, RN

John J. Schaefer III, MD

The future is bright for simulation, providing numerous possibilities to enhance clinical education for health care providers; improve patient safety; and create safer, more efficient systems of care through process improvement and risk management. Simulation is being used today to teach clinical judgment, problem solving, and decision-making skills. In academic settings, clinical simulations are increasingly substituting for actual clinical hours and creating the opportunity for all learners to experience a set of standardized clinical scenarios that prepare them for complex clinical situations. Educators, leaders, and researchers are identifying best practices when designing and implementing simulations and developing the research that will provide the evidence of value in the future. The technical advances and health policy decisions that are emerging today will help dictate the future of simulation in health care.

This chapter discusses how simulation, simulation-based education, and gaming will be used in future courses and curricula; the programmatic changes that may occur within the health professions as simulation-based education continues to escalate; the emerging technologies and how these will be integrated

OBJECTIVES

- Describe the issues, challenges, and new opportunities that are evolving around the use of simulation in health care.
- Discuss programmatic changes that may occur in health professions education as the use of simulation pedagogy escalates.
- Explore how the emerging technologies will be integrated and used in the clinical simulation experiences.

within the simulation environment; the issues, challenges, and new opportunities, such as required certification and accreditation of simulation centers, that are evolving around clinical simulations; and the integration of simulation as a process improvement methodology.

How Simulation, Simulation-Based Pedagogy, and Gaming Will Be Used in the Future

As the use of simulation in health care increases, innovative types of simulation are being developed that rely on greater use of technology. Simulations using gaming and virtual reality platforms are now being utilized to teach and evaluate clinical skills and decision-making.

Today's millennial learners are not only technologically savvy but also accustomed to learning through video games that require learners to try multiple strategies in order to reach their goals by quickly searching and manipulating the virtual environment throughout the process (Mangold, 2007). Gaming is an active learning strategy that requires the learner to use skills and knowledge to reach a specific goal (Peddle, 2011). The goal of gaming in health care is to provide an authentic clinical environment in which either individuals or a group of learners can experiment without risk to the patient. When used in the education of health professionals, gaming can help to reinforce knowledge and skills. Kopp and Hanson (2012) used gaming to effectively teach baccalaureate nursing students how to provide end-of-life care. Not every learner responds to this learning strategy, however, as motivation and enjoyment may be dependent upon individual learner styles (Blakely, Skirton, Cooper, Allum, & Nelmes, 2008).

Games and applications, particularly those that can be accessed, engaged in, or played on mobile devices, offer an interesting paradigm shift in the way a participant or learner can access information. Massive Open Online Courses (MOOCs) are providing access to academic content to millions of people who until just a few years ago had little or no access to college-level or professional training. Very prestigious academic institutions are engaging educational technology like MOOCs as a way to provide a distributed educational experience that transcends the challenges of time, place, and socioeconomic status. The future may well include that mobile devices with quick and efficient access to just-in-time learning through clinical simulations that demonstrate certain procedures, communication techniques, and/or clinical reasoning be readily available as a tool used and required by all health care professionals.

War games, used by the military since the 1950s (Jackson, 2004), are strategy games in which teams of stakeholders are faced with a particular challenge and must work together to identify both strengths and threats in order to find an optimal solution. As with all games, participants are given a set of rules within which to operate. In health care, this type of simulation format has been utilized for various clinical simulation scenarios in which a team must work together to face a critical event, such as a disaster. Hedrick and Young (2008) studied whether the use of repeated simulations in the war game format would improve the performance of medical students verses postgraduate residents in the care of an unstable patient within the surgical intensive care unit. The researchers found that although the medical students initially performed worse than the residents, after participation in multiple war game sessions those with the least amount of experience demonstrated the most improvement (Hedrick & Young, 2008). Given the need to reduce failure to rescue events, simulations using a war game format hold promise for the future.

Another innovation within simulation that is used now and will be integrated more in the future is the use of virtual reality platforms, also known as a Massively Multiplayer Virtual World (MMVW), serious gaming, or virtual worlds (Hansen, 2008). These are three-dimensional (3D) Internet-based environments in which participants interact via the use of an avatar. An example is *Second Life* (www.secondlife.com) (Linden Research Inc., n.d.), an online world that allows interactions between users in various settings. Virtual worlds used in simulation are unique environments constructed so that learners can accomplish specific learning objectives. They allow for interaction and feedback among avatars in the environment so that the learner may modify or change behaviors to adapt to the specific demands of the clinical scenario (Hansen, 2008). Because virtual reality platforms are accessed online, they are available around the clock and provide a means for learners to interact without being physically present. This is particularly useful when dealing with distance education (Bauman, 2010).

There are certainly drawbacks in using these new simulation formats. Serious gaming and virtual reality simulations require quite a bit of time, as well as financial and technological resources, to create the desired environment (Hansen, 2008). Ultimately, the desire for higher degrees of sophistication and realism will affect the costs to create simulations in the future.

Virtual simulations have been used in health care for skills training, knowledge acquisition, and clinical decision-making (Foronda, Godsall, & Trybulski, 2012). In a prospective cohort study, Burden et al. (2012) used an ultrasound virtual reality simulator to measure competency in obstetrical ultrasonography between trainees and experts. Although the trainees had significantly more deviation from the target measurements on the initial assessment and took significantly longer to conduct the ultrasonography than the expert cohort, there were no significant differences between the trainees and the experts in target ultrasonography measurements after the third repetition (Burden et al., 2012).

LeFlore et al. (2012) used a virtual pediatric hospital unit with virtual patients to determine if this environment was effective in teaching pediatric content. In this study, baccalaureate nursing students who were randomized to receive an experience with a virtual patient trainer had significantly higher knowledge acquisition and better knowledge application as compared to those students who received a traditional lecture (LeFlore et al., 2012). Virtual patients have also been used to measure clinical decision-making. Wendling et al. (2011) found that junior anesthesiology residents were more likely to suspect obstructive sleep apnea after interviewing a virtual patient when compared with those residents who interviewed a standardized patient. One can reasonably expect, therefore, to see more virtual patients being used in the future.

Virtual reality has not only been found to be effective in skill and knowledge acquisition but also in the retention of knowledge. Associate degree nursing students who received additional virtually simulated disaster experience in addition to a web-based module were significantly more likely to retain the knowledge 2 months after the training when compared with those students who only received the web-based module (Farra, Miller, Timms, & Schafer, 2013).

Further research is needed (1) to compare the effectiveness of these simulation methods compared to more traditional methods, (2) to determine whether these methods are a cost-effective method of educating health care personnel, and, more importantly, (3) to determine whether there is ultimate improvement in patient safety and outcomes because of this simulation (Agency for Healthcare Research and Quality [AHRQ], 2013). Future research efforts need to determine the most cost-effective methods of creating and delivering education using gaming and virtual reality platforms. Regardless, gaming and other virtual reality platforms will surely be powerful tools for health care education in the future.

Potential Curriculum and Programmatic Changes

Simulation has long been a part of the educational process for health professionals. With rapid advances in technology and the demand for high-quality care, it is gaining even more widespread adoption. The changing landscape of health care and the emphasis on improving safety and outcomes has increased the need to focus on innovative ways to transfer evidence and guidelines into clinical practice (McNeill, Parker, Nadeau, Pelayo, & Cook, 2012). As we move forward, we must address how knowledge and identified best practices can be translated into the clinical setting and how it can be done more effectively and efficiently. Simulation methodologies will certainly play a significant part in addressing this need.

Implementation of simulation into the health care curriculum is being viewed as an integral part to its effective use (Issenberg, McGaghie, Petrusa, Lee Gordon, & Scalese, 2005). This integration involves many factors that must be effectively and strategically implemented, including managing faculty expectations, student outcomes, and resources. Simulations across a curriculum should have outcomes consistent with improving skills, knowledge, confidence, and student satisfaction (Howard, Englert, Kameg, & Perozzi, 2011). Starkweather and Kardong Edgren (2008) use simulations to develop fundamental skills with entry level nursing students. Their simulations incorporate important aspects of professional role development including interprofessional interactions, cultural diversity, and bedside communications. The integration of these factors into simulations designed for skill acquisition minimizes the need for additional simulations. It is likely that in the future educators will be developing more of these types of nuanced, integrated simulations that will be used across the curriculum as well as in clinical sites. Some have suggested that simulation be incorporated early into programs, with a focus on matching simulation scenarios to course objectives (Henneman & Cunningham, 2005) although little research has been done on evaluating its implementation across an entire curriculum (Howard et al., 2011).

For nursing, the National Council of State Boards of Nursing (NCSBN) embarked on a national, multisite study in which clinical competency, clinical knowledge, and other outcomes are being evaluated with different doses of simulations being substituted across seven core clinical courses in five baccalaureate and five associate degree programs across the United States (NCSBN, 2013). In the fall of 2011, traditional nursing students enrolled in the ten selected schools were randomized into one of three groups in which hours in a clinical setting were substituted for hours in clinical simulation activities. The substitution of hours is done on an hour-for-hour basis, with one hour in simulation as an active participant or active observer substituted for one hour of clinical time. The three randomized groups are (1) a control group having less than 10% simulation; (2) a group with substitution of 25% of clinical time with clinical simulations; and (3) a group with substitution of 50% of clinical time with clinical simulations. Simulations occur in a simulation center managed by a simulation team trained to ensure the integrity of the simulations for the study. Students were evaluated throughout their nursing education and will be followed into their first year of practice. This sentinel study, which will be completed in December 2014, is being monitored closely and is likely to have significant implications in the future for the amount of simulation educators may incorporate or substitute for time spent in traditional clinical settings.

When implementing pedagogy of simulation across a program, whether in academia or a clinical setting, developing educator competence and acceptance are keys to appropriate and sustained implementation and use. Reluctance to adopt new technologies is a significant and complex barrier to effective implementation, and therefore, overcoming it is necessary to accommodate today's learners who are overall more savvy and comfortable with technology. In addition to the time and training needed to develop educator competence and confidence in the use of available technology, educators also need to be taught how to effectively develop and deliver simulation teaching strategies and how to debrief learners. This training time can be difficult to negotiate with current workloads and schedules. Workshops, "lunch and learn" sessions, and continuing education offerings tailored to both novice and experienced educators are a few ways to overcome some of the initial barriers to programmatic adoption of new technology and practice (McNeill et al., 2012). In the future, you have to wonder if, when hiring new educators, organizations will start to use competence in the use of simulation as a requirement for educators in the health professions.

As additional evidence is gathered, more educators are prepared to use simulation pedagogy, and more resources are available, schools, and organizations will need to decide how simulation will be incorporated into programs, ranging from skill development to high stakes testing. How much clinical time will be substituted with clinical simulations? Will this substitution happen because it improves learner or program outcomes or because we cannot find enough clinical sites to provide clinical placement for students? Will educators be required to integrate simulations across the curriculum in every core clinical course using a standardized approach to demonstrate specific, critical behaviors, skills, and competencies?

What about high stakes testing with simulations? Medical students are required to demonstrate competency by participating in high stakes simulations to evaluate their performance related to assessment, clinical reasoning, and professional behaviors. With emerging ethical and regulatory pressure to ensure health care providers are competent to provide care, will other health professions follow medicine's approach?

And what about demonstrating ongoing competency once a health care provider is out in practice? How will maintenance of competency be assessed? Whether in the academic or clinical setting, those involved in educating health care professionals are responsible for seeing these questions are answered. The answers to these questions will have a significant effect on the overall use of simulation in health care in the future.

The Integration of Emerging Technologies Into Simulation Experiences

Another aspect to consider for the future of simulation includes the integration of additional technologies, such as handheld devices, within the various simulation platforms. Clinical simulations and video games, particularly those that are accessible via mobile devices (for example, tablets and smartphones), represent not only opportunities for interactive knowledge acquisition traditionally obtained through static didactic teaching modalities, but also cognitive aids that can be accessed in other learning environments. In other words, the content embedded within these games and applications comes to represent more than just-in-time information. It also models the context of the content being accessed (Bauman, 2010; Bauman & Games, 2011; Games & Bauman, 2011). In this way, games and mobile applications can also be used in traditional simulation laboratories to support learning objectives during supervised clinical encounters and in independent practice.

Game-based and mobile application–based learning is being embraced as one of many pedagogical modalities available for clinical education of health care providers as well as a mechanism for patient education. Increasingly, game-based learning is being embraced as a complementary tool available to meet specific learning objectives. Examining fit prior to deploying game-based learning helps to ensure that both educators and learners are ready for this methodology. Without a carefully planned infrastructure, the introduction, integration, and evaluation of game-based learning will leave both learners and educators frustrated (Bauman, 2012). Determining how these modalities best fit alongside other teaching and learning techniques is still to be determined and an area ripe for future research.

Despite the challenges associated with reexamining the curricula and determining where new methods, such as game-based learning, can be best leveraged, organizations and educators need to meet this challenge quickly and efficiently. Today's learners are often much more comfortable with digital technology than their educators. Traditional students are *digital natives*, whereas their educators are often *digital immigrants.*

- The term *digital native* refers to those people who have always been part of the digital generation (Prensky, 2001). Smartphones and the Internet have always been part of digital natives' day-to-day experience, and journal articles have always been available online. Digital natives have an innate sense of media literacy (Bauman, 2012; Prensky, 2001).

- The term *digital immigrants* refers to individuals who adopted digital technology later in life (Prensky, 2001). For the digital immigrant, digital literacy is a second language.

The number of digital natives in academia and hospital settings will continue to increase as will the number of patients and health care consumers who are digital natives. Educators and other health care leaders will have to adapt in order to create effective learning environments that will certainly involve a full array of simulation methodologies.

Certification, Accreditation, and Value Recognition of Simulation

As the use of simulation becomes a best practice in academic and clinical settings in health care, there are ample opportunities for professional growth. There are now multiple organizations that are dedicated to advancing the use of simulation (see accompanying sidebar). These organizations assist both individuals and professional groups to employ best practices in the use of simulation in health care, including how to develop a simulation center, create a simulation scenario, or select valid and reliable tools for evaluation. Many of these organizations publish journals and offer annual conferences to help simulation novices and experts network, collaborate, and disseminate their experiences in simulation.

Examples of Simulation Organizations

Association of Standardized Patient Educators: http://www.aspeducators.org/

International Nursing Association for Clinical Simulation and Learning: https://inacsl.org/

National Center for Simulation: http://www.simulationinformation.com/

National League for Nursing Simulation Innovation Resource Center: http://sirc.nln.org/

Society for Simulation in Healthcare: http://ssih.org

Certification and Accreditation

As a means for improving patient safety, simulation technology, educational methods, practitioner assessment, and patient safety, the Society for Simulation in Healthcare (SSH) has launched two programs to set standards and recognize expertise in simulation. You can find additional information on these programs in Chapter 14.

- One program was established to certify individuals with expertise in simulation education in health care. Successful completion of the process results in the individual being granted recognition as a Certified Healthcare Simulation Educator (CHSE) (SSH, 2013a). A detailed overview of the process is available online in the SSH Certified Healthcare Simulation Educator Handbook (SSH, 2013b). The organization also is in the process of developing a certification process for those with advanced health care simulation educator experience and one for simulation technologists.

- The SSH also has developed another program that is designed to provide accreditation for programs dedicated to using simulation technologies and methodologies to improve patient safety and outcomes (SSH, 2013c). Interested simulation programs submit a self-study application demonstrating compliance and fulfillment in each of the seven core standards and participated in a one-day, on-site survey. Accreditation is granted for a 3-year period with required submission of an annual program report. More than 25 simulation programs have been accredited within the United States, Australia, and Canada.

Educators who are enthusiastic about the use of simulation technology in their courses and curriculum should consider the best method for their professional growth in the pedagogy of simulation. Initial steps may be to join a simulation organization, become immersed in the simulation literature, and participate in an annual simulation conference. Those who have developed an expertise should consider becoming certified as a CHSE. Educators who practice in settings that have actualized their mission to improve patient outcomes and safety through the use of simulation technology should consider undergoing the process of program accreditation.

In the future, will certification be required for educators who are engaged in health care–related simulations? Will simulation programs be required to be accredited? With an emphasis on documenting competency, this could be a next step in the integration of simulation into the health care industry.

Value

Another consideration for the future of simulation includes the changes in health care reform and government regulations within the United States. The Patient Protection and Affordable Care Act and the Health Care and Education Reconciliation Act of 2010 each have three main goals. They seek to expand health care coverage by providing affordable health care for more than 95% of all Americans while reducing health care costs and improving the health care delivery system (American Public Health Association, 2012).

With the constant change in health care, the question is how will simulation-based strategies be positioned as part of the solution to the economic pressures and training challenges? In order to be relevant in the future, those who embrace and advocate simulation in health care will have to ensure that the message to decision-makers is clear. Simulation saves lives and improves efficiency. If this message is not transmitted, the question becomes, "What will happen to simulation programs?" Will they be viewed as an expensive luxury or part of the value equation of affordable, safe patient care with the necessary expansion of a well-trained nursing and physician workforce? Successful simulation programs need to demonstrate that the value of simulation-based strategies is significantly greater than the cost. This will require a "4-box mentality" (see Figure 16.1) directed toward programmatic investment of courses in schools for health professionals as well as in the clinical setting. There are myriad potentially valuable training topic areas with the adoption of this paradigm.

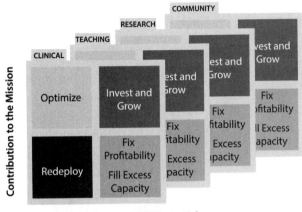

Figure 16.1   4-Box Mentality

In the future, it will not be sufficient to just perform "valuable" training; it must be communicated to stakeholders through translational and economic-based research. To survive, simulation programs might need to diversify their revenue streams as well as work with industry to decrease costs while increasing the ability to report value.

Integration of Simulation as a Process Improvement Methodology

As more and more focus is being placed on improving health care systems, simulation for that purpose is becoming increasingly popular. In earlier chapters, in situ simulations have been discussed as efficient and effective ways to not only improve performance but also identify opportunities for improvements in patient flow, unit design, equipment use, and the development of procedures (Gaba, 2004; SSH, 2013c). Industrial approaches to system analysis and improvement (for example, Lean and Six Sigma) are being adopted in health care organizations to help manage complex processes (for example, scheduling) or develop flow for time-sensitive processes (such as stroke or trauma team response) (Henriksen, Battles, Keyes, & Grady, 2008). Simulation provides a unique way to assess an existing system or evaluate a proposed new one (Dunn et al., 2013).

In the future, will simulation-based assessment of in-place and proposed systems become an accepted part of all performance improvement programs in health care? One can only hope so.

Conclusion

Simulation continues to evolve and redefine itself. Gaba (2004) discussed the power of immersive fidelity by comparing the authenticity of future simulation laboratories to the *Star Trek* "holodeck." In the fictional holodeck, participants are unable to distinguish the difference between a simulation occurring in a created environment (Bauman, 2007) and reality. Created environments are those spaces existing in either a real-time fixed physical space, such as a simulation laboratory, or within a digital environment (Bauman, 2007, 2010, 2012).

As technology continues to rapidly evolve, so will simulation. Simulation-based technology is already becoming more mobile, so where will it be in the future? In the evolution of modern clinical simulation we began with mannequin-based simulation laboratories. As the simulators themselves became increasingly more portable, educators began to leverage in situ simulation to increase the authenticity and fidelity of the learners' experiences. Game-based learning is the natural evolution of screen-based simulation. Early screen-based simulators were often based on decision trees that resembled active multiple-choice scenarios that evolved to some fixed endpoint based on the participants' selection of provided menu choices. Modern game-based learning environments strive to provide immersive experiences. These experiences are often based on situated and unfolding narratives in which players or learners are encouraged to explore their environments and to leave no stone unturned (Bauman, 2010; Gee, 1991, 2003). In the future, as new simulation platforms are developed, gaming and other technology-mediated technologies will increasingly be used to educate health professionals in skills and concepts as well as measure performance.

Academic and clinical expectations are rapidly changing and evolving. Learners have a whole host of expectations about how content will be delivered and accessed and how clinical competence will be acquired and maintained. If educators fail to acknowledge these expectations, the best and brightest students and providers will simply embrace those institutions that are able to meet their expectations (Bauman, 2010). Furthermore, clinical practice is increasingly steeped in digital technology. Embracing teaching methods that include designed experiences that authentically mirror practice settings provide meaningful, situated learning experiences that prepare students for future practice (Squire, 2006).

Using different types of technologies, simulators, and platforms has many future implications in clinical practice. Health care professionals must learn to use the technology associated with contemporary patient care from patient monitoring systems to electronic medical records. Just as higher education is revolutionizing through the use of MOOCs, clinical practice is also transforming through the use of a variety of technologies, platforms, and types of simulations. The value of simulations will need to continue to be addressed as educators and practitioners adopt these new technologies for education, training, skill-competency, and translating the outcomes of clinical simulations into clinical practice.

References

Agency for Healthcare Research and Quality (AHRQ). (2013). *Making health care safer II: An updated critical analysis of the evidence for patient safety practices. Comparative Effectiveness Review No. 211.* (Prepared by the Southern California RAND Evidence-based Practice Center under Contract No. 290-2007-10062-I.) AHRQ Publication No. 13-E001-EF. Rockville, MD: Author. Retrieved from www.ahrq.gov/research/findings/evidence-based-reports/ptsafetyuptp.html

American Public Health Association. (2012). *Affordable Care Act overview: Summaries of selected provisions.* Retrieved from http://www.apha.org/advocacy/Health+Reform/ACAbasics

Bauman, E. B. (2007). *High fidelity simulation in healthcare.* (Doctoral dissertation) The University of Wisconsin–Madison, United States. Dissertations & Theses @ CIC Institutions database. (Publication no. AAT 3294196 ISBN: 9780549383109 ProQuest document ID: 1453230861)

Bauman, E. B. (2010). Virtual reality and game-based clinical education. In K. B. Gaberson & M. H. Oermann (Eds.), *Clinical teaching strategies in nursing education* (3rd ed.) (pp. 183-212). New York, NY: Springer.

Bauman, E. B. (2012). *Game-based teaching and simulation in nursing & healthcare.* New York, NY: Springer.

Bauman, E. B., & Games, I. A. (2011). Contemporary theory for immersive worlds: Addressing engagement, culture, and diversity. In A. Cheney & R. Sanders (Eds.), *Teaching and learning in 3D immersive worlds: Pedagogical models and constructivist approaches* (pp. 248-270). Hershey, PA: IGI Global.

Blakely, G., Skirton, H., Cooper, S., Allum, P., & Nelmes, P. (2008). Educational gaming in the health sciences: Systematic review. *Journal of Advanced Nursing, 65*(2), 259-269.

Burden, C., Preshaw, J., White, P., Draycott, T., Grant, S., & Fox, R. (2012). Validation of virtual reality simulation for obstetric ultrasonography: A prospective cross-sectional study. *Simulation in Healthcare: Journal of the Society for Simulation in Healthcare, 7*(5), 269-273. Retrieved from http://journals.lww.com/simulationinhealthcare/Abstract/2012/10000/Validation_of_Virtual_Reality_Simulation_for.1.aspx doi:10.1097/SIH.0b013e3182611844

Dunn, W., Deutsch, E., Maxworthy, J., Gallo, K., Dong, Y., Manos, J.,...Brazil, V. (2013). Systems integration: Engineering the future of healthcare delivery via simulation. In A. I. Levine, S. DeMaria, A. D. Schwartz, & A. Sim (Eds.), *The comprehensive textbook of healthcare simulation.* London: Springer.

Farra, S., Miller, E., Timms, N., & Schafer, J. (2013). Improved training for disaster using 3-D virtual reality simulation. *Western Journal of Nursing Research, 35*(5), pp. 655-671. doi:10.1177/0192945012471735

Foronda, C., Godsall, L., & Trybulski, J. (2012 in press). Virtual clinical simulation: The state of the science. *Clinical Simulation in Nursing, X,* e1-8. doi:10.1016/j.ecns.2012.05.005

Gaba, D. M. (2004). The future vision of simulation in health care. *Quality and Safety in Health Care, 13*(Suppl 1), i2-10.

Games, I., & Bauman, E. (2011). Virtual worlds: An environment for cultural sensitivity education in the health sciences. *International Journal of Web Based Communities, 7*(2), 189-205. doi: 10.1504/IJWBC.2011.039510

Gee, J. P. (1991). Memory and myth: A perspective on narrative. In A. McCabe & C. Peterson (Eds.), *Developing Narrative Structure* (pp. 1-26). Mahwah, NJ: Erlbaum.

Gee, J. P. (2003). *What videogames have to teach us about learning and literacy (1st ed.).* New York, NY: Palgrave-McMillan.

Hansen, M. (2008). Versatile, immersive, creative and dynamic virtual 3-D healthcare learning environments: A review of the literature. *Journal of Medical Internet Research, 10*(3), e26. doi:10.2196/jmir.1051

Hedrick, T. L., & Young, J. S. (2008). The use of "war games" to enhance high-risk clinical decision making in students and residents. *The American Journal of Surgery, 195*(6), 843-849.

Henneman, E. A., & Cunningham, H. (2005). Using clinical simulation to teach patient safety in an acute/critical care nursing course. *Nurse Educator, 30*(4), 172-177.

Henriksen, K., Battles, J. B., Keyes, M. A., & Grady, M. L. (Eds.) (2008). *Advances in patient safety: New directions and alternative approaches (Vol. 3: Performance and tools).* Rockville, MD: Agency for Healthcare Research and Quality. Retrieved from http://www.ncbi.nlm.nih.gov/books/NBK43665/

Howard, V. M., Englert, N., Kameg, K., & Perozzi, K. (2011). Integration of simulation across the undergraduate curriculum: Student and faculty perspectives. *Clinical Simulation in Nursing, 7*(1), e1-e10.

Issenberg,, S. B., McGaghie, W. C., Petrusa, E. R., Lee Gordon, D., & Scalese, R. J. (2005). Features and uses of high-fidelity medical simulations that lead to effective learning: a BEME systematic review. *Medical Teacher, 27*(1), 10-28.

Jackson, M. (2004). Making visible: Using simulation and game environments across disciplines. *On the Horizon, 12*(1), 22-25. doi:10.1108/10748120410540463

Kopp, W., & Hanson, M. A. (2012). High fidelity and gaming simulations enhance nursing education in end-of-life care. *Clinical Simulation in Nursing, 8*(3), e97-e102.

LeFlore, J., Anderson, M., Zielke, M., Nelson, K., Thomas, P. E., Hardee, G., & John, L. D. (2012). Can a virtual patient trainer teach student nurses how to save lives—Teaching nursing students about pediatric respiratory diseases. *Simulation in Healthcare: Journal of the Society for Simulation in Healthcare, 7*(1), 10-17.

Linden Research Inc. (n.d.) *Second life.* San Francisco, CA: Author. Retrieved from http://secondlife.com/

Mangold, K. (2007). Educating a new generation: Teaching baby boomer faculty about millennial students. *Nurse Educator, 32*(1), 21-23.

McNeill, J., Parker, R. A., Nadeau, J., Pelayo, L. W., & Cook, J. (2012). Developing nurse educator competency in the pedagogy of simulation. *Journal of Nursing Education, 51*(12), 685-691.

National Council of State Boards of Nursing (NCSBN). (2013). National Council of State Boards of Nursing national simulation study. Chicago, IL: Author. Retrieved from www.ncsbn.org/2094.htm

Peddle, M. (2011). Simulation gaming in nurse education: Entertainment or learning? *Nurse Education Today, 31*(7), 647-649.

Prensky, M. (2001). Digital natives, digital immigrants. *On the Horizon, 9*(5), 1-6.

Society for Simulation in Healthcare (SSH). (2013a). *Certification.* Wheaton, IL: Author. Retrieved from ssih.org/certification

Society for Simulation in Healthcare (SSH). (2013b). *SSH certified healthcare simulation educator handbook.* Wheaton, IL: Author. Retrieved from http://ssih.org/uploads/static_pages/PDFs/Certification/CHSE_Handbook.pdf

Society for Simulation in Healthcare (SSH). (2013c). *Accreditation.* Wheaton, IL: Author. Retrieved from ssih.org/accreditation

Squire, K. D. (2006). From content to context: Videogames as designed experience. *Educational Researcher, 35*(8), 19-29.

Starkweather, A. R., & Kardong-Edgren, S. (2008). Diffusion of innovation: Embedding simulation into nursing curricula. *International Journal of Nursing Education Scholarship, 5*(1), 1-21. doi:10.2202/1548-923X.1567

Wendling, A., Halan, S., Tighe, P., Le, L., Euliano, T., & Lok, B. (2011). Virtual humans versus standardized patients: Which leads residents to more correct diagnosis? *Academic Medicine, 86*(3), 384-388.

Resources

Accreditation for Simulation Programs

- **Society for Simulation in Healthcare:** http://ssih.org/accreditation

Certification for Simulation Educators in Healthcare

- **Certified Healthcare Simulation Educator (CHSE), the Society for Simulation in Healthcare:** http://ssih.org/certification

Journals

- **Clinical Simulation in Learning (Journal):** http://www.nursingsimulation.org
- **Simulation in Healthcare (Journal of the Society for Simulation in Healthcare):** http://journals.lww.com/simulationinhealthcare/pages/aboutthejournal.aspx

Organizations/Associations

- **Association of Standardized Patient Educators (ASPE):** http://aspeducators.org/
- **Australia Society for Simulation in Healthcare (ASSH):** http://www.simulationaustralia.org.au
- **International Pediatric Simulation Society (IPSS):** http://www.ipedsim.com
- **International Nursing Association for Clinical Simulation and Learning (INACSL):** www.inacsl.org

- **National League for Nursing (NLN) Simulation Innovation Resource Center (SIRC):** http://sirc.nln.org/
- **Society for Simulation in Healthcare (SSH):** www.ssih.org
- **Society in Europe for Simulation Applied to Medicine (SESAM):** http://www.sesam-web.org

A

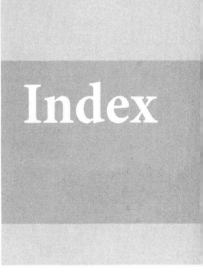

Index

D

T

U–V

W

X–Y–Z